CLINICAL NEUROLOGY

Prof. (Dr.) Sujata K. Das

ALLIED
HEALTH
PRESS

Clinical Neurology

Author: **Prof. (Dr.) Sujata K. Das**

Allied Health Press
4164 Lakeshore Road
Burlington ON L7L 1A4
Canada
www.alliedhealthpress.com
Email: orders@arclereducation.com

ISBN: 978-1-77956-221-0

Allied Health Press publishes wide variety of books and eBooks. For more information about Allied Health Press and its products, visit our website at www.alliedhealthpress.com

ABOUT THE AUTHOR

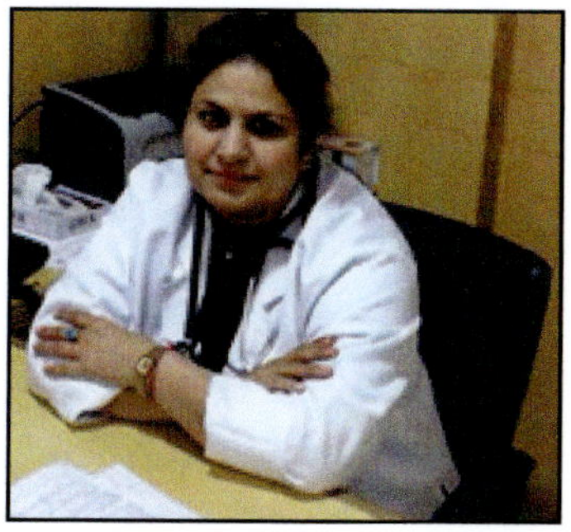

Prof (Dr) Sujata K. Dass, M.B.B.S, D.N.B, Ph.D. (Medicine) is a distinguished neuro-physician and academician, currently serving as an Attending Consultant in the Department of Neurology, B.L. Kapur Hospital, a renowned super-specialty medical institution in the New Delhi. Her illustrious career in medicine and research spans over three decades, characterized by her profound contributions to neurology and her unwavering commitment to medical education.

Dr. Dass began her educational journey at Flushing High School in New York, USA, and completed her High School Diploma thereafter she joined Queens College of the City University of New York as an undergrad student. With a passion for medicine, she pursued her MBBS degree at King George Medical College, Lucknow, U.P., India. Her academic prowess and dedication to medicine were evident early on, setting the stage for a remarkable career. Dr Dass worked under the supervision of Dr M.S. Bains, M.D. as a Visiting Fellow in cardio-thoracic surgery at Memorial Sloan Kettering Cancer Research Center, New York, USA.

Dr. Dass furthered her medical training by obtaining a D.N.B. (Family Medicine) and conducted significant research on hematological changes in malaria. Her quest for knowledge and excellence led her back to New York, where she completed her Ph.D. (Medicine) at the Department of Obstetrics & Gynecology, The New York Hospital-Cornell University Medical Center under the mentorship of Prof. Brij B. Saxena. Her groundbreaking work on Sn-Proto and Sn-Mesoporphyrin and the chemoprevention of neonatal jaundice culminated in the award of her D.Sc. (Medicine).

Dr. Sujata Dass joined as the BR Ambedkar Chair Professor in July 2002 in the Institute of Biomedical Sciences, Faculty of Medicine, Bundelkhand University, Jhansi. Her tenure was marked by her dedication to advancing medical research and education. She also served as UGC National Research Award (Professor) at V.P. Chest Institute, University of Delhi.

Throughout her career, Dr. Dass has received numerous awards and accolades on a global level. Notable among these are the UGC Research Award, the Fast Track Young Scientist Award from the Department of Science and Technology (DST), and the Women's Award of Highest Honour from Soka University, Japan. She has also received numerous research grants from DST, DBT and ICMR, UGC etc. These awards and grants underscore her exceptional contributions to medical science and research.

Dr. Dass is a respected member of various scientific and administrative bodies like Planning Board (IGNOU), Executive Council - Bhagat Phool Singh Mahila Vishwavidhlaya, Haryana (2008-2011) where she continues to influence the medical community with her insights and expertise. Her commitment to guiding and mentoring students in their master's and doctoral thesis highlights her dedication to nurturing the next generation of medical professionals.

Dr. Dass remains a beacon of excellence and a role model for aspiring medical professionals worldwide.

Word Roots, Prefixes, and Suffixes by Chapter

Chapter 1 Fundamentals of Neurology

Prefix: What It Means

Hemi-: Half

Pachy-: Thick

Para-: Beyond, around, beside

Polio-: Gray

Quadri-: Four

Sub-: Below, under

Suffix: What It Means

-algia: Pain

Chapter 2 Coma

Coma (from Greek “koma,” meaning deep sleep)

Somn/o (sleep)

Hypn/o (sleep)

Hyper- (excessive, above normal)

Hypo- (deficient, below normal)

A- (without, absence of)

-ose (full of, resembling)

-tion (process, state)

-ic (pertaining to)

Chapter 3 Apoptosis Implication in Neurodegenerative Disorders

A-, An-: negative, an absence of something.

Ab-: Away from,

Acantho-: Spine, spiny

Ad-: To, towards, near

Aer-: Air or gas

Chapter 4 Disorders of Equilibrium

Equilibr/o (balance)

-libr- (from Latin “libra,” meaning balance)

Balanc/o (balance)

Dys- (abnormal, difficult, painful)

Mal- (bad, abnormal, diseased)

Hyper- (excessive, above normal)

Chapter 5 Dementia and Amnestic Disorders

-ation: (process, state)

-ia: (condition, state)

-osis: (abnormal condition)

-pathy: (disease, disorder)

Un-: (not, opposite of)

-osis: (abnormal condition)

-ia: (condition, state)

Chapter 6 Headache and Facial Pain

Cephalad: (cephal-ad)

Cephalalgia: (cephal-algia)

Cephalic: (cephal-ic):

Cephalin; (cephal-in):

Cephalization: (cephal-ization):

Chapter 7 Neuro-Ophthalmic Disorders

Neur/o: (pertaining to nerves)

Nerv/o: (nerve)

Ophthalm/o: (pertaining to the eye)

Opt/o: (vision)

Optic/o: (optic nerve)

Peri-: (around)

Para-: (abnormal, beside)

Intra-: (within)

Exo-: (outside, away from)

Chapter 8 Seizures and Syncope

Pre- (before)

Post- (after)

Inter- (between)

Neo- (new)

Peri- (around)

Vas(o)- (vessel)

Hypo- (under, below)

Chapter 9 Sensory Disorders

Blephar/o: Eyelid

Core/o, cor/o: Pupil

Corne/o: Cornea

Dipl/o: Double

Glauc/o: Gray

Is/o: Equal

Lacrim/o: Tear, tear duct

Mi/o: Smaller, les

Mydri/o: Wide

Opt/o: Eye, vision

Phac/o, phak/o: Crystalline lens

Table of Contents

LIST OF FIGURES

LIST OF TABLES

PREFACE

The field of neurology is an extensive and multifaceted area within the field of clinical medicine, incorporating a wide array of research activities that span clinical, translational, and fundamental inquiries into the myriad disorders and physiological processes associated with the brain and the broader central nervous system. The depth and breadth of our comprehension of neurological diseases have significantly broadened in recent years. This expansion in knowledge and understanding is primarily attributable to the pioneering and rapid advancements in a variety of scientific and medical disciplines, including but not limited to, neuroscience, molecular biology, regenerative medicine, and computational biology.

Neurology holds a profound appeal not just for those specialized in the field, such as neurologists, but also for individuals outside the discipline. This widespread interest stems from the critical role of our nervous system, which orchestrates every function within our body. Furthermore, the brain, as the central component of the nervous system, is fundamental to our very essence—shaping how we think, perceive the world around us, experience emotions, engage in behavior, and retain memories. Conditions and diseases affecting the nervous system are relatively prevalent, yet it is reassuring to note that treatments are available for every such condition. These treatments vary widely in their objectives and outcomes; some may offer a complete cure, others aim to modify the progression of the disease, and there are always options to alleviate the symptoms, even if the underlying condition remains. The field of neurology has witnessed exceptional progress in the understanding of nervous system diseases, a development that continues to accelerate. Each passing year sees the introduction of an increasingly large number of new therapeutic options in neurology, surpassing the rate of new treatments available in nearly any other medical field. This constant evolution in the treatment landscape highlights the dynamic nature of neurology and underscores the ongoing advancements that contribute to improving patient care and outcomes.

This book, titled "Clinical Neurology;" is designed to encapsulate a comprehensive collection of the most crucial neurological topics, specifically tailored for individuals who are not specialized in neurology. The content within this book is meticulously organized to not only review but also illuminate the details of neuroscience and neuropathology. It aims to deliver content that is of high value, deeply clinically relevant, and immensely practical for the effective care of patients. In an era where neurological diseases are becoming more common, a diverse range of healthcare professionals, including physicians and various other healthcare providers, find themselves at the forefront, providing essential care to patients grappling with neurological issues. For these healthcare professionals, possessing a solid understanding of the epidemiology, pathophysiology, and methods of diagnosis, management strategies, and the prognosis of neurological conditions is of paramount importance.

This book goes beyond mere discussion to offer a detailed, insightful, and comprehensive perspective on how to accurately diagnose neurological conditions. The approach taken in this book is thoughtful and expansive, ensuring that healthcare providers are well-equipped with the knowledge and skills needed to navigate the complexities of neurologic diseases. By covering a broad spectrum of neurologic topics, the book facilitates a deeper understanding of the subject matter, enabling healthcare professionals to deliver high-quality, informed, and compassionate care to their patients. The aim is to enhance the reader's familiarity with various neurological conditions, improving their ability to diagnose, manage, and prognosticate effectively, which is critical in the landscape of modern healthcare where neurological conditions are increasingly encountered.

"Clinical Neurology;" is aimed at healthcare providers outside the field of neurology, including primary care physicians, medical students, nurses, and other allied health professionals. It seeks to equip these professionals with the necessary knowledge and tools to manage patients withneurological concerns effectively. The book is also valuable for non-specialists interested in gaining a comprehensive understanding of neurological diseases and their care.

Chapter 1

FUNDAMENTALS OF NEUROLOGY

Contents

Introduction

Neurology, an essential field in the medical sciences, delves into the inner workings of the nervous system to uncover the intricate mechanisms that govern human behavior, cognition, and bodily functions. Central to its study is the examination of the brain, spinal cord, peripheral nerves, and neuromuscular junctions, encompassing a wide range of physiological and pathological phenomena.

An insightful exploration of this complex field, Fundamentals of Neurology gives readers a thorough grasp of the anatomy, physiology, and pathology of the nervous system. It explores the basic ideas behind neural circuitry, synaptic transmission, and neural communication, setting the stage for investigating higher-order cognitive processes and motor abilities.

A wide range of neurological disorders is covered in this introductory course, from neurological emergencies like stroke and traumatic brain injury to neurodegenerative diseases like Parkinson's and Alzheimer's. It looks at the various neurology diagnostic modalities, such as clinical evaluation, electrophysiological studies like EEG and EMG, and neuroimaging methods like MRI and CT scans.

Fundamentals of Neurology also provides in-depth information on neuropharmacology, explaining how different drugs work in treating neurological disorders. The book highlights the importance of interdisciplinary collaboration in neurology, incorporating findings from genetics, molecular biology, psychology, and related fields to better understand the complexities of the nervous system. This approach ultimately leads to groundbreaking therapeutic approaches and advancements in neuroscience.

Orientation and Directional Terms

Term	Definition	Illustration
Neurotubules	Neurotubules are microtubules found in neurons in nervous tissues. Along with neurofilaments and microfilaments, they form the cytoskeleton of neurons.	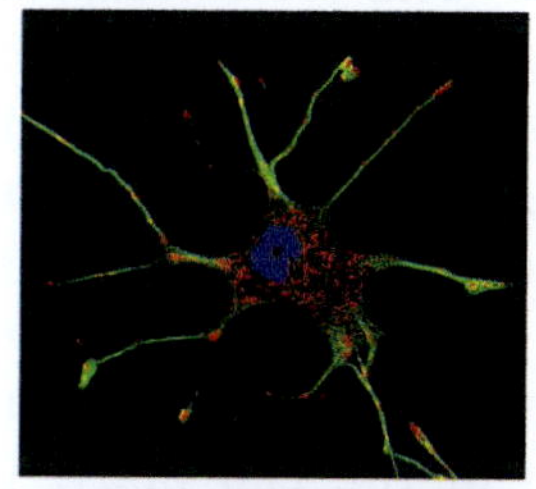
Neuroglial cell	Neuroglial cells, also known as glial cells or glia, are a diverse group of non-neuronal cells in the nervous system. They make up about half of the volume of the human brain.	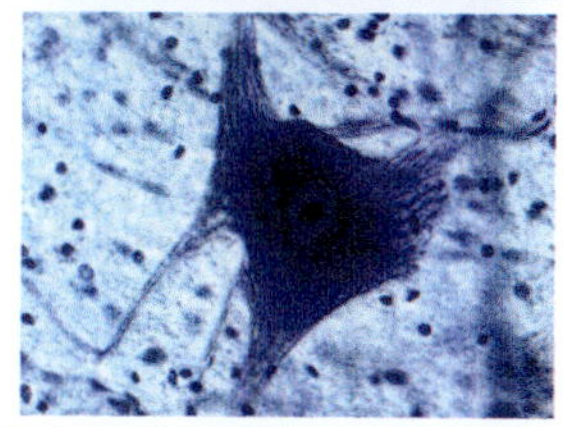
Axolemma	The axolemma is the cell membrane of an axon, the branch of a neuron through which signals (action potentials) are transmitted.	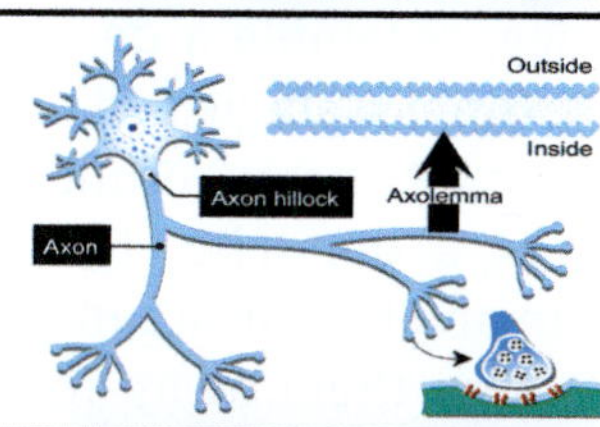
Saltatory conduction	Saltatory conduction describes the way an electrical impulse skips from node to node down the full length of an axon, speeding the arrival of the impulse at the nerve terminal in comparison with the slower continuous progression of depolarization spreading down an unmyelinated axon.	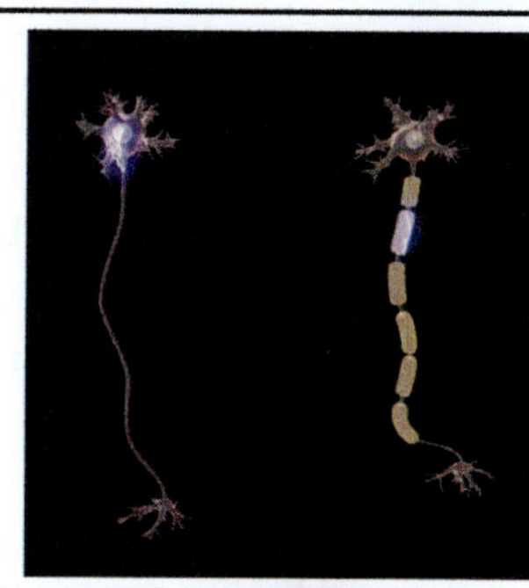
Lumbar lordosis	Lumbar lordosis is an exaggerated inward curve of the lumbar spine, which is the lower back.	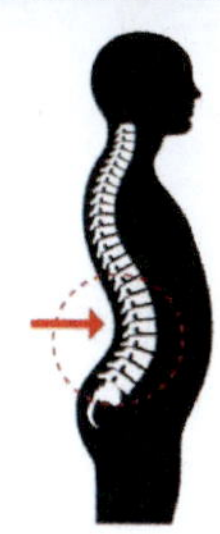

1.1. Microscopic Anatomy of the Nervous System

Neurons. The cell nucleus, mitochondria, endoplasmic reticulum, neurotubules, and neurofilaments are found in the cell body, or soma, of the neuron, which is surrounded by the cell membrane (Figure 1.1). Short, roughly widely branched cellular structures called dendrites carry afferent impulses in the direction of the cell body. They give the cell a far greater surface area than the cell body alone, which expands the area that can be used for cell membrane receptor deployment and intercellular contact. Dendrites of different neuronal species have distinct morphological types; the dendrites of cerebellar Purkinje cells, for instance, resemble a deer's antlers (Figure 1.2). The axon is a single cell process that leaves the cell body at the axon hillock. It is typically longer than a dendrite. It transfers efferent impulses to an effector organ or another neuron by conducting them away from the cell body. Every neuron, in general, consists of an axon, a soma, and one or more dendrites. Depending on the purpose of the neuron, different nerve cell processes—particularly the dendrites—have different shapes and sizes. Consequently, a variety of morphological subtypes of neurons can be distinguished (Figure 1.3).

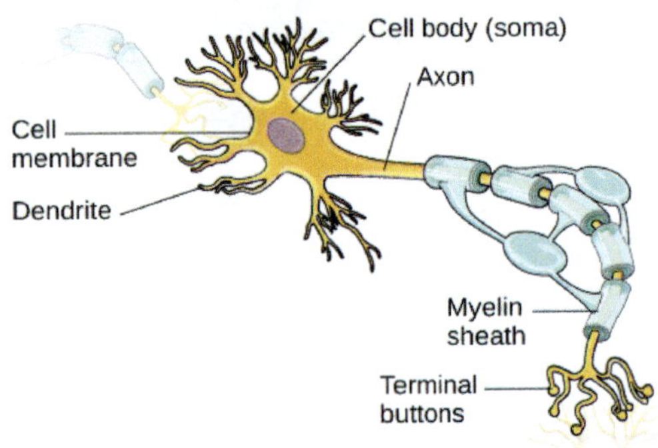

Figure 1.1. Fine structure of a neuron.

Source: https://courses.lumenlearning.com/waymaker-psychology/chapter/cells-of-the-nervous-system/.

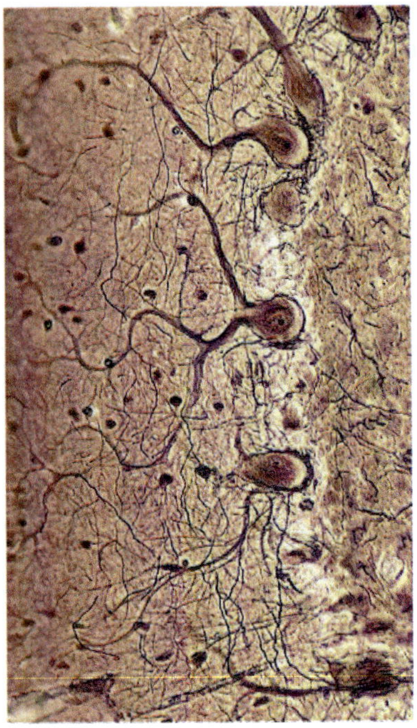

Figure 1.2. Cerebellar Purkinje cell (microphotograph). Note the numerous synapses on the dendrites.

Source: By Lennart Rikk – Own work, CC0, https://commons.wikimedia.org/w/index.php?curid=113361666.

- **Neuroglia:** The neurons, which make up the significant functional component of the nervous system, are encircled by neuroglia, a group of supporting cells. One specific type of neuroglial cell, called an astrocyte, resembles a star in appearance. They have perivascular foot processes that touch 85% of the nervous system's capillaries and make contact with nonsynaptic sites on the neuronal surface. Astrocytes are a crucial part of the blood-brain barrier and guarantee that neurons receive enough nutrition. In the central nervous system, oligodendrocytes, microglia, ependymal cells, and choroid plexus cells are additional forms of supporting cells.

- **Myelin Sheaths:** Axons with a diameter of less than 1 μm are typically myelinated, whereas axons with a greater thickness are covered in myelin. An axon "sinks" into an oligodendrocyte, also known as a Schwann cell in the peripheral nervous system, to form a mesaxon, which is made up of two sheets of cell membrane. This process creates the myelin sheath. The axon is wrapped around by the mesaxon several times (Figure 1.4c). The intervening nodes of Ranvier, which can be as long as 1 mm, divide individual segments of myelin and are crucial to the movement of nerve impulses along the axon. The 1–4 μm wide "naked" axonal segments at the nodes of Ranvier are partially covered by the processes of the nearby Schwann cells. Therefore, the neuronal cell membrane (neurilemma or axolemma) is the only thing separating them from the surrounding endoneural interstitium. Voltage-dependent sodium channels are primarily found in the nodal axolemma, whereas potassium channels are primarily found in the internodal segments.
- **Synapse:** Synapses are the locations where neurons exchange impulses with one another. The synaptic cleft, the postsynaptic membrane of the receiving neuron or effector organ, and the bulb-like expansion of the axon end, known as an axon terminal (or bouton), make up each synapse (Figure 1.5). The myelin sheath of myelinated axons is lost very close to the axon terminal. Synaptic input can come from one or more axons for a single neuron, and the impulses it gets can be either excitatory or inhibitory. An axon may synapse onto a dendrite, another axon, or the cell body. The nervous system's functional adaptability, or "plasticity," is derived from ongoing processes of structural and functional change at the synaptic connections between nerve cells, even after an individual has reached maturity. Chemical compounds known as neurotransmitters facilitate the transmission of neural impulses between synapses; dopamine, serotonin, acetylcholine, and γ-aminobutyric acid (GABA) are among the more significant ones in the central nervous system. The peripheral nervous system's axons are joined to effector organs like muscle or glandular cells by specialized synapses.

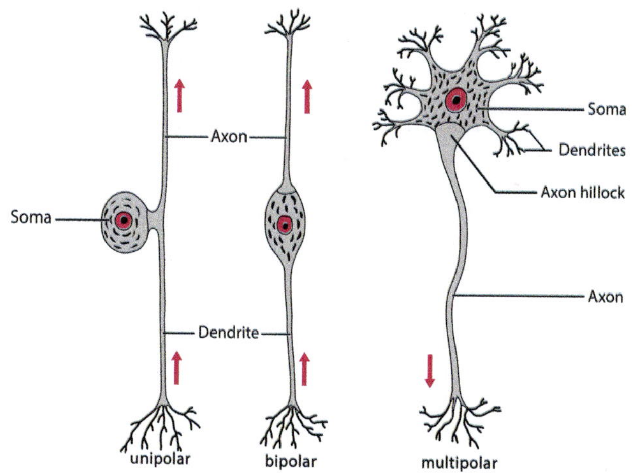

Figure 1.3. Three types of neurons. The arrows indicate the usual direction of impulse conduction.

Source: Wilkinson, J.L.: Neuroanatomy for medical students, 2nd ed, Butterworth-Heinemann, Oxford 1992.

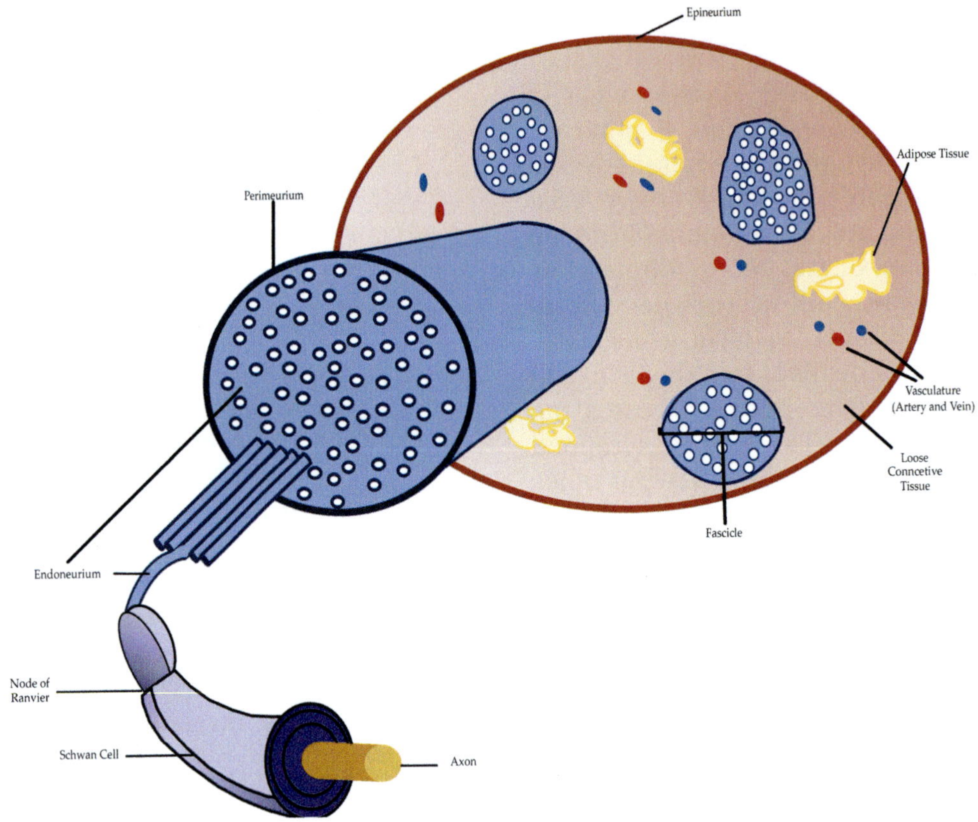

Figure 1.4. Peripheral nerve (schematic drawings).

Source: Lopes B, Sousa P, Alvites R, Branquinho M, Sousa AC, Mendonça C, Atayde LM, Luís AL, Varejão ASP, Maurício AC. Peripheral nerve injury treatments and advances: One health perspective. *International Journal of Molecular Sciences*. 2022; 23(2):918. https://doi.org/10.3390/ijms23020918.

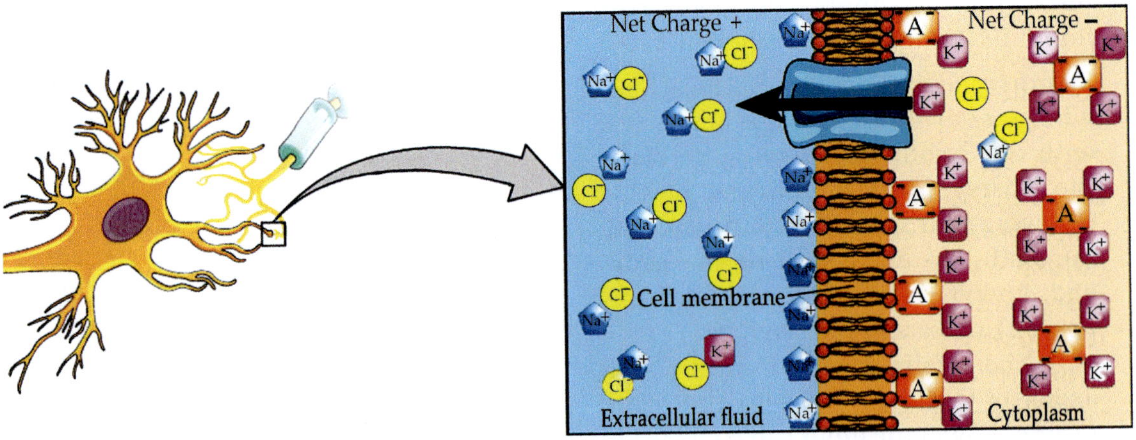

Figure 1.5. Fine structure of a synapse.

Source: https://courses.lumenlearning.com/waymaker-psychology/chapter/reading-neural-communication/.

1.2. Elements of Neurophysiology

A double-layered cell membrane with an outer layer of glycoprotein and an inner layer of phospholipid surrounds each neuron. Within the cell membrane, specialized protein molecules create channels that allow only sodium, potassium, or chloride ions to pass through. Certain ion channels (e.g., on the postsynaptic membrane) only become open upon the binding of a particular ligand, e.g., the chemical known as a neurotransmitter that transfers nerve impulses between cells. The term "ligand-dependent ion channels" refers to these channels. Conversely, voltage-dependent ion channels are primarily located on the axonal membrane. Depending on the transmembrane electrical potential, they open and close.

- **Resting Potential:** The uneven ion concentrations in the intracellular and extracellular spaces (ICS, ECS) along with the membrane's variable electrical conductivity to various ion types cause a difference in electrical potential across the neuronal membrane. Since the membrane is relatively impermeable to sodium ions while at rest and highly permeable to potassium ions, the ratio of intracellular to extracellular potassium concentration primarily determines the resting potential. Approximately 35 times more potassium is present in the ICS than in the ECS. Potassium ions therefore have a tendency to diffuse out of cells. As a result, the membrane's inner surface loses its positive charge and acquires a negative charge. A difference in electrical potential is created when the negative charge accumulates on the inner surface of the membrane, preventing additional potassium ions flow outward. A negative charge builds up until the potential difference precisely balances the force resulting from the variation in potassium ion concentration. The overall result is a stable, resting membrane potential with a value between -60 and -90 mV, indicating that there is no more net transfer of potassium ions across the membrane in either direction.
- **Action Potential:** In comparison to the ICS, the ECS has a sodium ion concentration that is about 20 times higher. So, a quick influx of sodium ions into the cell occurs after neurotransmitter-induced opening of ligandsensitive postsynaptic sodium channels. The all-or-nothing law of cellular excitation states that an action potential whose amplitude and time course are independent of the type and intensity of the depolarizing impulse is produced when the inner surface of the cell membrane becomes positively charged. Between + 20 and + 50 mV is the range at which the transmembrane potential difference reaches its maximum positive value. Following a brief interval, the cell membrane's potassium channels become more permeable than they are while at rest, leading to a net outflow of potassium ions. This repolarizes the membrane to its resting potential and makes up for the previous sodium influx. In this process, an active sodium pump also takes part. The membrane is momentarily incapable of conducting any more impulses until repolarization is finished; this absolute refractory period is succeeded by a relative refractory period.
- **Impulse Conduction:** At the axon hillock, voltage-dependent sodium channels open one after another, conducting the axon potential forward

along the axonal membrane. The local depolarization wave propagates along the axon at a velocity determined by the axon's thickness and the myelin sheath's thickness. Nodes of Ranvier are particularly significant in this process because of the isolating myelin sheaths, which increase the electrical resistance and decrease the capacitance of the axonal membrane. Because of this, the action potentials are only started at the nodes and "jump over" the internodal axon segments (a process known as saltatory conduction). Action potentials are conducted by myelinated nerve fibers substantially faster than by unmyelinated fibers due to this unique mechanism. Peripheral nerves typically have a conduction velocity of 50–60 m/s for motor and sensory functions.

1.3. Elements of Neurogenetics

1.3.1. General Genetics

An individual's physical traits, or phenotype, are influenced by their environment during and after pregnancy as well as the entirety of their genetic makeup, or genotype. DNA molecules found in the cell nucleus and mitochondria carry genetic information. The entirety of an organism's genes is referred to as its genome, and a gene is a segment of DNA that contains the instructions required for the synthesis of a protein molecule. Humans have 23 pairs of chromosomes that contain their nuclear genes: 22 pairs of autosomes and one pair of sex chromosomes, or gonosomes, which can be either XX (found in females) or XY (found in males).

- **Recombination of Genetic Material:** An enormous number of cell divisions, or mitoses, are necessary for the organism to grow. Nuclear genetic material doubles (replicates) during each mitosis and is subsequently divided between the two daughter cells, resulting in each daughter cell having a full (diploid) complement of chromosomes, just like the parent cell did. However, a reductive cell division known as meiosis takes place for the purpose of sexual reproduction, resulting in egg or sperm cells that only have a haploid set of chromosomes—i.e., as opposed to the 23 pairs present in all other cells, only one of each chromosome (22 autosomes and one sex chromosome). A complete (diploid) complement of chromosomes, half from the paternal and half from the maternal genomes, is restored when an egg cell and a sperm cell unite.

Mendelian inheritance dictates that features (genes) derived from both parents are randomly and independently distributed to the germ cells, and consequently to the progeny. Since entire chromosomes are passed on to the germ cells, genes on the same chromosome are typically transmitted together, which poses a significant limitation to this random and independent assortment. However, during a specific stage of meiosis, homologous chromatids' corresponding DNA segments can trade places (cross over), resulting in a reorganization of the genes on the chromatids involved in the exchange (genetic recombination). Recombination between two genes on a chromosome occurs more frequently the farther apart they are.

Apart from the natural physiological processes that cause genetic material to change and recombine (such as the random assortment of chromosomes during meiosis and fertilization, and gene recombination on homologous chromosomes), mutations can also spontaneously occur in the genome. These mutations in the germ line can be inherited by an individual's offspring.

- **Autosomal Dominant Inheritance:** Dominant genes are those that substantially alter or entirely dictate an individual's phenotype when they are heterozygous. A child has a 50% chance of being heterozygous and exhibiting the matching phenotypic trait if both the mother and father are heterozygous for the dominant allele.
- **Autosomal Recessive Inheritance:** Recessive autosomal genes are those that only show phenotypic expression in homozygotes and have no effect in the heterozygous state. 75% of the offspring will carry at least one copy of the recessive allele if both the mother and father are heterozygous for it. Of these, 25% will be homozygous and the remaining 50% will be heterozygous. The corresponding phenotypic trait will only be displayed by the homozygous offspring (e.g., a genetic illness that is recessively inherited). Neither the heterozygous offspring ("carriers") nor the 25% of offspring lacking the recessive allele will exhibit the phenotypic trait.
- **X-chromosomal Inheritance:** While females receive an X chromosome from both parents, males receive an X chromosome from their mother and a Y chromosome from their father. Thus, if a mother is heterozygous for an X chromosomal gene, she will pass it on to half of her children, male or female (provided the mother is also heterozygous for it), whereas fathers will pass it on to all of their daughters but not to their sons. Males and females are affected by dominantly inherited X-chromosomal diseases, whereas males are primarily affected by recessively inherited diseases, which only affect the infrequent females who are homozygous for the disease, i.e., only those who have received the faulty gene on their X chromosome from each of their parents. As long as his female partner is not a carrier of the disease, all of the affected male's daughters will be healthy carriers. Any affected male certainly inherited the gene from his mother. Half of the sons of female carriers whose male partners are not affected by the disease will also be affected; all of their daughters will be healthy, but half will carry the disease's gene.
- **Maternal Inheritance of the Mitochondrial Genome:** Because mitochondrial DNA is only passed down through mothers, fathers are never the carriers of mitochondrial genetic diseases, which affect both male and female children. It is possible for mitochondria with altered DNA to be present alongside mitochondria with healthy DNA in the same cell. The nuclear genome, found in all body cells, does not exhibit any counterpart to this phenomenon, known as heteroplasmia. With genetic diseases of the mitochondria, the phenotype, i.e., the quantity of defective mitochondria and the ratio of mutated to normal mitochondrial DNA determine how much damage is done to the affected cells and tissues.

Mutations play a vital role in evolution, as they are necessary for the existence of the human species. However, harmful mutations can result in genetic defects and diseases. Mutations can be categorized as genomic or intragenic.

There are two categories of genomic mutations: structural and numerical chromosomal abnormalities. The former kind of mutation results in an abnormally high number of chromosomes (e.g., trisomy, and monosomy); in the latter case, a chromosome's structure is abnormal. Chromosome segment deletions, translocations, and inversions are examples of structural abnormalities.

Mutations that occur within a gene are known as intragenic mutations. DNA within each chromosome is organized linearly. Genes, which code for proteins, are made up of DNA segments called exons, which are interspersed with noncoding sequences known as introns. Exons make up just 5% of human chromosomal DNA. During transcription, the primary RNA transcript includes copies of the introns, which are later removed in a process called splicing. This results in the production of mature mRNA.

An amino acid in a protein undergoing biosynthesis is coded for by each triplet, or group of three consecutive nucleotides, in the mRNA molecule. The length of the protein that needs to be synthesized is determined by the "stop codons" that are located between the exons and indicate the start and finish of the gene.

Missense mutations occur when a DNA nucleotide is substituted with a different nucleotide, changing the sense of the codon to which it belongs. This occurs when the incorrect amino acid is inserted into the gene product at this stage of protein biosynthesis.

The end result of this varies greatly in terms of how proteins function. However, an incomplete or overly long protein will be produced (nonsense mutations) if a nucleotide replacement occurs that results in the creation or destruction of a stop codon.

Frame-shift mutations are those that affect the rhythm of nucleotide triplets and involve the insertion of an extra nucleotide or the deletion of a nucleotide from the DNA. These typically result in seriously aberrant protein structure and function.

- **Expanded Repetitive DNA Sequences:** Another kind of mutation that is particularly significant in the field of neurology modifies the number of trinucleotides or triplets. Gene function and expression are impacted by the numerous repetitive trinucleotide sequences found in normal human DNA. Mutations involving abnormally long (expanded) triplet repeat sequences are responsible for a significant group of neurodegenerative diseases. These conditions are known as triplet repeat diseases or trinucleotide diseases. The afflicted sequence has dozens or even hundreds of triplets, whereas the normal repeat sequence may only have a few. The earlier the disease onset age and the more severe its symptoms, the longer the expansion. From generation to generation, the repeat sequences lengthen, causing the disease to manifest itself earlier and earlier (a condition known as "anticipation") and to worsen over time.

A variety of diseases, including mitochondrial encephalomyopathies, are caused by mutations in the mitochondrial DNA that affect the oxidative metabolism of the mitochondria.

1.3.2. Neurogenetics

Neurology is especially affected by triplet diseases. Table 1.1 lists the neurodegenerative disorders caused by expanded triplet repeats, and Table 1.2 summarizes the traits they have in common. Table 1.3 lists a few of the more prevalent inherited mitochondrial diseases.

Neurological and other diseases are being linked to an increasing number of genetic defects. For those looking for the most recent information, there are books and large tables available. The Internet provides the fastest way to quickly access the state of knowledge at any given time.

1.3.3. Genetic Counselling

DNA analysis can directly detect a large number of genetic mutations. The outcomes are quite particular. This means that a long-term prognosis can be provided for many diseases even before they exhibit symptoms. Unfortunately, most of these illnesses are incurable and progressively worsen over time.

Before any DNA analysis is performed, the treating physician should:

- perform a meticulous clinical examination;
- obtain a detailed family history and personally examine the patient's relatives, if possible;
- inform the patient and his or her relatives in detail about the suspected disease; and
- explain the consequences of the proposed DNA analysis to them in a readily understandable manner.

Table 1.1. Some Neurodegenerative Diseases Caused by Triplet Repeat Expansions

Disease	Major clinical manifestations	Triplet	Chromosomal localization
Fragile X-chromosome	diminished intelligence, sometimes facial dysmorphism, connective tissue dysplasia	CGG	Xq27
Myotonic dystrophy	progressive, mainly distal muscular dystrophy and myotonia	CTG	19q13.3
Friedreich ataxia	ataxia, areflexia, pyramidal tract signs, dysarthria	GAA	9q13–q21.1
Spinobulbar muscle atrophy (Kennedy syndrome)	muscle atrophy, dysarthria, fasciculations, gynecomastia	CAG	Xq13–q21
Huntington disease	chorea, rarely spasticity or rigidity, cognitive and behavioral disturbances	CAG	4p16.3
Spinocerebellar ataxia type 1 (SCA1)	cerebellar ataxia, sometimes chorea or dystonia, polyneuropathy, often pyramidal tract signs, sometimes dementia	CAG	6p24
Spinocerebellar ataxia type 2 (SCA2)	cerebellar ataxia, sometimes chorea or dystonia, myoclonus, polyneuropathy, sometimes pyramidal tract signs and dementia	CAG	12
Spinocerebellar ataxia type 3 (SCA3); Machado–Joseph disease	cerebellar ataxia, sometimes chorea or dystonia, polyneuropathy, sometimes pyramidal tract signs and dementia	CAG	14
Spinocerebellar ataxia type 6 (SCA6)	cerebellar ataxia, sometimes polyneuropathy and pyramidal tract signs	CAG	19p13
Spinocerebellar ataxia type 7 (SCA7)	cerebellar ataxia, sometimes chorea or dystonia, retinal degeneration, polyneuropathy, sometimes pyramidal tract signs	CAG	3p
Spinocerebellar ataxia type 8 (SCA8)	cerebellar ataxia, spasticity, impaired vibration sense	CTG	13q21
Dentato-rubro-pallido-luysian atrophy (DRPLA)	ataxia, myoclonus, epilepsy, choreoathetosis, dementia	CAG	12p

Source: Mumenthaler / Mattle, Fundamentals of Neurology © 2006 Thieme.

The patient may experience relief and anxiety-free living after a negative DNA analysis. A positive outcome, however, could send the patient into a deep depression because they will have to deal with the certainty of having an inherited disease, which usually has a poor prognosis, and they might not be able to handle this information. A marriage or other type of partnership may also be severely strained by learning of a genetic abnormality. Because people with inherited diseases are, regrettably, frequently treated like outcasts in our postindustrial society, social problems of yet other kinds may arise. They might experience issues at work, in part because they probably won't be covered by insurance. For all these reasons, waiting until the disease has manifested symptoms before undergoing genetic testing usually results in fewer issues. Even if the parents request it, genetic testing shouldn't be done on asymptomatic children. When they are old enough and have reached legal majority, they ought to be free to choose whether or not to have testing.

After being fully informed about the potential genetic disease they may have and the implications of DNA analysis, many patients and their families choose not to have testing done. People who are asymptomatic or presymptomatic, in particular, frequently prefer not to learn if they will eventually develop the disease. Their chances of having good health in the future would be destroyed by a positive test result.

In a private discussion, the doctor should notify the patient and any family members if the patient chooses to have a DNA test and results are positive. This will give them enough time to weigh all the options. Results from tests should never be given out in writing or over the phone. Long-term psychotherapy is frequently required for patients who tested positive. Furthermore, the doctor-patient relationship doesn't end with the test results; for many patients with genetic neurological diseases, ongoing symptomatic treatment and psychological support can be very beneficial.

Table 1.2. Common Features of Triplet Repeat Diseases

•	Autosomal dominant or X-chromosomal inheritance
•	Onset usually between the ages of 25 and 45
•	Gradual progression of disease
•	Symmetrical neuronal loss and gliosis in the brain
•	Anticipation
•	The number of triplet repeats is correlated with the age of onset and the severity of the disease
•	The diagnosis can be established by DNA analysis

Source: Mumenthaler / Mattle, Fundamentals of Neurology © 2006 Thieme.

Table 1.3. Mitochondrial Encephalomyopathies

•	Progressive external ophthalmopathy (PEO)
•	Kearns–Sayre syndrome (KSS)
•	Leber hereditary optic neuropathy (LHON)
•	Mitochondrial encephalomyopathy with lactic acidosis and stroke (MELAS)
•	Leigh disease
•	Neuropathy, ataxia, and retinitis pigmentosa syndrome (NARP)
•	Myoclonus epilepsy with ragged red fibers (MERRF)

Source: https://www.ruseducation.in/books/Fundamentals-Neurology.pdf.

1.4. The Clinical Interview in Neurology

1.4.1. General Principles of History Taking

In neurology, perhaps more than in any other medical specialty, the clinical history is crucial. It is an essential tool for diagnosis, helps to build a trusting relationship between the doctor and patient, and is necessary for any subsequent treatment to be successful. It is always important to take the history very carefully.

Even prior to a physical examination or other tests, the kind of neurological disturbance a patient is experiencing can typically be identified from a thoroughly documented clinical history. For many patients, the history by itself allows for a precise diagnosis to be made, but only if the doctor has been paying close attention to what the patient has to say.

Skillfully noting the history is the distinguishing mark of a good clinician.

- **General Prerequisites for Good History Taking:** A good history can only be taken in any area of clinical medicine—not just neurology—if the patient has faith in the treating physician. Make an introduction to the patient and obtain their history in a location that provides the appropriate level of discretion and privacy. As far as the situation permits, the patient should be seated comfortably, emotionally at ease, and not feel hurried. If another person is with you for the interview, e.g., a medical student, present this individual and ensure that the patient is genuinely in agreement with their presence. Other than the doctor taking the history, people should act discreetly and fade into the background. As far as feasible, the history should be taken by, or under the supervision of, a qualified clinician. It should also be thorough and detailed.
- **General Principles of the Clinical Interview:** When conducting an interview with a patient, remember these guidelines: at first, the patient should speak the most, and you should speak as little as possible. Yes, you must specifically ask questions to elicit all pertinent historical information, but only after the patient has completed explaining the issue in his or her own words. Even though the patient may be rambling or ambiguous in their story, you should be careful not to come across as agitated or impatient. It is your responsibility, then, to build upon and clarify this preliminary information by adamant or persistent questioning until, at last, you have a clear picture of the current condition. Never discount a patient's explanation for their symptoms, no matter how ludicrous or unlikely it may seem. The patient will no longer be able to communicate with you, and you will appear as a smug, arrogant know-it-all.
- **Your Demeanor Toward the Patient:** Each patient has the right to be given the physician's undivided attention for a suitably designated amount of time, as well as to be treated with tact and civility. It is best to conduct a thorough physical examination only after you have thoroughly listened to the patient's narrative and followed it up with more in-depth questions. The patient is entitled to a thorough explanation of your results and any implications for the patient's condition. It is important that you communicate these issues to the patient honestly, in an understandable way, and with

appropriate consideration for their feelings. It will frequently be necessary for you to choose carefully between being direct and using euphemisms.

Even though the patient is a child or teenager, you should still give them your whole attention if they are with someone else, like a spouse, parent, other relative, or friend. It is best to speak with the patient directly. During the clinical interview or physical examination, you may need to ask accompanying people to leave the room. However, do not ignore their needs; the people closest to the patient may need to play a significant role in the patient's treatment down the road. As the cornerstones of a trusting relationship between the patient and the doctor, courtesy and consideration for the patient as a fellow human being, tangible respect for his or her dignity, and sincere understanding and sympathy are necessary prerequisites for a successful course of treatment.

The clinical diagnostic assessment consists of two distinct but equally significant components: the history and physical examination. They ought to be carried out somewhat concurrently and in a way that enhances one another. As the skilled medical professional listens to the patient's history, they will already be considering what particular abnormalities to check for during the physical examination. The physician can elicit more details from the patient's history by asking more focused questions if the examination turns up any additional, possibly unexpected findings. The diagnosis should ideally be made by the physician based only on the patient's history and physical examination.

1.4.2. Special Aspects of History Taking

A comprehensive picture of the patient, including past medical history, current complaints, personality, and life circumstances, is intended to be provided by the "classic" history, which consists of a few standard elements.

1.4.2.1. The Present Illness

Always allow the patient to explain their current complaints and the reason for the consultation before beginning to take a clinical history. It is only after that, in accordance with the previously discussed principles, that you should start methodically questioning the patient to complete the history. All areas of clinical medicine follow a standard procedure for taking a systematic history; Table 1.4 provides a basic overview. However, there are additional significant concerns that frequently come up in each specialty and these should be specifically discussed. Table 1.5 provides a summary of the crucial inquiries to make when reviewing the neurological history.

Medical, family, and social history from the past. You can start by asking general questions about the patient's past symptoms and illnesses and work your way up to more in-depth inquiries once you have a clear and comprehensive picture of their current complaints. Always inquire about any issues that may be related to the current condition. For example, a patient experiencing an ischemic stroke should be questioned about heart disease, smoking, and hypertension. Find out how the patient's blood relatives are doing, especially in terms of neurological and other inherited conditions. Lastly, find out about the patient's social and familial background, including their occupation, children, marital status, and any possible issues or conflicts in these domains. Find out how the patient's medical issues, past or present, impact him or her in daily life, at home and at work. However, broach these topics as quietly as possible, as excessive probing may lead the patient to believe incorrectly that you consider the majority of their issues to be psychogenic. Of course, the patient should also be fully informed if a comprehensive diagnostic evaluation indicates that a psychogenic mechanism is most likely the cause.

Table 1.4. Outline of the General Clinical History

1 **The patient's spontaneous description of his or her current complaints** —more precise information can be elicited by direct questioning

2 **Systematic analysis of the current complaints** (see Table 2.2)

3 **Prior illnesses** (past medical and surgical history)
- information spontaneously provided by the patient
- specific questioning by the physician, particularly about earlier conditions of potential relevance to the current complaints
- gestational and birth history, when indicated

4 **Life Habits**
- alcohol and tobacco
- medications
- illicit drugs
- potentially toxic environmental influences

5 **Neurovegetative functions**
- sleep, digestion, urination, sexual dysfunction

6 **Personality and social situation**
- the patient's **personal and social setting:** education, occupation, familial/social/financial position, and any current problems or conflicts (information of this type enables the physician to assess all of the factors affecting the patient's ability to deal with his or her medical problems successfully)
- the patient's behavior, manner of speaking, gestures, facial expressions, emotional responses, and reactions to questions, etc., give the examiner an **overall impression of the patient's personality**

7 **Family history**

Source: https://www.ruseducation.in/books/Fundamentals-Neurology.pdf.

An experienced clinician should be able to make a rough diagnosis even before performing a physical examination with the help of a well-elicited clinical history. He or she can then focus especially on specific areas of the examination with the preliminary diagnosis in mind. Naturally, the physician must take care to ensure that no previous expectations cloud their findings to the point where they become untrustworthy. The physical examination should be guided by the tentative diagnosis rather than becoming a meaningless exercise.

Table 1.5. History of the Present Illness

Major symptom(s)

- The patient's spontaneous description, refined by specific questioning
- How long have the symptoms been present? Where are they located?
- How did they begin? (suddenly, gradually, or after a specific inducing event?)
- How have they developed over time? (constant, increasing, decreasing, fluctuating?)
- What influences the symptoms? (ameliorating/aggravating influences, medications?)
- Effects
  - How severe are the symptoms in terms of their effect on everyday life at home and at work, and on the patient's emotional well-being? Is treatment required?

Current accompanying symptoms

- Here it is particularly important to supplement the patient's spontaneous complaints with specific questioning. An experienced clinician knows what questions to ask even if the patient has provided very little information.

Relevant past medical history

- Did the patient already have **earlier symptoms** or conditions that might be relevant to the current complaints? (e. g., earlier transient ischemic attacks in a patient suffering from acute stroke?)
- Does the patient have any **predisposing factors** for conditions that might account for the current complaints? (e. g., cigarette smoking leading to a Pancoast tumor of the apex of the lung?)

Relevant family history

- This may lend support to a conjectural diagnosis: e. g., similar symptoms in blood relatives of the patient's parents, if a recessively inherited condition is suspected, or hemicranial headaches in the mother of a patient with suspected migraine

Source: https://www.ruseducation.in/books/Fundamentals-Neurology.pdf.

1.5. The Neurological Examination

1.5.1. Basic Principles of the Neurological Examination

When combined with a physical examination, a carefully elicited history aids in the diagnosis of neurological diseases. The examining physician should examine every patient using the same general scheme, with individual variations made as needed, to ensure completeness. The nervous system's individual components (cranial nerves, reflexes, motor, sensory, and autonomic function) can be tested in a specific order, or the examination can be oriented along topographic lines (head, upper limbs, trunk, lower limbs). This chapter's presentation is set up topographically.

Neurology is a distinct medical specialty and area of study in and of itself. The majority of neurological diseases solely impact the nervous system. However, neurological symptoms and signs are frequently present in general medical illnesses. Thus, a general physical examination must always be part of the clinical neurological examination.

While the neurological components of the physical examination should receive special attention, the practicing neurologist cannot ignore its general components. Below is a list of some fundamental concepts of physical examination.

The examiner should speak with the patient, providing concise explanations for each step of the examination when necessary. This is especially important for pediatric patients, but applies to individuals of all ages.

Although the examiner is free to follow any order they choose, a neurological examination should, in theory, always be comprehensive and conducted in the same order. Table 1.6 contains a list of each examination component. An exceptionally skilled clinician may decide to conduct only a partial examination in some extraordinary circumstances. However, this should usually be avoided because even the most skilled neurologist may overlook something crucial in this manner. Furthermore, a methodical and thorough examination helps reassure the patient that the doctor is knowledgeable and caring.

Patients should receive explicit instructions regarding what clothing to remove before being examined undressed; typically, this includes everything but their underwear. If the upper body is still clothed, it is impossible to examine the spine. Additionally, if the patient is wearing socks, it is impossible to test sensation in the feet or elicit the Babinski reflex.

As we've already emphasized, the examination should always be methodical and thorough; however, the clinician will focus more on specific areas of the examination depending on the preliminary diagnosis—or diagnoses—that the history suggests. The mindless, robotic performance of an exacting examination on each patient makes no sense.

The examiner should put the results in writing as soon as possible after the examination is finished. Claims that are generalized, like "Neuro unremarkable," are useless. An outline like the one shown in Table 1.6 can be used to summarize the results. The ability for the clinician to track the progression of a disease process from one examination to the next is the primary goal of accurate documentation. It is also unquestionably essential for medicolegal purposes.

Furthermore, some findings—like muscle strength, in particular—should be measured or assigned a numerical grade. It is important to accurately document the topography and extent of any sensory disturbances.

Table 1.6. The Neurological Examination

Head and cranial nerves		
Head freely mobile		No meningismus
Skull not tender to percussion		No bruits
No supra- or infraorbital point tenderness		No occipital point tenderness
Carotid pulsations strong bilaterally, without bruits		Perioral reflexes not exaggerated
Temporal artery pulsations strong bilaterally, without tenderness		
I	Coffee correctly identified by smell in both nostrils (spontaneously named/chosen from list)	
II	Corrected visual acuity (distance): R L	
	Visual fields full to confrontation	
	Optic discs normal bilaterally	
III, IV, VI	Eye movements full and coordinated	
	No pathological nystagmus	
	Pupils equal, round, midsized, and symmetrical, with prompt reaction to light and convergence	
V	Sensation in the face intact	
	Corneal reflex symmetrically elicitable	
	Masseter strong bilaterally	
VII	Facial expression normal (both voluntary and involuntary movements)	
VIII	Hearing subjectively normal	
	Whisper heard at a distance of m (R ear), m (L ear)	
	Weber not lateralized	
IX, X	Palatal veil symmetrical at rest, elevates symmetrically	
	Gag reflex intact	
	Swallowing subjectively unimpaired	
XI	Sternocleidomastoid strength full and symmetrical	
XII	Tongue symmetrical, protrudes in the midline, freely mobile	
Language Unremarkable		
Upper Limbs	right-handed	Left-handed
Bulk normal bilaterally		
Tone normal bilaterally		
Full mobility throughout		
Raw strength normal in all muscle groups		
Postural testing normal bilaterally, without sinking		
Rapid alternating movements performed well bilaterally		
No rebound phenomenon		
Finger–nose test accurate bilaterally, no intention tremor		
No finger tremor		
Reflexes:	Biceps reflex symmetrical, of medium strength	
	Triceps reflex symmetrical, of medium strength	
	Brachioradialis reflex symmetrical, of medium strength	
	Mayer reflex elicitable bilat	Hoffmann, Trömner not exaggerated bilat.
Sensation bilaterally intact to touch		
Pain sensation bilaterally intact		Two-point discrimination < 5 mm bilat.
Temperature sensation bilaterally intact		
Position sense in the fingers bilaterally intact		
Vibration sense bilaterally intact		
Stereognosis prompt bilaterally		Coin recognition good bilaterally
Trunk		
Spine unremarkable, without percussion tenderness anywhere		
Sensation on trunk intact		"Saddle" sensation intact
Abdominal skin reflex symmetrically intact		Finger-to-floor distance: .../... cm
Cremaster reflex bilaterally present (males only)		Small Schober .../... cm
Lower limbs		
Bulk normal bilaterally		
Tone normal bilaterally		
Full mobility throughout		
Raw strength normal in all muscle groups, incl. plantar flexors and dorsiflexors		
Lasègue negative bilaterally		No nerve trunk tenderness
Postural testing (supine position) normal bilaterally, without sinking		
Heel–knee–shin test accurate bilaterally		
Reflexes:	Quadriceps reflex symmetrical, of medium strength	Oppenheim negative bilaterally
	Achilles' reflex symmetrical, of medium strength	
	Babinski negative bilaterally	
	Gordon negative bilaterally	

Sensation bilaterally intact to touch
Pain sensation bilaterally intact
Temperature sensation bilaterally intact
Position sense in the toes bilaterally intact
Vibration sense bilaterally intact
Graphesthesia (number recognition) good on both legs

Stance and gait
Romberg negative (in various positions of the head)
Normal gait with normal accessory movements
Walks well on heels bilaterally | Walks well on tiptoes bilaterally
No unsteadiness in heel-to-toe walk

Mental status grossly unremarkable without further testing | **General physical examination:** blood pressure, pulse, heart, lungs, abdomen, lymph nodes, peripheral pulses

Source: https://www.ruseducation.in/books/Fundamentals-Neurology.pdf.

1.5.2. Stance and Gait

- **General Information:** Even though stance and gait are mentioned at the bottom of Table 1.6, we actually advise evaluating these abilities as the initial stage of the patient's examination while they are not clothed. A patient's standing posture alone may provide insight into the nature of their illness. E.g., atrophy of the muscles, spinal abnormalities, and scapular winging. The patient may have abnormal resting posture, e.g., the patient's hunched, rigid posture caused by Parkinson's disease, or the pronounced lumbar lordosis associated with muscular dystrophy. It is optimal to assess a patient's stance and gait while they are barefoot; insightful results can only be obtained when the patient has adequate space to move around. Testing one's stance and gait can often reveal crucial information about the kind of disease process that is going on. The tests' order is displayed in Figure 1.6a–g. The ability of the patient to walk normally and without a limp are the two most crucial aspects of their gait. The pathological side is the one that bears weight for a shorter period of time if the patient limps. The patient's stride length, the way their feet are placed on and rolled off the ground, and the accompanying arm swings should all be noted by the examiner. Table 1.7 describes a few typical gait disturbances.
- **Walking on Tiptoe and Walking on the Heels:** (Figs. 1.6b, c) Allow the medical professional to assess the extensors of the foot and toe as well as the calf muscles. The patient can still walk on tiptoe if their plantar flexors are only slightly weak. However, they won't be able to stand on one leg and hop repeatedly (10 times on one foot) or elevate themselves to a standing position.
- **The "Tightrope Walk" (Heel-to-Toe Walk):** (Figure 1.6d) is an extremely sensitive test used to assess equilibrium and gait stability. During this test, the patient is asked to place one foot firmly in front of the other, first looking at the floor, then looking straight ahead, and finally looking at the ceiling. The ability to walk heel-to-toe should be possible in all of these conditions. However, performing heel-to-toe walking with eyes closed is a more challenging task that many healthy individuals struggle to achieve.
- **The Romberg Test:** (Figure 1.6e) is an additional equilibrium test. For at least twenty seconds, the patient is

asked to stand with their feet parallel and together and their eyes closed. This should be completed with ease and composure, without any noticeable swaying. The patient can tilt their head to one side or turn to make the test more challenging. Additionally, it can be carried out in conjunction with arm position testing (see below).

There are several methods to assess the vestibular system and cerebellum, one of which is the Unterberger step test (Figure 1.6f). With closed eyes, the patient walks in place, lifting one knee to the horizontal or higher with each stride. The patient should have rotated no more than 45° from starting position after 50 steps.

A number of common gait abnormalities are illustrated in Figure 1.7.

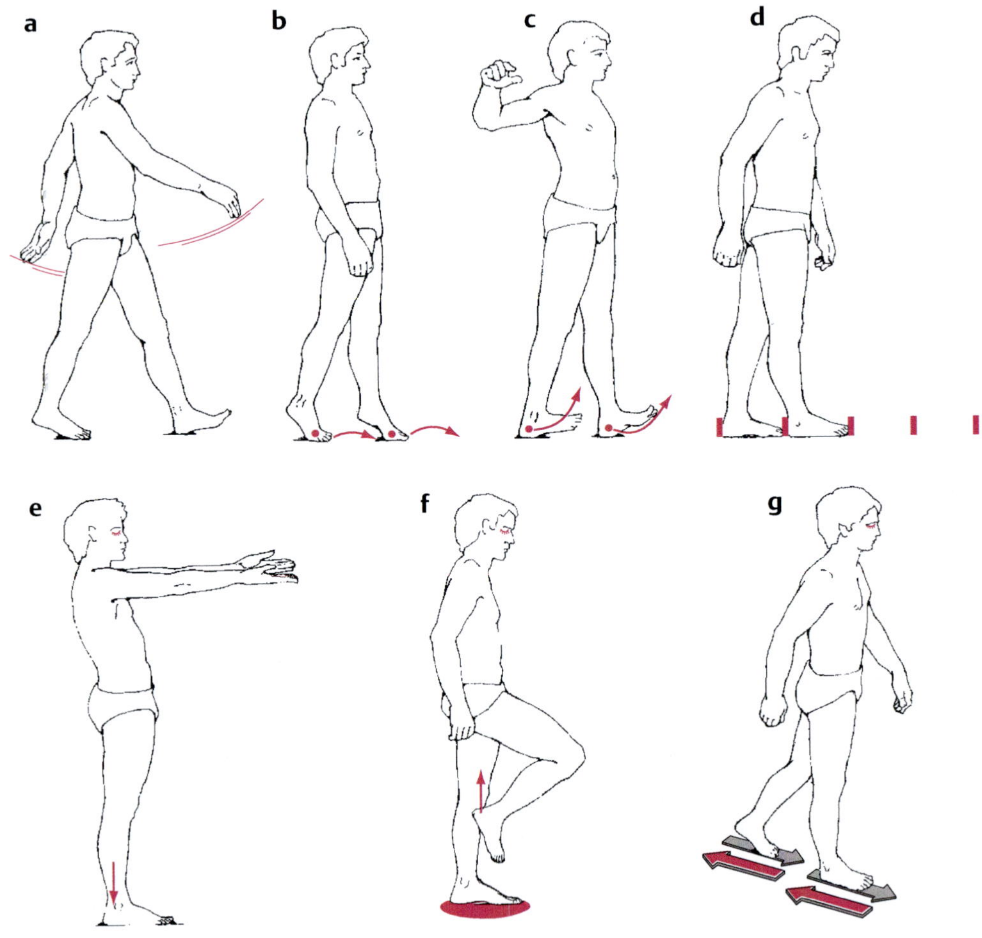

Figure 1.6. Tests of stance and gait. (a) normal gait. Note normal step length and arm swing. (b) Walking on tiptoes. c Walking on heels. (d) Heel-to-toe walking. One foot is placed precisely in front of the other. (e) Romberg test with eyes closed, combined with postural test of the upper limbs. (f) Unterberger step test: walking in place with eyes closed. See text for interpretation of results. (g) Babinski–Weil test with "star gait" (marche en étoile): the patient is asked to take two steps forward and two steps back, repeatedly, with eyes closed. For interpretation, see text.

Source: https://www.ruseducation.in/books/Fundamentals-Neurology.pdf.

Greater rotations indicate problems with either the cerebellar hemisphere or the vestibular apparatus on the side the patient has turned. Babinski and Weil's "star gait" test involves the patient repeatedly taking two steps forward and two steps back while keeping their eyes closed. An involuntary turn to the side of the lesion is an indication of vestibular dysfunction. When blind walking, the patient approaches the examiner from a distance after first glancing at him or her, closing their eyes. A deviation to the side of the lesion is caused by vestibular lesions.

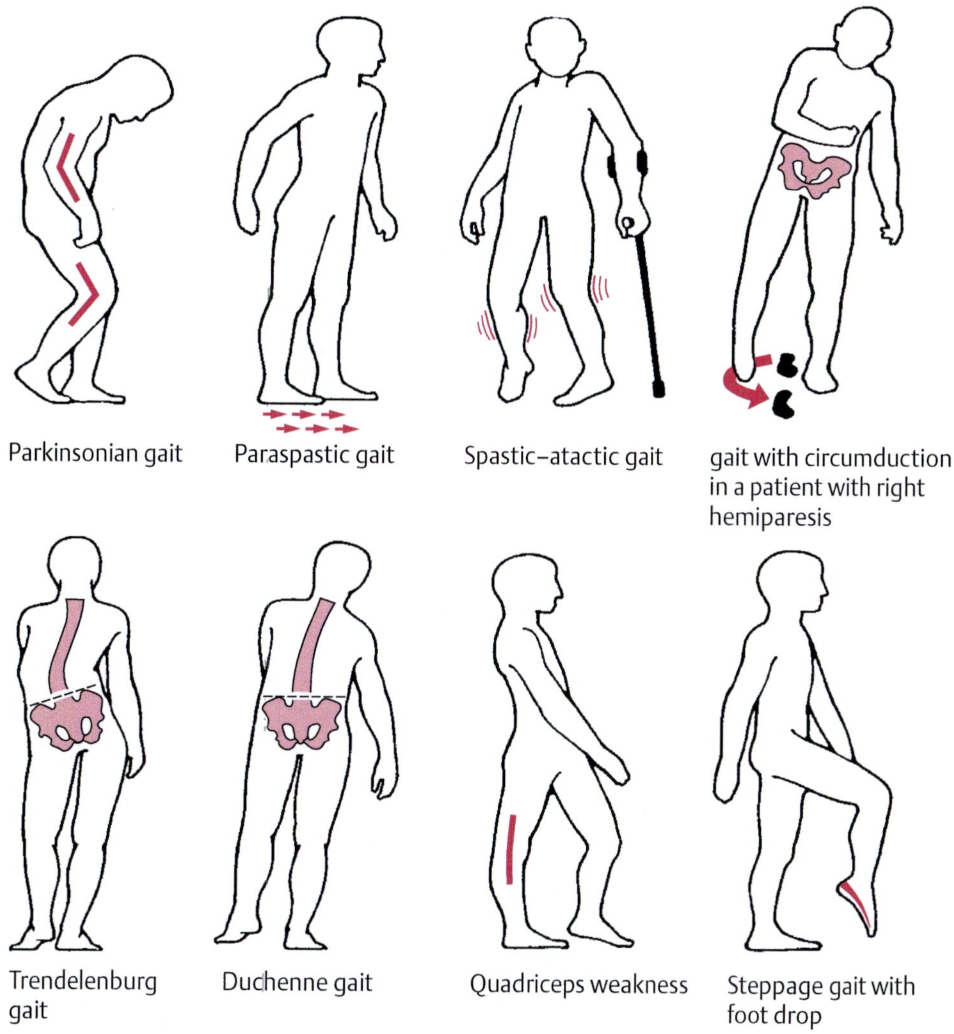

Figure 1.7. Common gait disturbances.

Source: Fundamentals of neurology © 2006 thieme.

Table 1.7. Characteristic Disturbances of Gait

Designation	Abnormalities of gait	Causes, remarks
Spastic gait	Slow, stiff, with audible dragging of the soles of the feet across the ground	Bilateral pyramidal tract lesion
Ataxic gait	Uncoordinated, stamping, unsteady, deviating irregularly from a straight line; heel-to-toe walking impossible	Cerebellar dysfunction, posterior column dysfunction, peripheral neuropathy
Spastic–ataxic gait	Combination of the two above disorders; jerky, stiff, inharmonious gait	Most commonly seen in multiple sclerosis
Dystonic gait	Uncontrollable additional movements interfering with the normal course of gait	Basal ganglionic disease causing choreoathetosis or dystonia
Hypokinetic gait	Slow gait, stiff, bent posture, small steps, lack of accessory arm movements; turning requires multiple small steps	Most commonly seen in parkinson's disease; similar picture in the lacunar state
Small-stepped gait	Small steps, unsteady, resembles hypokinetic gait but with more normal accessory movements	"Old person's gait" most commonly seen in the lacunar state, i.e., multiple small infarcts in the basal ganglia and along the corticospinal tracts, generally caused by atherosclerosis; distinguishable from parkinsonian gait mainly by the different accompanying signs
Circumduction	Increased tone in the extensors of the paretic leg, which comes forward in a gentle outward arc, with a strongly plantar-flexed foot; hardly any accompanying movement of the flexed and adducted ipsilateral arm	Central (spastic) hemiparesis
Steppage gait	The advancing leg is raised high and then placed on the ground toe first, often with an audible slap	Unilateral: foot drop, e.g., in peroneal nerve palsy; bilateral: e.g., polyneuropathy or steinert myotonic dystrophy
Hyperextended knee	With each step, the knee of the stationary leg is hyperextended	Prevents buckling of the knee when the knee extensors are weak—unilaterally, e.g., in quadriceps weakness due to a lesion of the femoral n.; bilaterally, e.g., in muscular dystrophy

Hyperlordotic gait	Exaggerated lumbar lordosis	E.g., in muscular dystrophy affecting the pelvic girdle, in boys with duchenne muscular dystrophy
Trendelenburg gait	With each step, the pelvis tilts downward on the side of the swinging leg	Severe hip abductor weakness—unilaterally, e.g., in lesions of the superior gluteal n.; bilaterally, e.g., in muscular dystrophy affecting the pelvic girdle and in bilateral hip dislocation
Duchenne gait	With each step, the upper body tilts to the side of the stationary leg	Mild or moderate weakness of the hip abductors (as in trendelenburg gait, but less severe), or as a painreducing maneuver in disorders of the hip joint

Source: Mumenthaler / Mattle, Fundamentals of Neurology © 2006 Thieme.

1.6. Examination of the Head and Cranial Nerves

1.6.1. Head and Cervical Spine

The head and cervical spine's overall appearance should be noted by the examiner first (e.g., sunken temples in Steinert myotonic dystrophy) as well as the look on the patient's face (e.g., lack of expression on the face in Parkinson's disease). Individuals who are young and in good health should be able to turn their head and neck nearly 90 degrees in either direction so that the eye that is further away from the examiner is hidden behind the patient's nose root. Furthermore, when the neck is maximally flexed, the patient should be able to rotate their head 60 degrees to the right or left and incline it laterally 45 degrees in either direction (this rotation occurs only at the atlantoaxial and atlanto-occipital joints). The patient is tested for meningismus while they are lying supine. If this finding is present, it typically indicates meningeal irritation from meningitis or subarachnoid hemorrhage, but it can also occasionally be a reflexive reaction to posterior fossa lesions that occupy space. Meningismus is characterized by a singular inhibition of cervical flexion, leaving the head free to rotate. The examiner bends the head forward in the supine patient's neck to check for meningismus. The Lasègue sign is typically positive in cases of true meningismus as well. A positive cervical Brudzinski sign occurs when attempted passive flexion of the neck also causes flexion of the lower limbs at the hip or knee joint. This sign is frequently accompanied by a positive Kernig sign, which indicates that the patient cannot passively extend their knee while seated and that passive straight leg raising causes reflex knee flexion when the patient is supine.

A pulse-synchronous bruit over an arteriovenous fistula or an arteriovenous malformation may be audible upon auscultation of the skull. Stenosis could be the cause of a carotid bruit.

- **The Intrinsic Reflexes of the Facial Musculature Should Always be Examined:** The ipsilateral orbicularis oculi reflex is typically triggered by tapping a finger placed over the patient's lateral canthus. If this reflex does not weaken (habituate) after repeated tapping, there is likely a bilateral lesion of the corticobulbar pathways. A bilateral corticobulbar lesion is also suggested by an excessively strong, bilateral contraction of the orbicularis oculi when the examiner taps on the patient's glabella (also known as the nasopalpebral reflex). Positive snout reflex (lip protrusion) can be caused by tapping on a tongue depressor positioned on the patient's lips. When a patient's mouth is half open, a gentle tapping motion from above can trigger the masseter reflex, also known as the jaw jerk reflex. Applying pressure to a tongue depressor placed on the patient's mandibular teeth can also trigger this reflex. When the cornea is touched, the jaw will deviate, causing the "winking jaw phenomenon" or corneomandibular reflex. The pontomesencephalic reticular formation is the termination point of ascending and descending brainstem pathways, which are disrupted if it is present on only one side or exhibits significant asymmetry.

1.6.2. Cranial Nerves

The individual cranial nerves are then examined. An overview of the structure and operation of the 12 cranial nerves can be found in Figure 1.8 and Table 1.8. We will go over the primary examination methods and a few of the significant abnormal results that each one can produce.

The olfactory and optic nerves are the first two cranial nerves, actually represent areas of the brain that have been moved to the periphery. In terms of both structure and function, the remaining ten cranial nerves are similar to the body's other peripheral nerves. They perform autonomic, somatosensory, motor, and special sensory functions.

- CN I: Olfactory N:
    - **Testing the Sense of Smell**: Every nostril's ability to smell is tested separately. After closing their eyes, the patient is instructed to identify—or at the very least, perceive—fragrant materials held beneath their open nose, such as coffee, cinnamon, or vanilla. 75% of average people can correctly identify coffee grounds. Asafetida, or onion extract, is a smelly substance that is used when a patient's ability to smell is questioned. Neurological significance only applies to total loss of smell (anosmia), not to a partial reduction in smell. The most common cause of anosmia is severe traumatic brain injury, but it can also result from postinfectious abnormalities of the nasal mucosa, e.g., olfactory groove meningioma, or frontal tumors. E.g., either in ozena or following an upper respiratory "cold."

Patients who are unsure if their anosmia is neurological in nature are given a diluted ammonia solution to sniff. It is not the olfactory nerve that mediates the unpleasant irritation that results from this, but through the trigeminal nerve. Should the patient not respond, it is likely that they are experiencing either an acute process that affects the nasal mucosa (e.g., either from a psychogenic disturbance (e.g., acute rhinitis). In either scenario, the anosmia is not neurogenic.

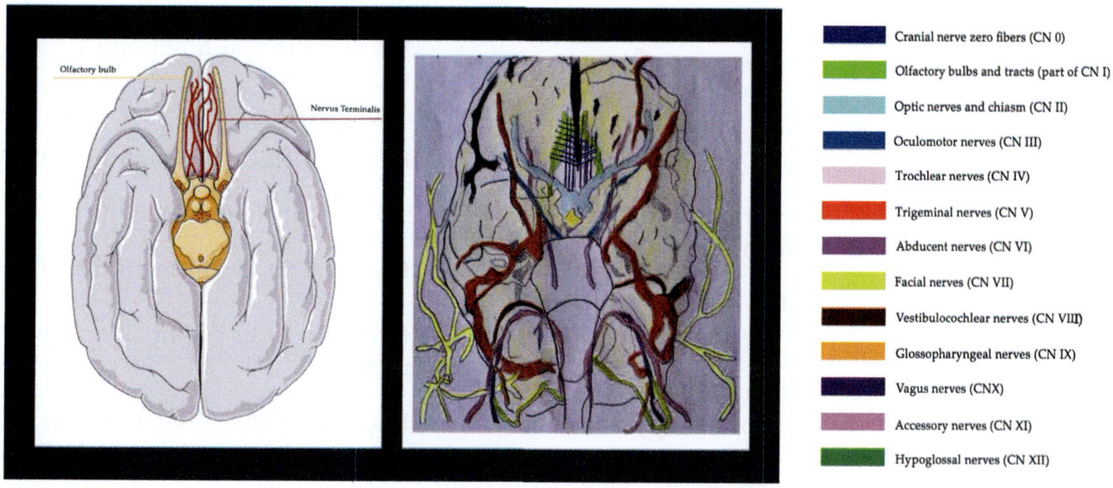

Figure 1.8. Overview of the topographical relations of the cranial nerves and their sites of exit from the skull. ACP = anterior clinoid process, OA = ophthalmic a., PCommA = posterior communicating a., pit. = pituitary gland. III = oculomotor n., IV = trochlear n., V = trigeminal n., VI = abducens n., VII = facial n., VIII = vestibulocochlear n., IX = glossopharyngeal n., X = vagus n., XI = accessory n., XII = hypoglossal n.

Source: Ruqa WA, Pennacchia F, Rusi E, Zoccali F, Bruno G, Talarico G, Barbato C, Minni A. Smelling TNT: Trends of the Terminal Nerve. *International Journal of Molecular Sciences*. 2024; 25(7):3920. https://doi.org/10.3390/ijms25073920.

Table 1.8. The 12 Cranial Nerves, Their Nuclei, and Their Functions

Cranial Nerve	**Ganglion and Type**	Origin of Neurons
CNI – olfactory (Ensheating glia of olfactory nerves)		Telencephalon/olfactory placode; NCCs at forebrain
CNIII – oculomotor (m)	Ciliary, visceral efferent	NCCs at forebrain– midbrain junction (caudal diencephalon and the anterior mesencephalon)
CNV – trigeminal (mix)	Trigeminal, general afferent	NCCs at forebrain– midbrain junction (from r2 into 1st PA), trigeminal placode
CNVII – facial (mix)	– Superior, general and special afferent – Inferior: geniculate, general and special afferent – Sphenopalatine, visceral efferent – Submandibular, visceral efferent	– Hindbrain NCCs (from r4 into 2nd PA), 1st epibranchial placode – 1st epibranchial placode (geniculate) – Hindbrain NCCs (2nd PA) – Hindbrain NCCs (2nd PA)

CNVIII – Vestibulocochlear (s)	– Acoustic: cochlear, special afferent; and vestibular, special afferent	– Otic placode and hindbrain (from r4) NCCs
CNIX – glossopharyngeal (mix)	– Superior, general and special afferent – Inferior, petrosal, general and special afferent – Otic, visceral efferent	– Hindbrain NCCs (from r6 into 3rd PA) – 2nd epibranchial placode (petrosal) – Hindbrain NCCs (from r6 into 3rd PA)
CNX – vagus (mix) Superior laryngeal branch; and recurrent laryngeal branch	– Superior, general afferent – Inferior: nodose, general and special afferent – Vagal: parasympathetic, visceral efferent	– Hindbrain NCCs (from r7– r8 to 4th & 6th PA) – Hindbrain NCCs (4th& 6th PA); 3rd (nodose) and 4th epibranchial placodes – Hindbrain NCCs (4th & 6th PA)
CNXI – accessory (m)	No ganglion *	Hindbrain (from r7– r8 to PA 4); NCCs (4th PA)

Source: *https://en.wikipedia.org/wiki/Cranial_nerves.*

- CN II: Optic N
  - **Ophthalmoscopy:** An essential method for evaluating the optic nerve is to examine the optic discs, or optic nerve papillae, using an ophthalmoscope. A lesion to the optic nerve is indicated by abnormal pallor (Figure 1.9). Examining the eye grounds can also reveal signs of increased intracranial pressure because papilledema causes the papillae to become raised, hyperemic, and blurry around their margins. Increased retinal veins are a sign of intracranial hypertension-related poor venous drainage. A blurred margin and elevated papilla may also indicate an inflammatory process affecting the optic nerve.

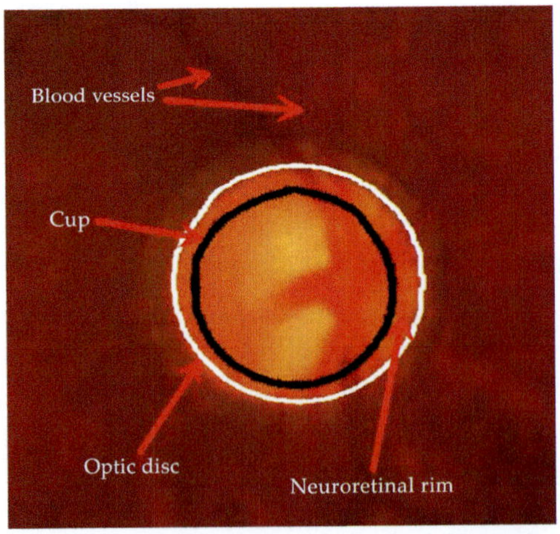

Figure 1.9. Optic disc (papilla) of the eye.

Source: Gao Y, Yu X, Wu C, Zhou W, Wang X, Zhuang Y. Accurate Optic Disc and Cup Segmentation from Retinal Images Using a Multi-Feature Based Approach for Glaucoma Assessment. *Symmetry*. 2019; 11(10):1267. https://doi.org/10.3390/sym11101267.

When testing visual acuity for neurological purposes, a wall chart viewed from a distance is typically used. Glasses are used to correct refractive errors when needed (Figure 1.10).

- o **Perimetry:** Neurology places a great deal of importance on visual field testing. Using a technique known as finger perimetry, the visual fields can be roughly evaluated in the neurologist's office or at the patient's bedside. The patient fixes one eye on the examiner's nose as the examiner sits squarely in front of them. Next, in order to test each eye independently, the examiner places a finger in each of the four visual field quadrants. When asked if they can see the finger, the patient responds positively. Using this technique can make a significant visual field defect, e.g., either quadrantanopsia or bitemporal hemianopsia. Figure 1.11 shows a variety of visual field defects along with the locations of the lesions that cause them. One point twelve.

The next step for the examiner should be double simultaneous stimulation of the visual field if visual neglect is suspected. This involves moving both index fingers simultaneously in corresponding quadrants in the two halves of the field (left and right hemifields). Both fingers should be visible to the patient. Visual neglect may be the cause if both fingers are perceived during individual testing but only one is visible during double simultaneous stimulation. When a finger is placed in the periphery of each eye and moved gradually toward the center, one can test each quadrant of the visual field separately to detect defects in monocular vision.

Smaller (monocular or binocular) defects in the visual field are typically only detectable through formal testing using devices like the Goldmann perimeter or octopus, though they can occasionally be found by confrontational perimetry with a red object.

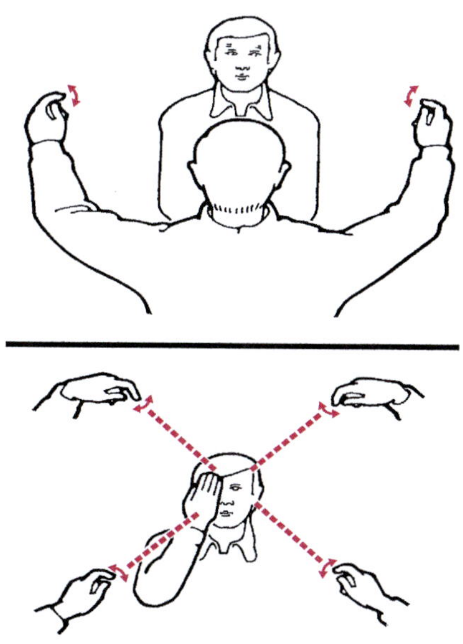

Figure 1.10. Testing the visual fields by digital confrontation. Above: double simultaneous testing for the detection of visual hemineglect. Below: individual testing of all four quadrants of the visual field of each eye.

Source: https://www.ruseducation.in/books/Fundamentals-Neurology.pdf.

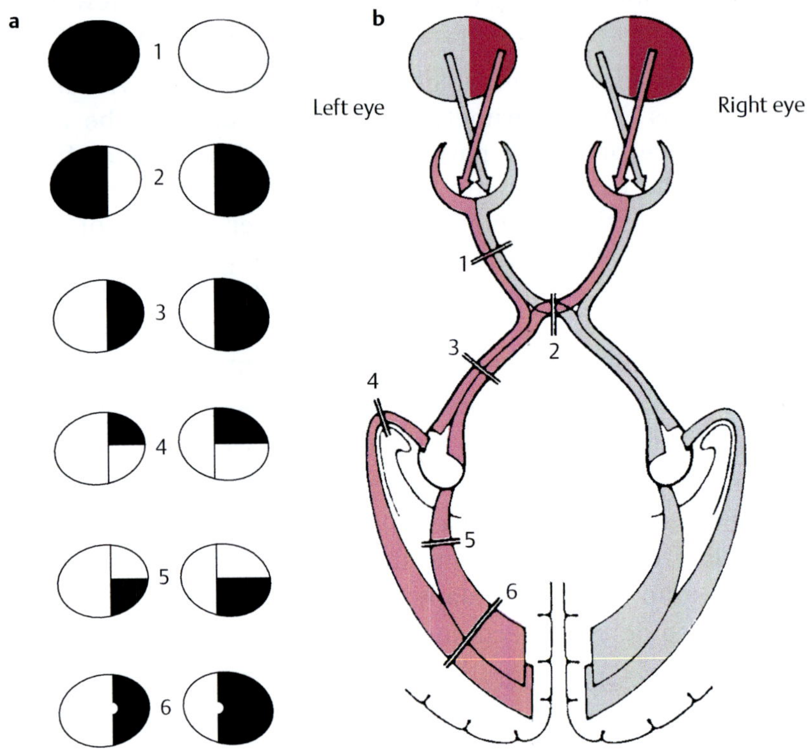

Figure 1.11. *Visual field defects and the sites of the lesions that cause them. (1) Blindness in the left eye due to a left optic nerve lesion. (2) Bitemporal hemianopsia due to a lesion of the optic chiasm. (3) Right homonymous hemianopsia due to a lesion of the left optic tract. (4–6) Lesions at various sites in the left optic radiation: 4 Right upper quadrantanopsia due to a left temporal lobe lesion. (5) Right lower quadrantanopsia due to a left parietal lobe lesion. (6) Right homonymous hemianopsia, sparing macular vision, due to a left occipital lobe lesion.*

Source: https://www.ruseducation.in/books/Fundamentals-Neurology.pdf.

- CN III, IV, and VI: Oculomotor, Trochlear, and Abducens Nn:

o **Inspection**: First, the examiner should record the resting positions of the eyes, focusing on the following details: the eyes' parallel alignment, any potential eye prominence, and the symmetry of the pupils and palpebral fissures. The best way to determine the patient's eyes' parallel position is to look at the tiny, reflected images of the light sources in the examination room in each eye. These images should be positioned similarly on each cornea. Occasionally, looking at the eyes tangentially from above will allow one to see a prominent globe (exophthalmos) (Figure 1.12).

o **Ocular Motility Testing:** The patient's ability to follow the examiner's finger with his or her eyes while maintaining a still head is tested. The vertical and horizontal axes are used to evaluate the globes' motility. The manner in which eye movement is restricted (including any abnormality of the eyes' resting position) and the type of double vision allow the examiner to determine which muscle (or muscles) is/are paretic and, consequently, which cranial nerve is dysfunctional (paralytic strabismus) if the examiner can see the abnormalities directly or if the patient reports double vision (diplopia).

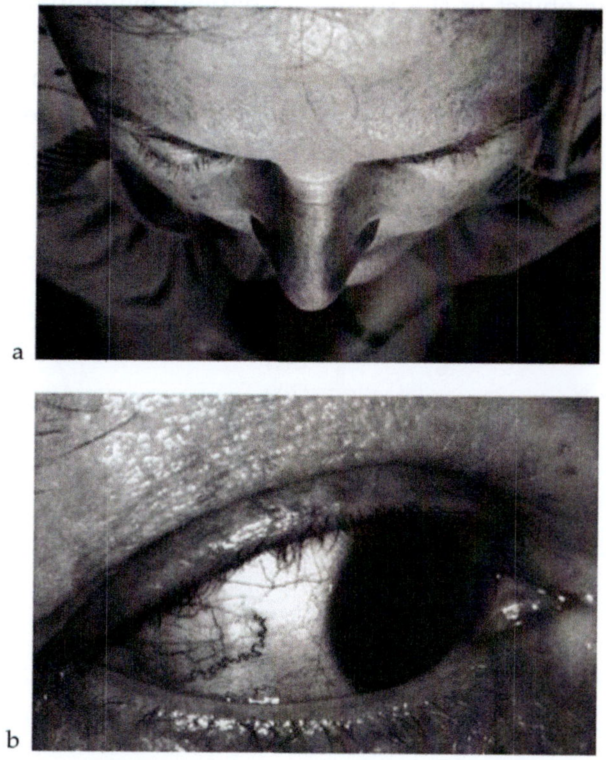

Figure 1.12. A patient with a right carotid–cavernous fistula (i.e., a fistula between the right internal carotid a. and the cavernous sinus). (a) the tangential photograph reveals exophthalmos. (b) Conjunctival venous stasis is caused by elevated venous pressure.

Source: Fundamentals of Neurology © 2006 Thieme.

On the other hand, intrinsic muscle lesions, as opposed to cranial nerve palsies, may weaken the eye muscles. A general rule for interpreting the results is that when the patient looks in the direction of the paretic muscle's function, their eyes are the furthest apart, and their diplopia is at its worst.

The incapacity to execute a conjugate eye movement to aim the gaze in a specific direction, either vertically or horizontally, is known as conjugate gaze palsy. In these patients, the lesion is centrally located within the brain (a supranuclear lesion, i.e., not in the peripheral segment of a cranial nerve). e.g., one situated above the cranial nerve nuclei responsible for innervating the extraocular muscles. The eyes stay parallel and double vision is absent, in contrast to peripheral lesions.

Nystagmus should be checked for by the examiner in addition to eye movements. The best way to identify deviations from the parallel axis is to look at the reflected images on the patient's cornea. A patient with concomitant strabismus—a condition caused by long-term vision impairment in one eye—is assumed to have nonparallel (skewed) positions of the two eyes without diplopia. (usually from birth or early childhood). There is no cranial nerve palsy. One useful tool for demonstrating concurrent strabismus is the cover test. While the examiner covers one eye and instructs the patient to focus on a specific object in the room, the patient maintains open eyes. After that, the covering is quickly moved to the other eye, requiring the covered eye to quickly adjust in order to maintain the same fixation. By putting the cover back on, it is possible to demonstrate how the previously uncovered eye, which is now covered, deviates to one side (alternating concomitant strabismus; usually divergent, but sometimes convergent).

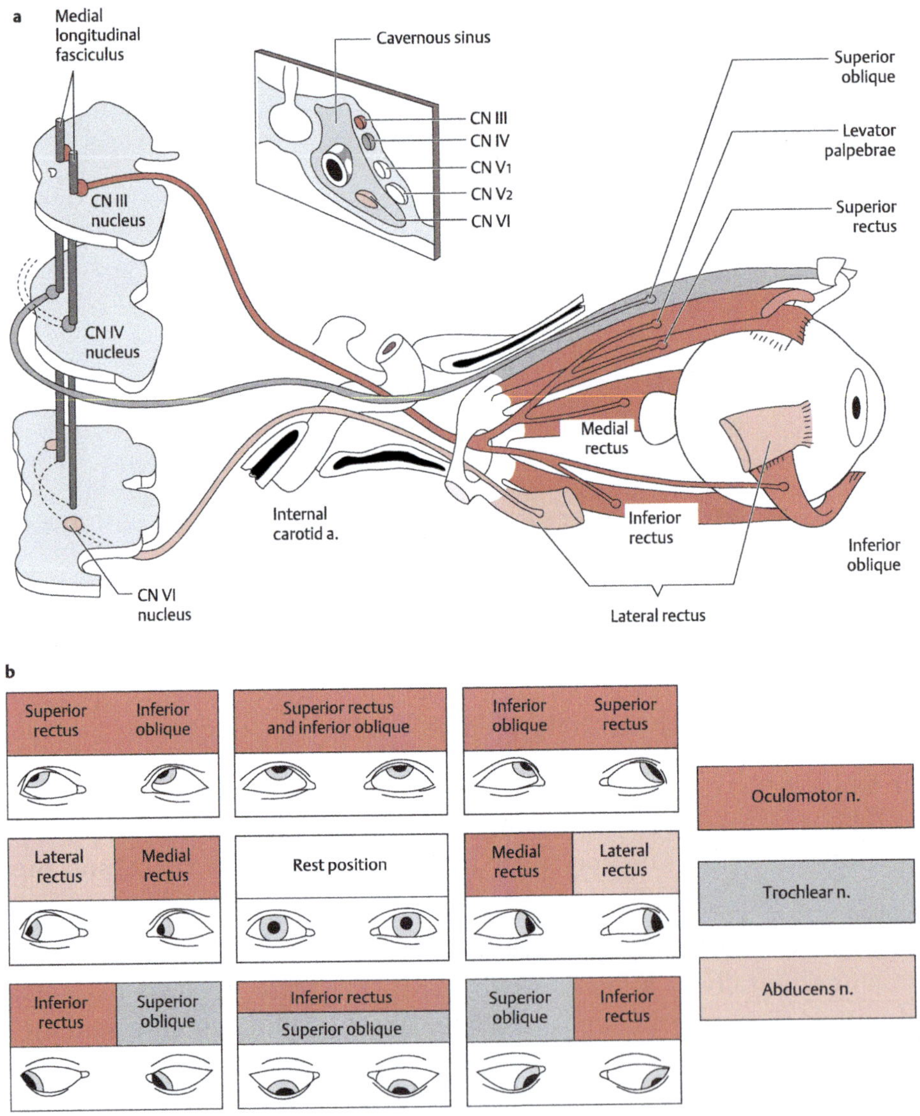

Figure 1.13. (a) the three nerves to the extraocular muscles and the muscles innervated by each. (b) Scheme according to Hering, indicating the direction of gaze in which the main function of each eye muscle is most strongly in evidence.

Source: https://www.ruseducation.in/books/Fundamentals-Neurology.pdf.

- **Assessment of the Pupils:** The size and form of the pupils—round or oblong—should be noted by the examiner. Normal pupils typically have equal sizes and respond to light in the same ways. Anisocoria, or pupil inequality, is a small amount of which is normal in certain people. One pupil should reflexively constrict (the direct light response) when the examiner illuminates it, and the other pupil should reflexively constrict (the consensual light response). Examiners shine a flashlight on one eye and use their own hand, held in the midline over the patient's nose root, to block light from the other eye, ensuring that only one pupil is illuminated. The examiner holds his or her finger close to the patient's face while the patient fixes their gaze on a distant point to test convergence. Adduction of both eyes (convergence) and concurrent reflex pupil constriction (the near response) are the typical reactions (Figure 1.14).

- **CN V: Trigeminal N:**

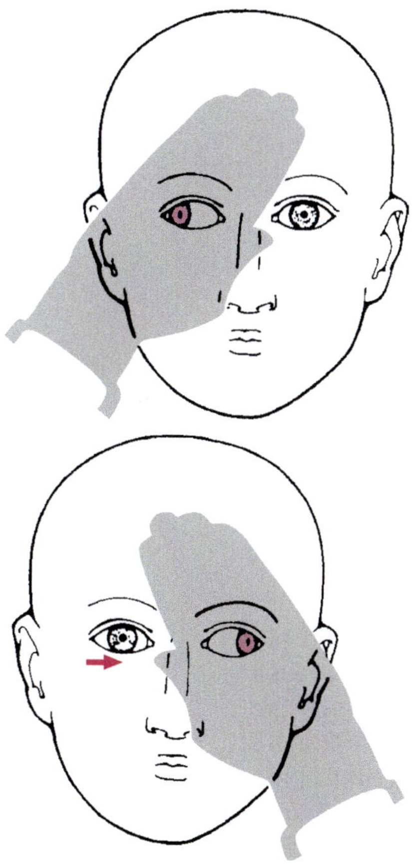

Figure 1.14. Cover test. In concomitant, alternating, divergent strabismus, the covered eye (i.e., the one that is not fixating) deviates outward. When the cover is rapidly switched to the other eye, the newly uncovered eye moves to the fixating position, while the covered other eye now deviates outward with a positioning saccade (→).

Source: https://www.ruseducation.in/books/Fundamentals-Neurology.pdf.

- **CN V: Trigeminal N**
  - **Testing Sensation in the Face:** The ganglion cells of the Gasserian ganglion are the source of the somatosensory portion of this mixed cranial nerve. The areas innervated by the trigeminal nerve that are cutaneous and mucosal. are displayed in Figure 1.15. Using a cotton swab or a piece of tissue paper, sensation should be tested. In order to prevent a visually induced fright reaction, the tactile stimulus is applied to the lower edge of the cornea while the patient is asked to look upward. This method can also be used to test the corneal reflex. The reflex reaction is to close the eyes right away.
  - **Assessment of the Muscles of Mastication:** The part of the trigeminal nerve that is motor. runs in the mandibular nerve, which is its third branch.) to provide the masticatory muscles, i.e., the temporalis mm and masseter mm. as well as the lateral and medial pterygoid mm. By placing both of his or her fingers in front of the jaw's angle and asking the patient to clamp their jaw tightly, the examiner can determine how well these muscles are working. In unilateral trigeminal neural net. paresis, the affected side's masseter contraction is palpably weaker, and there may be a decrease in the masseter reflex as well. The pterygoid muscles' dominant action on the healthy side causes the mandible to deviate to the side of the lesion when the patient opens their mouth.
- **CN VII: Facial N**
  - **Evaluation of the Facial Expression Muscles:** The examiner should record any asymmetry in the face, spontaneous facial expressions (mimesis), and contractions of the facial muscles during movement when evaluating its function. The patient should be methodically asked to clench their eyes, grin, whistle, and furrow their brow. When there are facial lesions. because the efferent arm of the reflex arc is disrupted (as opposed to the afferent arm, as in trigeminal lesions), the corneal reflex is weak. The clinical manifestations of facial nerve palsy and the distinction between central and peripheral facial weakness.
  - **Assessment of Taste, Lacrimation, and Salivation:** This includes gustatory fibers that provide taste to the front two-thirds of the tongue. Taste in this area can be tested by applying substances with the four basic modalities of taste—sweet, salty, sour, and bitter—to the corresponding half of the tongue when a facial nerve lesion is suspected. For instance, 20% glucose, 10% sodium chloride, 5% citric acid, and one percent quinine are suitable solutions to use. (Note: The glossopharyngeal nerve mediates the sensation of "bitterness," which is perceived in the mucosa of the posterior third of the tongue. not the n in the face.). facial lesions on the periphery. also result in decreased salivation and lacrimation, which are typically undetectable to the patient and need to be confirmed by specific testing. Additionally, hypersensitivity to sound (hyperacusis) could exist.
- **CN VIII: Vestibulocochlear N**
  - **Assessment of Hearing:** Figure 1.16 shows the anatomical structure of the vestibulocochlear nerve. The neurologist's evaluation of the patient's hearing is typically restricted to determining whether the patient has a hearing loss (uni- or bilateral) and, if so, whether the cause is a sensorineural deficit (affecting the

inner ear or the cochlear portion of the eighth cranial nerve) or impaired sound conduction (middle ear process, obstruction of the external auditory canal). The patient must physically rub their finger back and forth in the external auditory canal to deactivate the hearing in the ear that is not being tested. The examiner tests each ear independently by speaking or whispering words at a distance of five to six meters. Complete deafness, that is. deafness, even from extremely loud noises, is never the result of a middle ear problem on its own.

Distinguishing between hearing loss caused by electric current and vibration. The Rinne and Weber tests (Figure 1.17) can be used to distinguish between these two types of hearing loss.

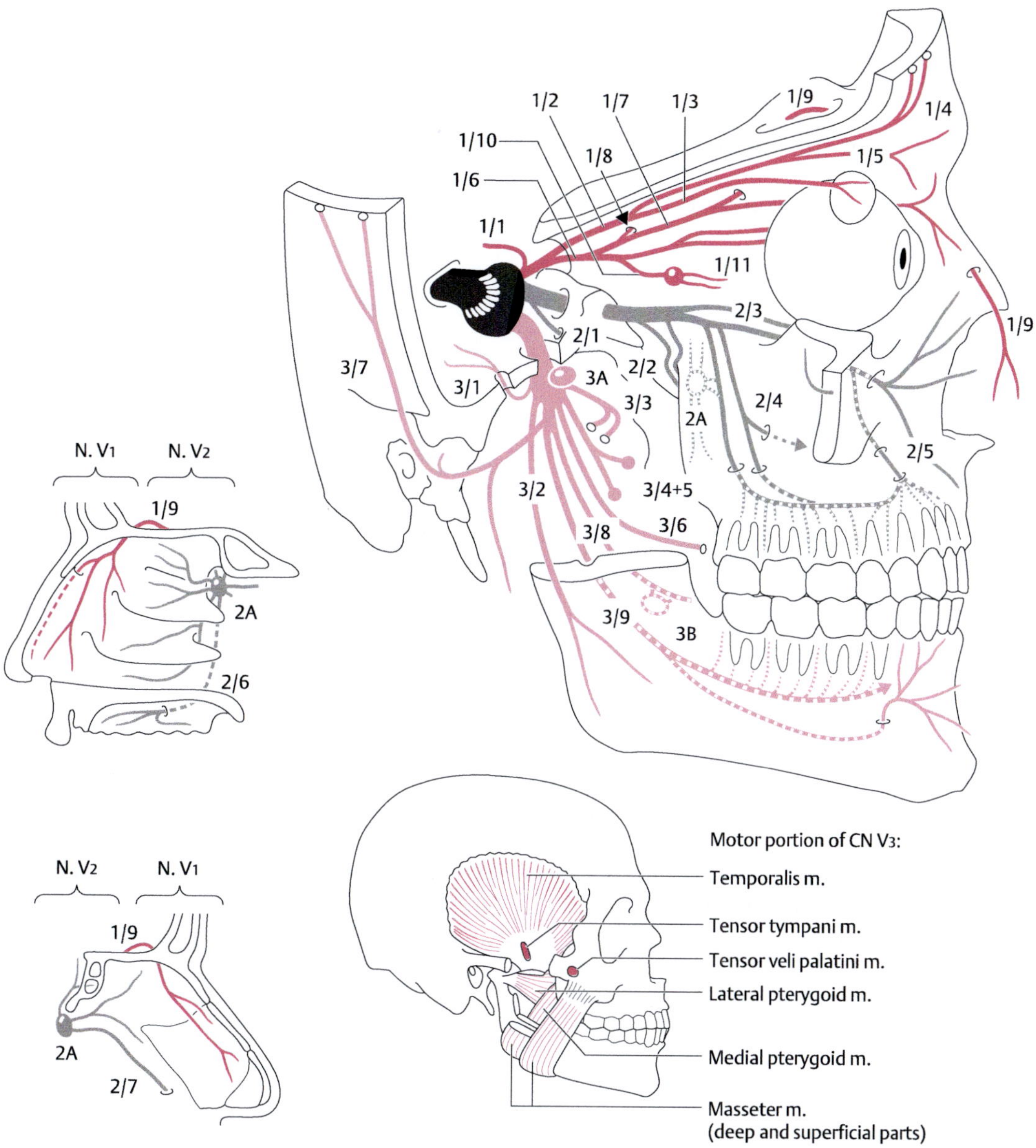

Ophthalmic n.

1/1 Tentorial branch
1/2 Frontal n.
1/3 Lacrimal n.
1/4 Supraorbital nn.
1/5 Supratrochlear n.
1/6 Nasociliary n.
1/7 Infratrochlear n.
1/8 Posterior ethmoidal n.
1/9 Anterior ethmoidal n. with external nasal branch
1/10 Ramus communicans → ciliary ganglion
1/11 Ciliary nn.

Maxillary n.

2/1 Middle meningeal branch
2/2 Pterygopalatine nn.
2A Pterygopalatine ganglion with:
Orbital branches
Nasal branches
Palatine nn.
2/3 Zygomatic n.
2/4 Superior alveolar nn.
2/5 Infraorbital n.
2/6 Greater palatine n.
2/7 Nasopalatine n.

Mandibular n.

3/1 Meningeal branch
3/2 Masseteric n.
3/3 Deep temporal n.
3/4+5 Medial and lateral pterygoid nn.
3/6 Buccal n.
3/7 Auriculotemporal n.
3/8 Lingual n.
3/9 Inferior alveolar n.
3A Otic ganglion
3B Submandibular ganglion

Figure 1.15. Anatomy of the somatosensory and motor portions of the trigeminal n.

Source: Fundamentals of Neurology © 2006 Thieme.

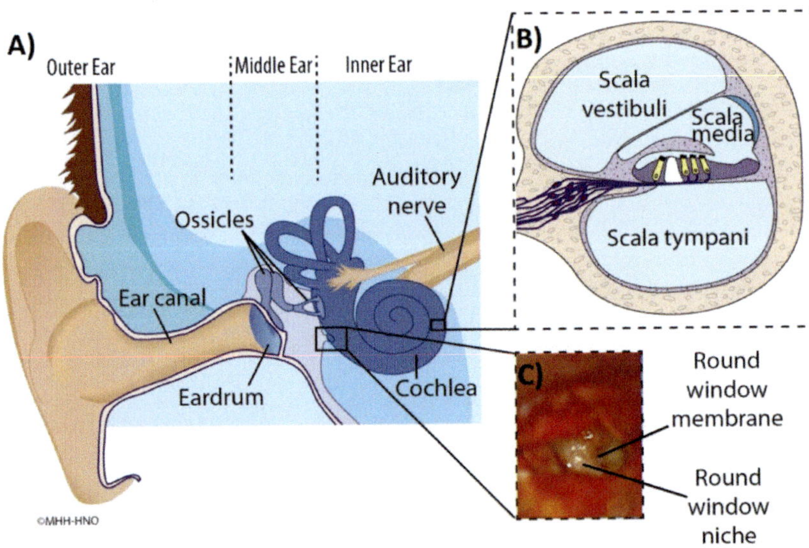

Figure 1.16. Anatomy of the internal ear and vestibulocochlear nerve. (schematic drawing).

Source: Matin F, Gao Z, Repp F, John S, Lenarz T, Scheper V. Determination of the round window niche anatomy using cone beam computed tomography imaging as preparatory work for individualized drug-releasing implants. *Journal of Imaging*. 2021; 7(5):79. https://doi.org/10.3390/jimaging7050079.

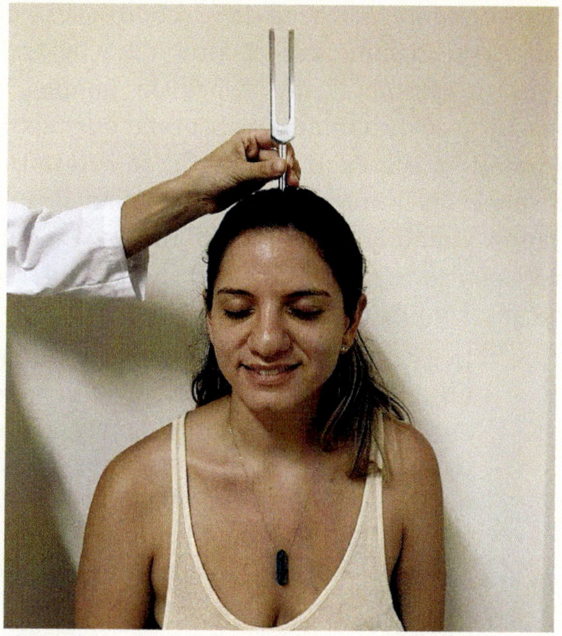

Figure 1.17. Weber and Rinne hearing tests. a Weber test: in a patient with right-sided conductive hearing loss (picture at left), the tuning fork cannot be heard when held next to the ear (1). If the tuning fork is placed on the forehead (2), however, it is heard, and the tone is localized to the side of the hearing loss, i.e., to the right ear. In contrast, in a patient with right-sided sensorineural hearing loss (picture at right), the tone is localized to the normally hearing (left) ear. b Rinne test: the tuning fork is first placed on the mastoid process (1). As soon as the tone is no longer heard, the tuning fork is held next to the ear. If hearing is normal, the tone will now be heard again (2). In right-sided conductive hearing loss (middle picture), the tone will not be heard again when the tuning fork is held next to the ear (negative Rinne test). In right-sided sensorineural hearing loss, however, the tone will be heard, though for a shorter time than normal, both by bone conduction and with the tuning fork held next to the ear (positive, i.e., normal Rinne test).

Source: By Dr SaltMD – Own work, , https://commons.wikimedia.org/w/index.php?curid=77951860.

- o **Rinne Test:** In healthy individuals, air conduction of sound is superior to bone conduction. This is illustrated by placing a vibrating tuning fork on the mastoid process first. Removing the tuning fork from the mastoid process and placing it next to the ear occurs as soon as the subject loses the ability to hear the tone. The tone should then be audible once more, and it should fade away roughly twice as quickly as it did on the mastoid process. We refer to this as a "positive," i.e., e. normal, Rinne examination. The Rinne test is negative and indicates conductive hearing loss (i.e., a middle ear process or obstruction of the external auditory canal) if the duration of the tone's air conduction hearing is shorter than usual or if the tone is not heard in this way at all. The Rinne test results in a positive (normal) result in patients with sensorineural hearing loss.
- o **Weber Test:** The tuning fork vibrates, and then is positioned on either the middle of the forehead or the vertex. In a typical scenario, the sound is heard evenly in both ears and is located at the center. In cases of conductive hearing loss, the sound is more noticeable in the affected ear, while in sensorineural hearing loss, it's more pronounced in the unaffected ear. When one ear has experienced prolonged hearing loss, the Weber test may no longer reveal a difference in sound localization.
- o **Assessment of Vestibular Function**: Vertigo is the most typical sign of a lesion affecting the vestibular portion of the vestibulocochlear nerve, or the labyrinth. Patients typically describe a specific kind of vertigo, such as directional or systematic vertigo that rotates ("like on a merry-go-round"), a sensation of turning, or a sensation

similar to that of an elevator. They are frequently able to pinpoint the direction of the vertigo. On the other hand, dizziness originating from nonvestibular sources, such as a brainstem lesion, is frequently less distinct. These patients may report feeling giddy, swaying, or having dark spots appear in front of their eyes.

Nystagmus is an objective indicator of a lesion in the vestibular portion of the vestibulocochlear nerve. This condition, known as "jerk nystagmus," is characterized by a quick, rhythmic jerking motion of both eyes in the same direction. The cycle repeats itself with a slow conjugate deviation in one direction followed by a quick conjugate movement that puts the eyes back in the starting position. The genuinely pathological aspect of nystagmus is the slow deviation, while the quick component is a reflexive correction meant to maintain fixation. The direction of the rapid phase is typically used to determine the direction of nystagmus. Nystagmus can be rotatory (clockwise or counterclockwise), vertical (upbeat or downbeat), or horizontal (toward the right or left). Vestibular nystagmus can sometimes be observed even when the patient is looking directly ahead (this type of spontaneous nystagmus is known as spontaneous nystagmus); in other situations, it is only visible when the patient is asked to look to the side. Regardless of whether the patient looks straight ahead, to the right, or to the left, nystagmus of vestibular origin always beats in the same direction (away from the side of the lesion).

It is important to distinguish between gaze-evoked and physiological end-gaze nystagmus when dealing with spontaneous nystagmus of vestibular origin. When a patient looks entirely to one side or the other (into the monocular visual field), end-gaze nystagmus occurs. It is characterized by rapid phase beats in the gaze direction, equal visibility in both eyes and spontaneous disappearance after a few beats. It is present symmetrically in healthy people. In case end-gaze nystagmus is observed during the examination, the examiner ought to rotate the test object back into the binocular visual field by approximately 10°. Only if the nystagmus persists following this maneuver is it considered clinically significant.

- **Instruments for Assessing Vestibular Function:** The use of Frenzel goggles enhances the observation of nystagmus by making it easier to see. These goggles have powerful magnifying lenses that prevent the patient from fixing their gaze, along with a built-in lamp to light up the eyes. When nystagmus is present, it can often be hidden by fixation but becomes visible when the patient wears Frenzel goggles (head shaking can further provoke the movement). Additionally, the magnification of the Frenzel lenses allows the examiner to more clearly see subtle eye movements.

  By measuring the corresponding labyrinth's rotational and caloric excitability, vestibular lesions can be objectively evaluated. When warm water is used to irrigate the external auditory canal, nystagmus is typically induced, with the rapid phase directed toward the irrigated ear (when cold water is used, the rapid phase is directed toward the opposite ear). The induced nystagmus is lessened or does not occur in the presence of a vestibular lesion.

- **Tests of Balance and Coordination.** Anomalies in some of the stance and gait tests (such as the heel-to-toe walking, Babinski-Weil, and Unterberger step tests) point to vestibular apparatus malfunction. In an additional assessment known as the Bárány pointing test, the patient is required to extend their arm forward and then bring it down to a target that the examiner has provided, such as e.g., the finger of the examiner. After that, the patient is instructed to repeat the motion while keeping their eyes closed and attempting to hit the target as precisely as they can. When there is a unilateral vestibular lesion, the arm veers to one side during the descent. On the other hand, ipsilateral cerebellar hemisphere lesions exhibit the same characteristics.

- **CN IX and X: Glossopharyngeal and Vagus Nn**

Through the glossopharyngeal and vagus nerves, the efferent fibers from the nucleus ambiguus to the muscles of the larynx, pharynx, and palate reach these structures. The superior laryngeal nerve and the recurrent laryngeal nerve are the two vagal branches that innervate the larynx.

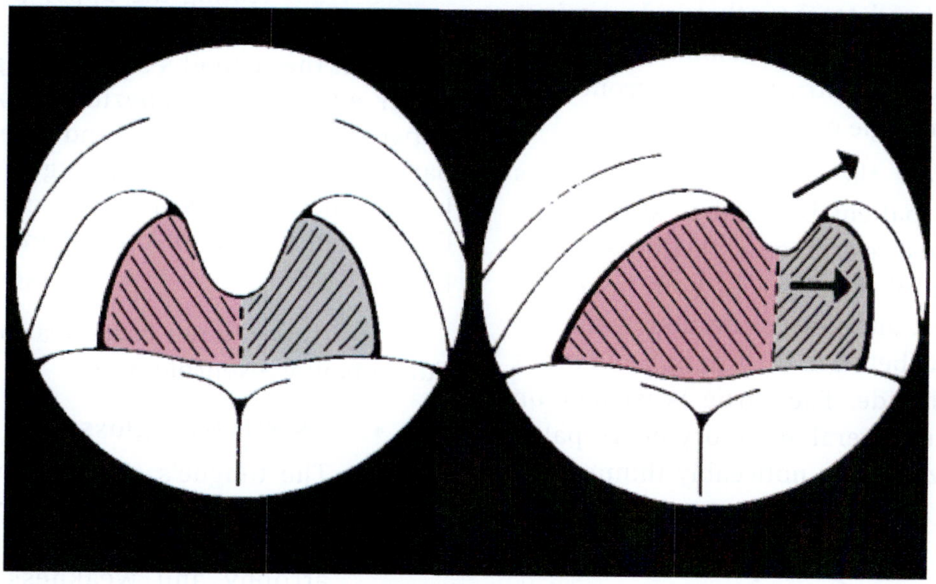

Figure 1.18. Palatal deviation. In right glossopharyngeal nerve palsy, the palate and posterior pharyngeal wall deviate to the normal left side when the patient gags.

Source: https://www.ruseducation.in/books/Fundamentals-Neurology.pdf.

The nasal glossopharynx. carries gustatory fibers from the posterior third of the tongue and somatosensory fibers from the tonsillar fossa, the middle ear, the posterior pharyngeal wall, and the soft palate. The vagus nerve. transports somatosensory fibers from the meninges of the posterior fossa, the external auditory canal, and a portion of the external ear. It also transports parasympathetic efferent fibers to the viscera of the thoracic and abdominal cavities.

- o **Examination of the Pharynx and Larynx.** Examining the palate and throat and, more crucially, observing how these structures move during phonation ("a–aa–ah.") are two ways to measure the motor function of the ninth and tenth cranial nerves. and following the induction of the gag reflex through the use of, e.g., touching the posterior pharyngeal wall, e.g., a cotton swab. As illustrated in Figure 1.18, unilateral weakness of the pharyngeal muscles and the palatal veil causes these structures to deviate laterally away from the side of the lesion. Sometimes the patient's unilateral recurrent laryngeal nerve palsy causes hoarseness that is only audible when they sing.

- **CN XI: Accessory N**

The sternocleidomastoid and trapezius mm are examined. The purely motor accessory n's external (final) branch. supplies the upper part of the trapezius muscle and the sternocleidomastoid muscle. To test the sternocleidomastoid muscle on one side, the examiner asks the patient to turn their head to the other side against resistance. After that, the examiner feels and watches the muscle contraction at the front edge of the lateral triangle of the neck (Figure 1.19).

This is how the upper trapezius m. is examined: the patient is asked to shrug their shoulders against resistance while the examiner stands in front of them, places both hands on their shoulders, and grasps the upper edge of the trapezius m. between their thumb and index finger on each side. The shrug is weaker on the side with unilateral accessory nerve palsy, and the trapezius m. is noticeably thinner and weaker (Figure 1.20).

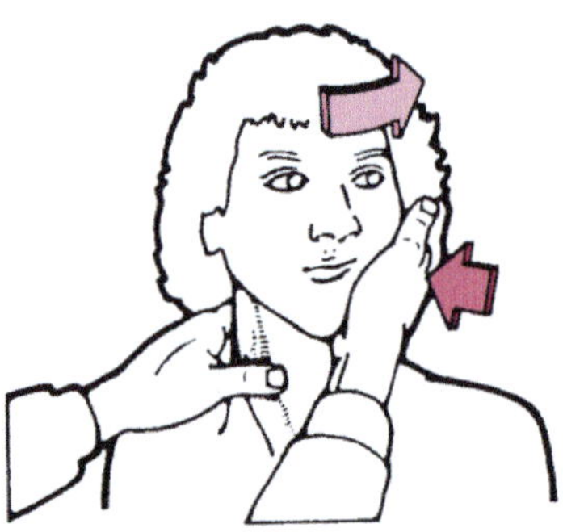

Figure 1.19. Testing the sternocleidomastoid m. The patient attempts to turn the head to the left against the examiner's resistance. The right sternocleidomastoid m. contracts.

Source: https://www.ruseducation.in/books/Fundamentals-Neurology.pdf.

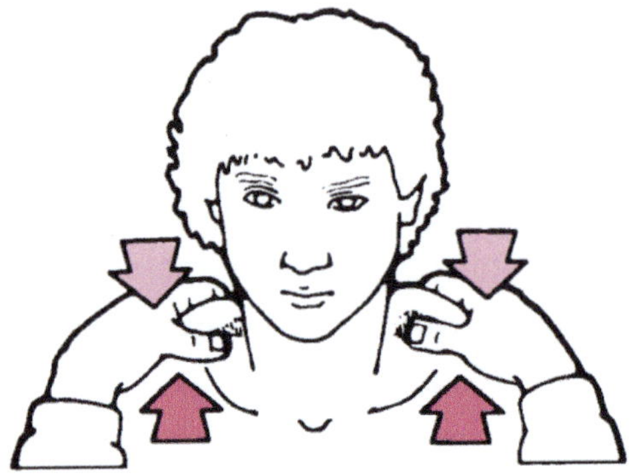

Figure 1.20. Testing the upper portion of the trapezius m. The examiner places his or her hands on the patient's shoulders, grasping the upper edge of the trapezius m. on each side between his or her thumb and index finger. The patient is then asked to shrug the shoulders. Unilateral weakness, reduced contraction, or diminished volume of the trapezius m. can be palpated.

Source: https://www.ruseducation.in/books/Fundamentals-Neurology.pdf.

- **CN XII: Hypoglossal N**

  The tongue's muscles are controlled solely by the twelfth cranial nerve, which is a motor nerve. The tongue atrophy and weakness are caused by lesions of this nerve. The tongue deviates to the weaker side when a unilateral lesion is protruded due to the dominant force of the intact contralateral genioglossus m., which "pushes" the tongue across the midline (Figure 1.21).

- **Phonation, Articulation, and Speech**

A mandatory component of the neurological examination is the evaluation of the patient's speech and voice. The examiner should be aware of any potential hoarseness, speech volume (e.g., hypophonia in Parkinson's disease), of potential articulation abnormalities (dysarthria), speech tempo, and linguistic form and content.

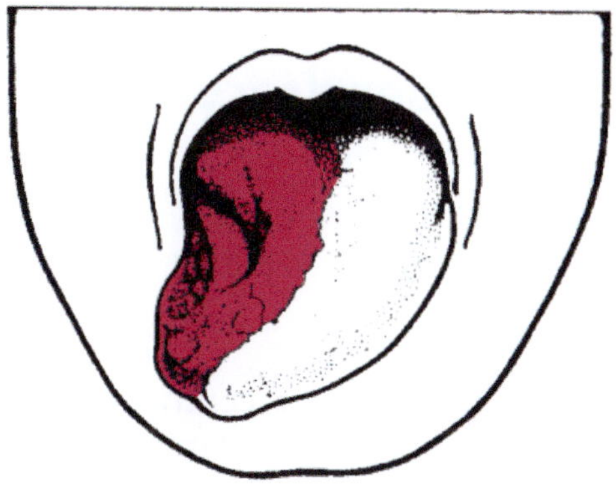

Figure 1.21. Atrophy and weakness of the right half of the tongue in a lesion of the right hypoglossal n.

Source: https://www.ruseducation.in/books/Fundamentals-Neurology.pdf.

A Closer Look

Oligodendrocyte

Oligodendrocyte, a type of neuroglia found in the central nervous system of invertebrates and vertebrates that functions to produce myelin, an insulating sheath on the axons of nerve fibers.

Oligodendrocytes are subdivided into interfascicular and perineuronal types and have few cytoplasmic fibrils but a well-developed Golgi apparatus. They can be distinguished from the type of neuroglia known as an astrocyte by the greater density of both the cytoplasm and the nucleus, the absence of fibrils and of glycogen in the cytoplasm, and large numbers of microtubules in the processes. Interfascicular oligodendrocytes are aligned in rows between the nerve fibers of the white matter of the central nervous system. In gray matter, perineuronal oligodendrocytes are located near the somata of neurons. In the peripheral nervous system, neuroglia that are equivalent to oligodendrocytes are called Schwann cells.

The type of axon determines whether loose or tight myelination is needed. In tight myelination, an oligodendrocyte wraps itself like a rolled sheet around a length of axon until the fiber is covered by several layers. Between segments of myelin wrapping are exposed sections called nodes of Ranvier, which are important in the transmission of nerve impulses. The role of oligodendrocytes after injury is unclear, but they may proliferate and form myelin sheaths.

Oligodendrocytes are a type of glial cell. They arise during development from oligodendrocyte precursor cells (OPCs), which can be identified by their expression of several antigens, including the ganglioside GD3, the NG2 chondroitin sulfate proteoglycan, and the platelet-derived growth factor-alpha receptor subunit (PDGF-alphaR). Mature oligodendrocytes are broadly classified into either myelinating or non-myelinating satellite oligodendrocytes. Precursors and both mature types are typically identified by their expression of the transcription factor OLIG2.

Most oligodendrocytes develop during embryogenesis and early postnatal life from restricted periventricular germinal regions. Oligodendrocyte formation in the adult brain is associated with glial-restricted progenitor cells, known as oligodendrocyte progenitor cells (OPCs). Subventricular zone cells migrate away from germinal zones to populate both developing white and gray matter, where they differentiate and mature into myelin-forming oligodendrocytes. However, it is not clear whether all oligodendrocyte progenitors undergo this sequence of events.

Between midgestation and term birth in human cerebral white matter, three successive stages of the classic human oligodendrocyte lineage are found: OPCs, immature oligodendrocytes (non-myelinating), and mature oligodendrocytes (myelinating). It has been suggested that some undergo apoptosis and others fail to differentiate into mature oligodendrocytes but persist as adult OPCs. Remarkably, the oligodendrocyte population originating in the subventricular zone can be dramatically expanded by administering epidermal growth factor (EGF).

Diseases that result in injury to oligodendrocytes include demyelinating diseases such as multiple sclerosis and various leukodystrophies. Trauma to the body, e.g., spinal cord injury, can also cause demyelination. The immature oligodendrocytes, which increase in number during mid-gestation, are more vulnerable to hypoxic injury and are involved in periventricular leukomalacia. This largely congenital condition of damage to the newly forming brain can therefore lead to cerebral palsy. In cerebral palsy, spinal cord injury, stroke and possibly multiple sclerosis, oligodendrocytes are thought to be damaged by excessive release of the neurotransmitter, glutamate. Damage has also been shown to be mediated by N-methyl-D-aspartate receptors. Oligodendrocyte dysfunction may also be implicated in the pathophysiology of schizophrenia and bipolar disorder.

Oligodendrocytes are also susceptible to infection by the JC virus, which causes progressive multifocal leukoencephalopathy (PML), a condition that specifically affects white matter, typically in immunocompromised patients. Tumors of oligodendrocytes are called oligodendrogliomas. The chemotherapy agent Fluorouracil (5-FU) causes damage to the oligodendrocytes in mice, leading to both acute central nervous system (CNS) damage and progressively worsening delayed degeneration of the CNS. DNA methylation may also have a role in the degeneration of oligodendrocytes.

Summary

- Neurology, an essential field in the medical sciences, delves into the inner workings of the nervous system to uncover the intricate mechanisms that govern human behavior, cognition, and bodily functions.
- The neurons, which make up the significant functional component of the nervous system, are encircled by neuroglia, a group of supporting cells.
- A double-layered cell membrane with an outer layer of glycoprotein and an inner layer of phospholipid surrounds each neuron.
- Mendelian inheritance dictates that features (genes) derived from both parents are randomly and independently distributed to the germ cells, and consequently to the progeny.
- Neurology is a distinct medical specialty and area of study in and of itself. The majority of neurological diseases solely impact the nervous system.
- The head and cervical spine's overall appearance should be noted by the examiner first (e.g., sunken temples in Steinert myotonic dystrophy) as well as the look on the patient's face (e.g., lack of expression on the face in Parkinson's disease).
- An essential method for evaluating the optic nerve is to examine the optic discs, or optic nerve papillae, using an ophthalmoscope.
- Nystagmus should be checked for by the examiner in addition to eye movements. The best way to identify deviations from the parallel axis is to look at the reflected images on the patient's cornea.

References

1. Adams, R. D., Victor, M., & Ropper, A. H. (Eds.). (2014). *Principles of Neurology* (10th ed.). McGraw-Hill Education.
2. Blumenfeld, H. (2010). *Neuroanatomy through Clinical Cases* (2nd ed.). Sinauer Associates, Inc.
3. Bradley, W. G., Daroff, R. B., Fenichel, G. M., & Jankovic, J. (Eds.). (2016). *Bradley's Neurology in Clinical Practice* (7th ed.). Elsevier.
4. Brazis, P. W., Masdeu, J. C., & Biller, J. (2011). *Localization in Clinical Neurology* (6th ed.). Lippincott Williams & Wilkins.
5. Campbell, W. W. (2012). *DeJong's The Neurologic Examination* (7th ed.). Lippincott Williams & Wilkins.
6. Fitzgerald, M. J. T., Gruener, G., & Mtui, E. (2012). *Clinical Neuroanatomy and Neuroscience* (6th ed.). Saunders.
7. Greenberg, D. A., Aminoff, M. J., & Simon, R. P. (Eds.). (2015). *Clinical Neurology* (10th ed.). McGraw-Hill Education.
8. Haan, J., & Thijs, R. D. (Eds.). (2017). *Handbook of Clinical Neurology* (Vol. 140). Elsevier.
9. Kandel, E. R., Schwartz, J. H., Jessell, T. M., Siegelbaum, S. A., & Hudspeth, A. J. (2012). *Principles of Neural Science* (5th ed.). McGraw-Hill Education.

10. LeBlond, R., Brown, D., & Sunija, M. (2014). *DeGowin's Diagnostic Examination* (10th ed.). McGraw-Hill.
11. Martin, J. H. (2019). *Neuroanatomy: Text and Atlas* (5th ed.). McGraw-Hill Education.
12. O'Brien, M. (2010). *Aids to the Examination of the Peripheral Nervous System* (5th ed.). Saunders.
13. Sidman, R. L., & Sidman, M. (2006). *The Neuroanatomy Laboratory* (6th ed.). Harvard University Press.
14. Waxman, S. G. (2013). *Clinical Neuroanatomy* (27th ed.). McGraw-Hill.
15. Waxman, S. G. (2016). *Clinical Neuroanatomy* (28th ed.). McGraw-Hill Education.

Chapter 2

COMA

Contents

Introduction

Comas may arise from a blow to the head during a traumatic event, from an infection, from complications of diabetes, or from low oxygen levels. Sometimes a coma is put on a patient by doctors to shield them from discomfort and problems while they heal.

A deep state of unconsciousness is called a coma. It's comparable to a deep sleep, except that the person is unable to wake up or react to their surroundings normally. The degree of brain function will determine their level of awareness and reactivity.

A person may be in a coma for a few days or several weeks. The cause and any existing brain damage will determine the result.

It is a medical emergency if someone goes into a coma after experiencing trauma or a medical event. In order to save their lives and maintain brain function, doctors might need to act quickly.

A physician may occasionally use medicine to put a patient into a coma. For instance, they might take this action to shield the patient from excruciating pain while the body heals or to maintain higher brain function after a brain injury.

In severe situations, though, a person's condition might not improve over time. They might be placed in a persistent vegetative state by medical professionals. It's possible that someone won't wake up if this state persists for several months.

A coma is a sleep-like state from which a patient cannot be awakened and in which they are not responding purposefully to their surroundings. The closed eyes do not open on their own. The patient shows no intention to move their limbs or face, and they remain silent. There is no reaction when spoken to. In response to painful stimulation, the brainstem or spinal cord may mediate involuntary reflex movements or no response at all. A disruption in the functioning of both cerebral hemispheres or the brainstem reticular activating system above the mid pons causes coma (Figure 2.1).

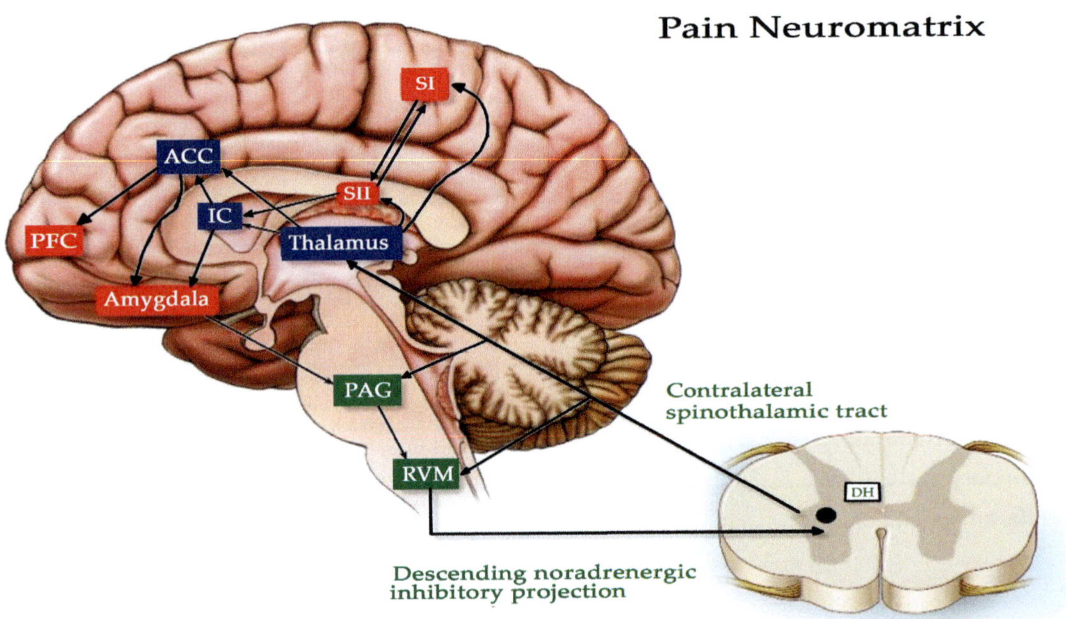

Figure 2.1. Anatomic basis of coma. Consciousness is maintained by the normal functioning of the brainstem reticular activating system above the mid pons and its bilateral projections to the thalamus and cerebral hemispheres. Coma results from lesions that affect either the reticular activating system or both hemispheres.

Source: Zasler ND, Formisano R, Aloisi M. Pain in Persons with Disorders of Consciousness. *Brain Sciences*. 2022; 12(3):300. https://doi.org/10.3390/brainsci12030300.

Orientation and Directional Terms

Term	Definition	Illustration
Hypoglycemic coma	Hypoglycemic coma, also known as diabetic hypoglycemic coma, is a serious complication of diabetes that occurs when blood sugar levels are too low.	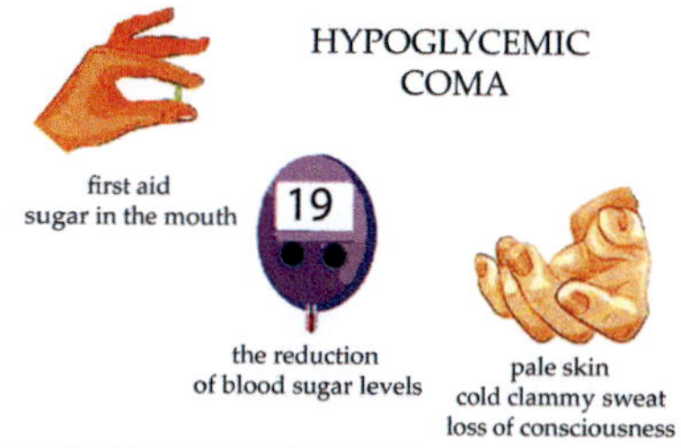
Intracerebral hemorrhage	Intracerebral hemorrhage (ICH), a subtype of stroke, is a devastating condition whereby a hematoma is formed within the brain parenchyma with or without blood extension into the ventricles.	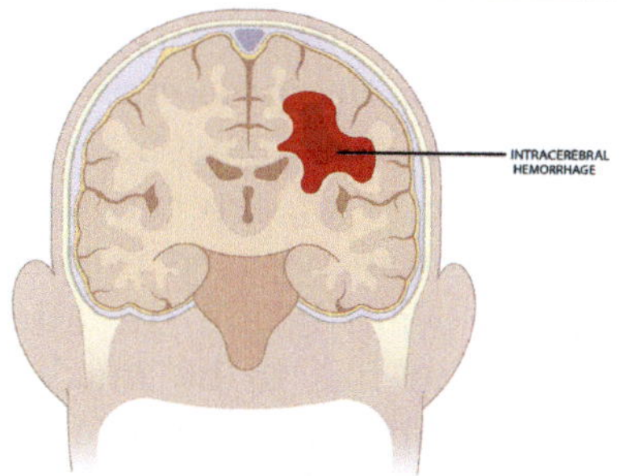
Chronic subdural hematoma	Chronic subdural hematoma (CSDH) is a collection of blood and blood breakdown products that builds up between the brain and its outermost covering, the dura.	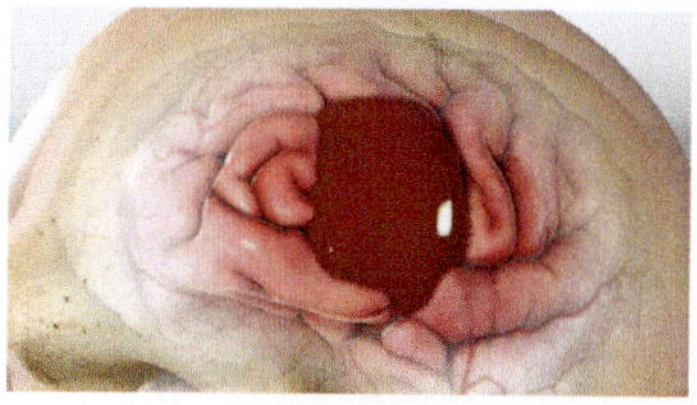
Pontine lesions	Pontine lesions are hyperintense lesions that appear on T2-weighted MRIs in the pons.	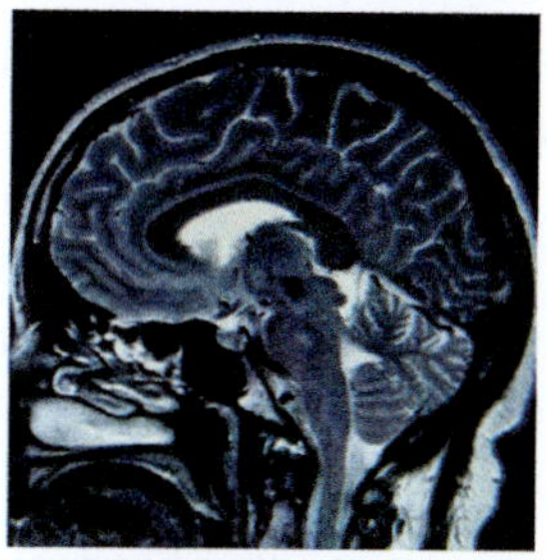
Agnosia	Agnosia is a rare disorder that prevents people from identifying objects, people, sounds, or smells using one or more of their senses, even though their senses are working normally.	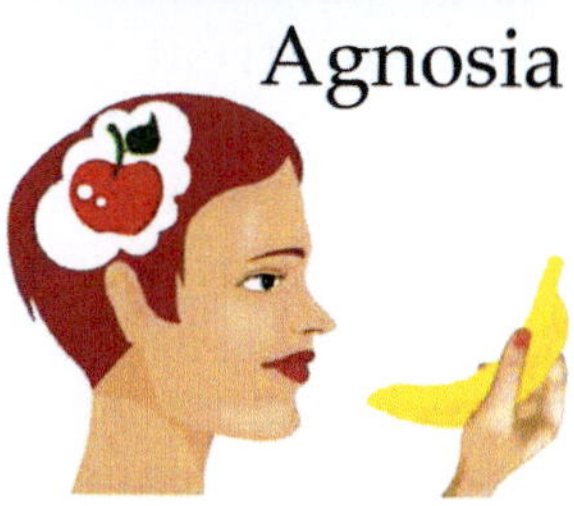

2.1. Approach to Diagnosis

When diagnosing a comatose patient, emergency care is provided to stabilize the patient and treat suspected life-threatening conditions. Subsequently, an etiologic diagnosis is attempted.

2.1.1. Emergency Management

1. Make sure the airway is open and that there is enough ventilation and circulation (Table 2.1). The absence of cyanosis, a respiratory rate higher than 8/min, the presence of breath sounds on chest auscultation, and the outcomes of arterial blood gas studies can all be used to determine whether ventilation is adequate. The patient has to be mechanically ventilated if any of these indicate insufficient ventilation. Blood pressure and pulse measurements allow for a quick evaluation of the circulation's health. As indicated, intravenous fluid replacement, pressors, and antiarrhythmic medications should be used to treat circulating embarrassment.
2. To determine serum glucose and electrolyte levels, hepatic and renal function tests, prothrombin time, partial thromboplastin time, complete blood count, and drug screen, insert an intravenous catheter and draw blood.
3. Administer naloxone, thiamine, and dextrose as part of an intravenous infusion. To treat a possible hypoglycemic coma, every comatose patient should receive 25 g of intravenous dextrose, usually in the form of 50 mL of a 50% dextrose solution. All comatose patients should also receive an intravenous dose of 100 mg of thiamine, as the administration of dextrose alone may exacerbate or cause Wernicke encephalopathy in thiamine-deficient patients. Naloxone, an opiate antagonist, should also be regularly given intravenously to comatose patients at a dose of 0.4 to 1.2 mg to treat possible opiate overdose. When a benzodiazepine overdose causes coma, the benzodiazepine antagonist flumazenil, administered intravenously at doses of 1 to 10 mg, may be helpful. Patients with a history of seizures, long-term benzodiazepine addiction, or suspected co-ingestion of tri-or tetracyclic antidepressants should not use it, though. If the electrocardiogram (ECG) reveals sinus tachycardia at a rate of 130 beats per minute or higher, a QTc interval longer than 0.5 seconds, and a QRS duration longer than 0.1 seconds, the latter should be suspected.
4. Collect arterial blood samples for blood gas analysis and pH determination. These tests can help evaluate ventilation status and also offer insights into the potential metabolic factors contributing to coma (refer to Table 2.2 for more information).
5. If seizures are present, start treatment. Seizures and syncope should be treated as seizures and status epilepticus in comatose patients exhibiting persistent or recurrent seizures.

2.1.2. History and Examination

2.1.2.1. History

The most crucial aspect of the history is the time over which coma develops.

1. A sudden onset of coma suggests a vascular origin, especially a brainstem stroke or subarachnoid hemorrhage.
2. Rapid progression from hemispheric signs, such as hemiparesis, hemisensory

deficit, or aphasia, to coma within minutes to hours is characteristic of intracerebral hemorrhage.

3. A more protracted course leading to coma (days to a week or more) is seen with tumor, abscess, or chronic subdural hematoma.
4. Coma preceded by a confusional state or agitated delirium, without lateralizing signs or symptoms, is probably due to a metabolic derangement or infection (meningitis or encephalitis).

Table 2.1. Emergency Management of the Comatose Patient

Immediately	Next	Later
Ensure adequacy of airway, ventilation, and circulation	If signs of meningeal irritation are present (see Figure 1-5), perform LP to rule out meningitis. Obtain a history if possible	ECG
Draw blood for serum glucose, electrolytes, liver and renal function tests, PT, PTT, and CBC	Perform detailed general physical and neurologic examination	Correct hyper- or hypothermia
Start IV and administer 25 g of dextrose, 100 mg of thiamine, and 0.4-1.2 mg of naloxone IV	Order CT scan of head if history or findings suggest structural lesion or subarachnoid hemorrhage	Correct severe acid–base and electrolyte abnormalities
Draw blood for arterial blood gas determinations		Chest x-ray
Treat seizures (see Chapter 12, Seizures & Syncope)		Blood and urine toxicology studies; EEG

Abbreviations: CBC, complete blood count; IV, intravenous; LP, lumbar puncture; PT, prothrombin time; PTT, partial thromboplastin time.

Source: https://dl.mehrsys.ir/pdf-books/Clinical%20Neurology%209%20Edition%20(www.myuptodate.com).pdf.

2.1.2.2. General Physical Examination

- Signs of Trauma

1. Inspection of the head may reveal signs of basilar skull fracture, including the following:
   - **Raccoon eyes:** Periorbital ecchymoses (Figure 2.4).
   - **Battle sign:** Swelling and discoloration overlying the mastoid bone behind the ear (Figure 2.4).
   - **Hemotympanum:** Blood behind the tympanic membrane.

iv. **Cerebrospinal Fluid (CSF) Rhinorrhea or Otorrhea:** Leakage of CSF from the nose or ear. CSF rhinorrhea must be distinguished from other causes of rhinorrhea, such as allergic rhinitis. Glucose concentration does not reliably distinguish CSF from nasal mucus, but beta-2 transferrin is unique to CSF, and its presence documents a CSF source of rhinorrhea.

Table 2.2. Metabolic Coma: Differential Diagnosis by Acid–Base Abnormalities

Respiratory acidosis
Sedative drug intoxication
Pulmonary encephalopathy
Respiratory alkalosis
Hepatic encephalopathy
Salicylate intoxication
Sepsis
Metabolic acidosis
Diabetic ketoacidosis
Uremic encephalopathy
Lactic acidosis
Methanol intoxication
Ethylene glycol intoxication
Isoniazid intoxication
Salicylate intoxication
Sepsis (terminal)
Metabolic alkalosis
Coma unusual

Source: Data from Plum F, Posner JB. The Diagnosis of Stupor and Coma. 3rd ed. Vol 19: Contemporary Neurology Series. Philadelphia, PA: Davis; 1980.

2. Palpation of the head may demonstrate a depressed skull fracture or swelling of soft tissues at the site of trauma.
   - **Blood Pressure:** High blood pressure in a comatose patient could indicate chronic hypertension, increasing the risk of a brain hemorrhage or stroke. In cases of hypertensive encephalopathy, blood pressure can spike to over 250/150 mm Hg in patients with long-term hypertension, though it may be lower in children or those with a sudden increase in blood pressure due to conditions like acute renal failure. Elevated blood pressure could also be caused by the underlying condition leading to the coma, such as brain hemorrhage, subarachnoid hemorrhage, or brainstem stroke.
   - **Temperature:** Intoxication with ethanol or sedative drugs, hypoglycemia, Wernicke encephalopathy, hepatic encephalopathy, and myxedema can all result in hypothermia in a coma. Coma with hyperthermia can occur in patients with heat stroke, status epilepticus, anticholinergic drug intoxication, malignant hyperthermia associated with inhalational anesthetics, pontine hemorrhage, and specific hypothalamic lesions.
   - **Signs of Meningeal Irritation:** The early diagnosis of meningitis or subarachnoid hemorrhage can be greatly aided by signs of meningeal irritation, such as nuchal rigidity or the Brudzinski sign (Figure 2.5). However,

these signs disappear in deep comas, so their absence does not rule out these conditions.

- **Optic Fundi:** When the optic fundi are examined, papilledema, retinal hemorrhages consistent with either acute or chronic hypertension, or an increase in intracranial pressure, may be seen (Figure 2.11). Adult subarachnoid hemorrhages are strongly suggestive of subhyaloid (superficial retinal) hemorrhages.

2.1.3. Neurologic Examination

The key to determining the etiologic diagnosis in a comatose patient is the neurologic examination. A thorough evaluation should be conducted of the motor response to pain, the size and reactivity of the pupillary, and the reflex eye movements (oculocephalic and oculovestibular reflexes) (Figure 2.2).

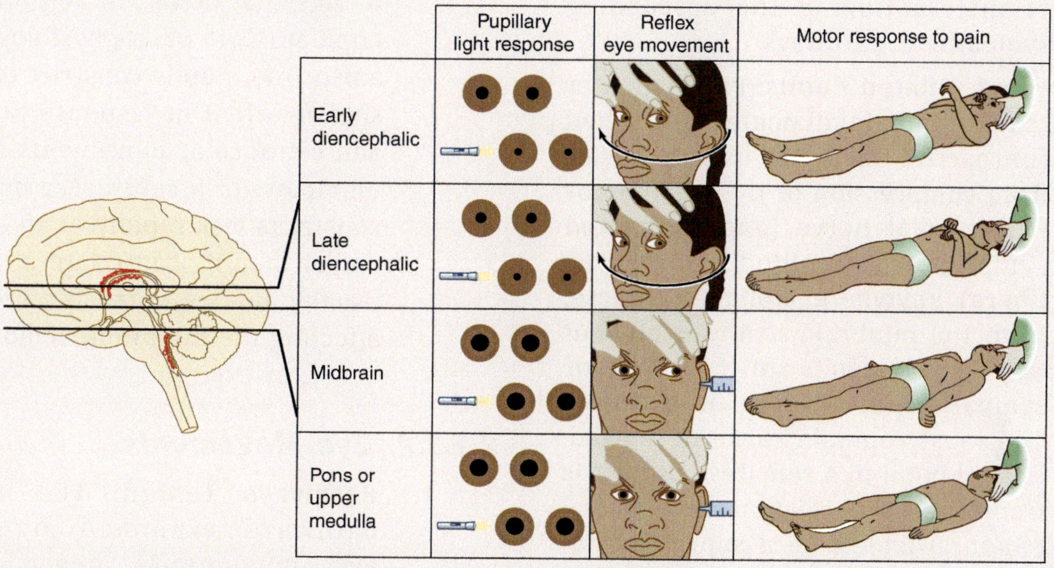

Figure 2.2. Neurologic signs in coma with downward transtentorial herniation. In the early diencephalic phase, the pupils are small (approximately 2 mm in diameter) and reactive, reflex eye movements are intact, and the motor response to pain is purposeful or semipurposeful (localizing) and often asymmetric. The late diencephalic phase is associated with similar findings, except that painful stimulation results in decorticate (flexor) posturing, which may also be asymmetric. With midbrain involvement, the pupils are fixed and midsized (approximately 5 mm in diameter), reflex adduction of the eyes is impaired, and pain elicits decerebrate (extensor) posturing. Progression to involve the pons or medulla also produces fixed, midsized pupils, but these are accompanied by loss of reflex abduction as well as adduction of the eyes and by no motor response or only leg flexion upon painful stimulation. Note that although a lesion restricted to the pons produces pinpoint pupils as a result of the destruction of descending sympathetic (pupillodilator) pathways, downward herniation to the pontine level is associated with midsized pupils. This happens because herniation also interrupts parasympathetic (pupilloconstrictor) fibers in the oculomotor (III) nerve.

2.1.3.1. Pupils

1. **Normal Pupils:** Normal pupils are typically 3 to 4 mm in diameter (but larger in children and smaller in the elderly) and equal in size bilaterally; they constrict briskly and symmetrically in response to light. Normally reactive pupils in a comatose patient are characteristic of a metabolic cause.
2. **Thalamic Pupils:** Slightly smaller (~2 mm) reactive pupils are present in the early stages of thalamic compression from mass lesions, perhaps because of interruption of the descending sympathetic pathways.
3. **Fixed, Dilated Pupils:** Pupils greater than 7 mm in diameter and fixed (unreactive to light) usually result from compression of the oculomotor (III) cranial nerve (and associated sympathetic, pupillodilator nerve fibers) anywhere along its course, from the midbrain to the orbit, but may also be seen in anticholinergic or sympathomimetic drug intoxication. The most common cause of a fixed, dilated pupil in a comatose patient is transtentorial herniation of the medial temporal lobe from a supratentorial mass.
4. **Fixed, Midsized Pupils:** Pupils fixed at approximately 5 mm in diameter are the result of brainstem damage at the midbrain level, which interrupts both sympathetic, pupillodilator and parasympathetic, pupilloconstrictor nerve fibers.
5. **Pinpoint Pupils:** Pinpoint pupils (1–1.5 mm in diameter) in a comatose patient usually indicate opioid overdose or, less commonly, a focal structural lesion in the pons. These causes can be distinguished by the administration of naloxone (see earlier) or by the associated defects in horizontal eye movements that usually accompany pontine lesions. Pinpoint pupils may appear unreactive to light except when viewed with a magnifying glass. Pinpoint pupils can also be caused by organophosphate poisoning, miotic eye drops, or neurosyphilis (Argyll Robertson pupils).

- 6. **Asymmetric Pupils**: Asymmetry of pupillary size (anisocoria) with a difference of 1 mm or less in diameter is a normal finding that occurs in 20% of the population. In such physiologic anisocoria, pupils constrict to a similar extent in response to light, and extraocular movements are unimpaired. In contrast, a pupil that constricts less rapidly or to a lesser extent than its contralateral fellow usually implies a structural lesion affecting the midbrain, oculomotor nerve, or eye.

2.1.3.2. Eye Movements

1. **Pathways Tested:** The neuronal pathways examined by testing eye movements begin at the pontomedullary junction (vestibular [VIII] nerve and nucleus), synapse in the caudal pons (horizontal gaze center and abducens [VI] nerve nucleus), ascend through the central core of the brainstem reticular activating system (medial longitudinal fasciculus), and arrive at the contralateral midbrain (oculomotor [III] nucleus and nerve; Figure 2.3).
2. **Methods of Testing:** In the comatose patient, eye movements are tested by stimulating the vestibular system (semicircular canals of the middle

ear) by passive head rotation (the oculocephalic reflex, or doll's-head maneuver) or using the stronger stimulus of ice-water irrigation against the tympanic membrane (oculovestibular reflex, or cold-water caloric testing) (Figure 2.3). The doll's-head (oculocephalic) maneuver is performed by rotating the head horizontally to elicit horizontal eye movements and vertically to elicit vertical movements. The eyes should move in the direction opposite to that of head rotation. This may be an inadequate stimulus for inducing eye movements, however, and the reflex may be overridden in conscious patients.

A more powerful stimulus is known as cold-water caloric stimulation, or oculovestibular stimulation, which is applied by irrigating the tympanic membrane with ice water. This maneuver should never be attempted without first undergoing an otoscopic examination because it is not recommended in cases where the tympanic membrane is perforated. Unilateral cold-water irrigation causes nystagmus in conscious patients, with the fast phase directed away from the irrigated side. Unilateral ice water irrigation causes the eyes of comatose patients with intact brainstem function to tonicly deviate toward the irrigated side. A structural lesion involving the posterior fossa (cerebellum or brainstem) or sedative drug intoxication are the likely causes of an absent or impaired response to caloric stimulation with large volumes (e.g., 50 mL) of ice water.

3. **Normal Movements:** A comatose patient with intact brainstem function has full conjugate horizontal eye movements, which occur either spontaneously (as "roving eye movements") or during the doll's-head maneuver, as well as tonic conjugate deviation of both eyes toward the side of the ice-water irrigation during cold-water caloric testing. Full horizontal eye movements in a comatose patient exclude a structural lesion in the brainstem as the cause of coma and suggest either a nonstructural (e.g., metabolic) cause or, less commonly, bilateral hemispheric lesions.
4. Abnormal Movements:
    - With lesions affecting the oculomotor (III) nerve or nucleus, such as hemispheric mass lesions causing downward transtentorial herniation at the midbrain level (Figure 2.2), cold-water caloric testing fails to produce adduction of the contralateral eye, whereas the ipsilateral eye abducts normally.
    - Complete unresponsiveness to cold-water caloric testing in a comatose patient implies either a structural lesion of the brainstem affecting the pons or a metabolic disorder that affects the brainstem preferentially, such as sedative drug intoxication.
    - Downward deviation of one or both eyes in response to unilateral cold-water caloric testing also suggests sedative drug intoxication.

2.1.3.3. Motor Response to Pain

Strong pressure is applied to the sternum, nail beds, or supraorbital ridge in order to evaluate the motor response to pain. The way the brain reacts to these stimuli can reveal if the illness that is causing the coma is affecting it symmetrically, as is common with diffuse disorders like metabolic ones, or asymmetrically, as is the case with unilateral structural lesions. The motor reaction to pain may also serve as a marker for the depth of coma or a means of localizing the anatomical level of cerebral dysfunction.

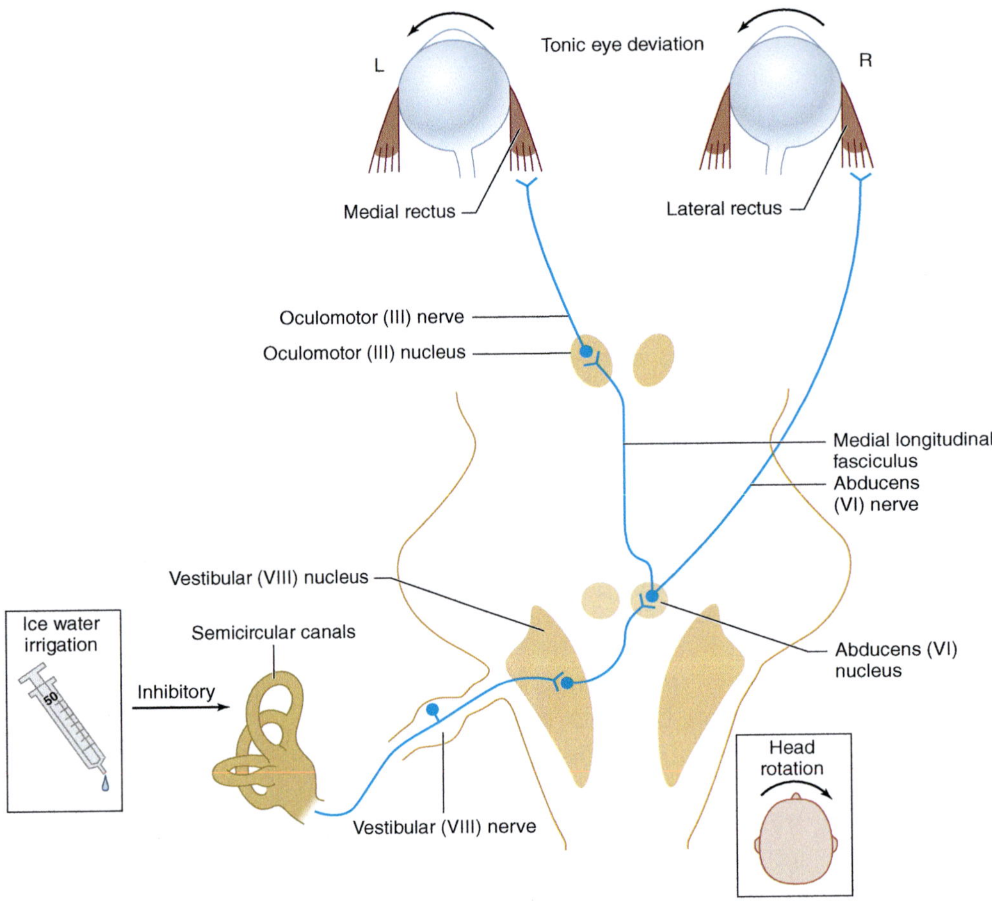

Figure 2.3. Brainstem pathways mediating reflex conjugate horizontal eye movements. In a comatose patient with intact brainstem function, irrigation of the tympanic membrane with ice water inhibits the vestibuloocular pathways shown, resulting in tonic deviation of both eyes toward the irrigated side; head rotation causes eye deviation away from the direction of rotation.

Source: https://dl.mehrsys.ir/pdf-books/Clinical%20Neurology%209%20Edition%20(www.myuptodate.com).pdf.

1. With cerebral dysfunction of only moderate severity, patients may localize an offending stimulus by reaching toward the site of stimulation. Although such "semipurposeful" localizing responses can be difficult to distinguish from the reflex responses described later, movements that involve limb abduction rarely represent reflex movements.
2. A decorticate response to pain (flexion of the arm at the elbow, adduction at the shoulder, and extension and internal rotation of the leg and ankle) is classically associated with

lesions that involve the thalamus directly or large hemispheric masses that compress the thalamus from above.

3. A decerebrate response (extension at the elbow, internal rotation at the shoulder and forearm, and leg extension) tends to occur when brain dysfunction has descended to the level of the midbrain. Thus decerebrate posturing generally implies more severe brain dysfunction than decorticate posturing, although neither response localizes the site of dysfunction precisely.
4. Bilateral symmetric posturing may be seen in both structural and metabolic disorders.
5. Unilateral or asymmetric posturing suggests structural disease in the contralateral cerebral hemisphere or brainstem.
6. In patients with pontine and medullary lesions, there is usually no response to pain, but occasionally some flexion at the knee (a spinal reflex) is noted.

Table 2.3. Glasgow Coma Scale

Test	Not Testable (NT): Examples	1	2	3	4	5	6
Eye (ocular response)	Severe trauma to the eyes, enucleation	Does not open eyes	Opens eyes in response to pain[a]	Opens eyes in response to voice	Opens eyes spontan-eously	N/A	N/A
Verbal (oral response)	Intubation, non-oral language disability, linguistic barrier	Makes no sounds	Incompreh-ensible sounds	Inappropriate words	Confused and disoriented, but able to answer questions	Oriented to time, person, and place, converses normally	N/A
Motor (motoric response)	Paralysis/ hemiparesis (acquired causes such as post-stroke, post-neurological injury; congenital/ innate such as cerebral palsy)	Makes no movements	Abnormal extension (decerebrate posture)[b]	Abnormal flexion (decorticate posture)	Flexion / Withdrawal from painful stimuli	Moves to localize pain	Obeys comma

Source: https://en.wikipedia.org/wiki/Glasgow_Coma_Scale: Teasdale G, Jennett B (1976). "Assessment and prognosis of coma after head injury." Acta Neurochirurgica. 34 (1–4): 45–55. doi:10.1007/BF01405862. PMID 961490. S2CID 32325456.

2.1.3.4. Glasgow Coma Scale

In order to facilitate changes in the examination over time and comparisons between examiners, the previously described pupillary, eye movement, and motor responses are occasionally converted to a numerical scale (Table 2.3).

2.2. Pathophysiologic Assessment

Selecting whether the cause of a comatose patient is a diffuse disorder due to a metabolic disturbance, meningitis, or seizures (for which immediate medical treatment may be required) or a structural brain lesion (for which emergency neurosurgical intervention may be required) is the most crucial step in evaluating the patient.

2.2.1. Supratentorial Structural Lesions

When a supratentorial mass lesion causes a coma, one cerebral hemisphere's dysfunction is typically indicated by the early physical findings and medical history. Contralateral hemiparesis, contralateral hemisensory loss, aphasia (due to dominant, typically left, hemisphere lesions), and agnosia (denial or indifference to the deficit, resulting from damage to the nondominant hemisphere) are among the symptoms and indicators.

Compression of the contralateral hemisphere or thalamus results in the patient becoming more and more lethargic as the mass grows (usually from associated edema). Coma develops from stupor, but examination results are frequently still asymmetric. The thalamus, midbrain, pons, and medulla become sequentially involved with rostral–caudal (downward) progression of brain injury, and the neurologic examination reveals dysfunction at successively lower anatomic levels (Figure 2.2). The diagnosis of a supratentorial mass with downward transtentorial herniation is strongly supported by this segmental pattern of rostral-caudal involvement (Figure 2.4), which also determines the necessity of neurosurgical intervention.

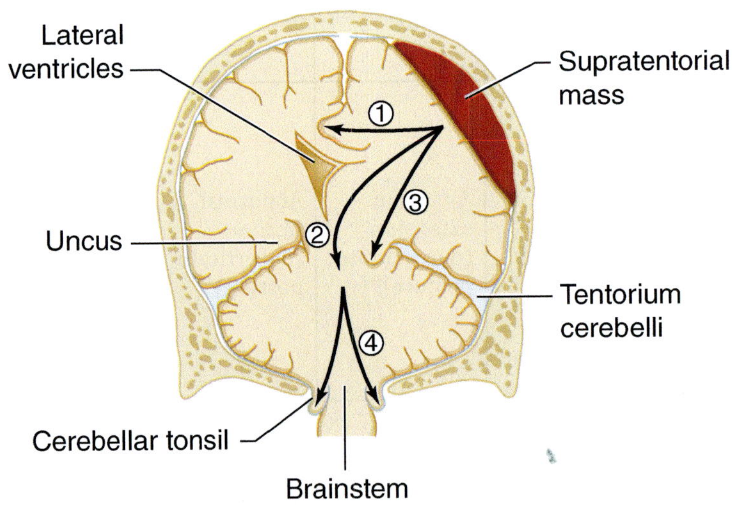

Figure 2.4. Anatomic basis of herniation syndromes. An expanding supratentorial mass lesion may cause brain tissue to be displaced into an adjacent intracranial compartment, resulting in (1) cingulate herniation under the falx, (2) downward transtentorial (central) herniation, (3) uncal herniation over the edge of the tentorium, or (4) cerebellar tonsillar herniation into the foramen magnum. Coma and ultimately death result when (2), (3), or (4) produces brainstem compression.

Source: https://dl.mehrsys.ir/pdf-books/Clinical%20Neurology%209%20Edition%20(www.myuptodate.com).pdf.

The likelihood of surviving without significant neurologic impairment rapidly declines at the fully developed midbrain level (midsized, unreactive pupils), particularly in adults. A fatal outcome is guaranteed once the pontine level of dysfunction is reached (unreactive pupils, absent horizontal eye movements).

Herniation of the uncus, or medial portion of the temporal lobe, over the edge of the cerebellar tentorium can result from supratentorial mass lesions (Figure 2.4). In addition to producing symptoms of oculomotor (III) nerve and midbrain compression, such as ipsilateral pupillary dilatation and impaired adduction of the eye (uncal syndrome), this directly presses on the upper brainstem and may even cause a loss of consciousness. If functional recovery is to occur, neurosurgical decompression must take place early in the course of oculomotor (III) nerve involvement.

2.2.2. Subtentorial Structural Lesions

Sudden onset coma strongly suggests a subtentorial structural lesion, as do focal signs of brainstem dysfunction. The most suggestive findings of a subtentorial structural lesion are abnormal pupillary function and impaired eye movement, particularly if these abnormalities are asymmetric. Loss of pupillary function results from midbrain lesions; the pupils are unresponsive to light and midsized, measuring about 5 mm in diameter. Pinpoint pupils are caused by pontine hemorrhage, pontine infarction, or compression of the pons by nearby cerebellar hemorrhage or infarction.

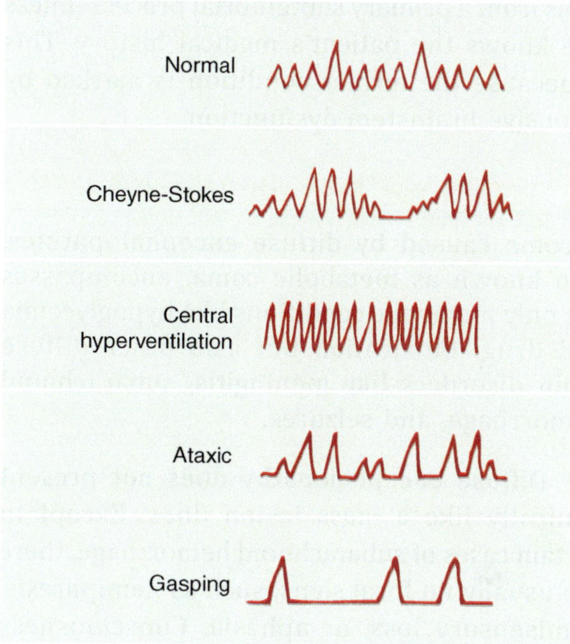

Figure 2.5. Ventilatory patterns in coma. Cheyne stokes respiration and central hyperventilation are seen with metabolic disturbances and with structural lesions at a variety of sites in the brain. They are therefore not useful for anatomic localization of disorders producing coma. Ataxic and gasping ventilatory patterns are most commonly seen with pontomedullary lesions.

Source: Edlow JA, Rabinstein A, Traub SJ, Wijdicks EF. Diagnosis of reversible causes of coma. Lancet. 2014; in press.

Additionally, conjugate gaze deviation toward a hemiparesis and away from the lesion's side, as well as disconjugate eye movements like internuclear ophthalmoplegia (selective impairment of eye adduction), may be linked to brainstem lesions. In general, motor responses are not useful in differentiating between lesions that are supratentorial and subtentorial. Subtentorial lesions are linked to abnormal, varying ventilation patterns, which can be ataxic or gasping (Figure 2.5). It may be impossible to distinguish the fully developed syndrome of transtentorial herniation from a supratentorial mass from a primary subtentorial process unless one knows the patient's medical history. This is because the former condition is marked by extensive brainstem dysfunction.

2.2.3. Diffuse Encephalopathies

A coma caused by diffuse encephalopathies, also known as metabolic coma, encompasses not only metabolic conditions like hypoglycemia and drug intoxication but also other diffuse brain disorders like meningitis, subarachnoid hemorrhage, and seizures.

Diffuse encephalopathy does not present clinically like a mass lesion does. Except in certain cases of subarachnoid hemorrhage, there are usually no focal signs, such as hemiparesis, hemisensory loss, or aphasia. Consciousness is lost gradually, usually following a period of progressive somnolence or agitated delirium.

Generally, a symmetric neurologic examination is performed; however, focal signs, such as hemiparesis, may occasionally accompany hypoglycemia, hyperosmolar nonketotic hyperglycemia, and hepatic encephalopathy. The presence of asterixis, myoclonus, and tremor prior to coma are crucial indicators of metabolic illness. In comas caused by sedative drugs, liver disease, uremia, anoxia, hypoglycemia, or other conditions, symmetric decorticate or decerebrate posturing may be observed.

Metabolic encephalopathy is characterized by reactive pupils when brainstem function is otherwise compromised. While early transtentorial herniation can also result in a coma with intact pupillary reaction (Figure 2.2), the latter is linked to asymmetric neurologic findings like hemiparesis. Acute anoxia, marked hypothermia, massive barbiturate overdose with apnea and hypotension, anticholinergic poisoning (large pupils), and opioid overdose (pinpoint pupils) are a few metabolic causes of coma that can also impair pupillary light reflexes. However, even in these situations, completely unreactive pupils are rare.

The ventilation patterns can vary greatly (refer to Figure 2.5), but assessing the pH and arterial blood gases can aid in determining the cause of the condition. Table 2.2 lists the abnormalities in arterial blood gas in coma patients.

Table 2.4 provides an overview of the connection between neurologic symptoms and the pathophysiology of coma. Determining whether brain function is disrupted at a discrete anatomic level (structural lesion) or in a diffuse manner (metabolic coma) is aided by testing reflex eye movements, the motor response to pain, and pupil size and reactivity.

The brain is progressively compromised by supratentorial structural lesions, resulting in dysfunction at progressively lower anatomic levels. Such localization is not possible in patients in metabolic coma, and findings may be sporadic and anatomically inconsistent. The retention of pupillary reactivity in the face of otherwise depressed brainstem functions—such as paralysis of eye movements, respiratory depression, flaccid muscle tone, and unresponsiveness to painful stimuli—after sedative drug overdose is an impressive example of the anatomically discordant findings characteristic of metabolic coma. The more rostrally located midbrain structures that mediate pupillary reactivity would first be compromised by the same degree of low brainstem dysfunction caused by a supratentorial mass lesion, before having an impact on the lower brainstem centers.

Table 2.4. Pathophysiologic Assessment of the Comatose Patient

	Supratentorial Structural Lesion	Subtentorial Structural Lesion	Diffuse Encephalopathy/Meningitis
Pupil size and light reaction	Usually normal size (3-4 mm) and reactive; large (>7 mm) and unreactive with transtentorial herniation	Midsized (about 5 mm) and unreactive with midbrain lesion; pinpoint (1-1.5 mm) and unreactive with pontine lesion	Usually normal size (3-4 mm) and reactive; pinpoint (1-1.5 mm) and sometimes unreactive with opiates; large (>7 mm) and unreactive with anticholinergics
Reflex eye movements	Normal (gaze preference toward side of lesion may occur)	Impaired adduction with midbrain lesion; impaired adduction and abduction with pontine lesion	Usually normal; impaired by sedative drugs or Wernicke encephalopathy
Motor responses	Usually asymmetric; may be symmetric after transtentorial herniation	Asymmetric (unilateral lesion) or symmetric (bilateral lesion)	Usually symmetric; may rarely be asymmetric with hypoglycemia, hyperosmolar nonketotic hyperglycemia, or hepatic encephalopathy

Source: https://dl.mehrsys.ir/pdf-books/Clinical%20Neurology%209%20Edition%20(www.myuptodate.com).pdf.

2.3. Causes of Coma

2.3.1. Supratentorial Structural Lesions

2.3.1.1. Subdural Hematoma

A collection of blood in the subdural space between the arachnoid and dura mater is called a subdural hematoma. Any comatose patient with a suspected supratentorial mass lesion should always have a subdural hematoma evaluated as soon as possible because it is a resectable condition. Because cerebral atrophy stretches bridging cortical veins and makes them more vulnerable to laceration from shearing injury or seemingly spontaneous rupture, subdural hematomas are more common in older patients.

The most frequent cause is trauma, and focal neurologic deficits are frequently noticeable in the acute phase following a head injury. With age, the extent of injury required to cause a subdural hematoma decreases; in about 25% of cases, a history of trauma is not present.

The most typical clinical findings are headache and altered consciousness; however, in certain cases, particularly in cases of chronic subdural hematomas that manifest months or years after injury, symptoms and signs may be absent, nonspecific, or nonlocalizing (Table 2.5). The traditional history of waxing and waning symptoms and signs is too rare to be useful in making a diagnosis. In about 70% of cases, hemiparesis is contralateral to the lesion when it occurs. 90% of the time, ipsilateral pupillary dilation is present. Localization may be challenging due to the frequency of bilateral hematomas and the presence of concurrent cerebral contusion.

Magnetic resonance imaging (MRI) or computed tomography (CT) scans are used for diagnosis (Figure 2.6). Surgery is used to remove a subdural hematoma that has put the patient in a coma.

Table 2.5. Clinical Features of Subdural Hematoma

	Acute[2] (82 Cases) (%)	Subacute[3] (91 Cases) (%)	Chronic[4] (216 Cases) (%)
Symptoms			
Depressed consciousness	100	88	47
Vomiting	24	31	30
Weakness	20	19	22
Confusion	12	41	37
Headache	11	44	81
Speech disturbance	6	8	6
Seizures	6	3	9
Vertigo	0	4	5
Visual disturbance	0	0	12
Signs			
Depressed consciousness	100	88	59
Pupillary inequality	57	27	20
Motor asymmetry	44	37	41
Confusion and memory loss	17	21	27
Aphasia	6	12	11
Papilledema	1	15	22
Hemianopia	0	4	3
Facial weakness	0	3	3

Source: [1]Data from McKissock W, Richardson A, Bloom WH. Subdural hematoma, a review of 389 cases. Lancet. 1960;1:1365–1370.

[2]Within 3 days of trauma.

[3]4–20 days after trauma.

[4]More than 20 days after trauma.

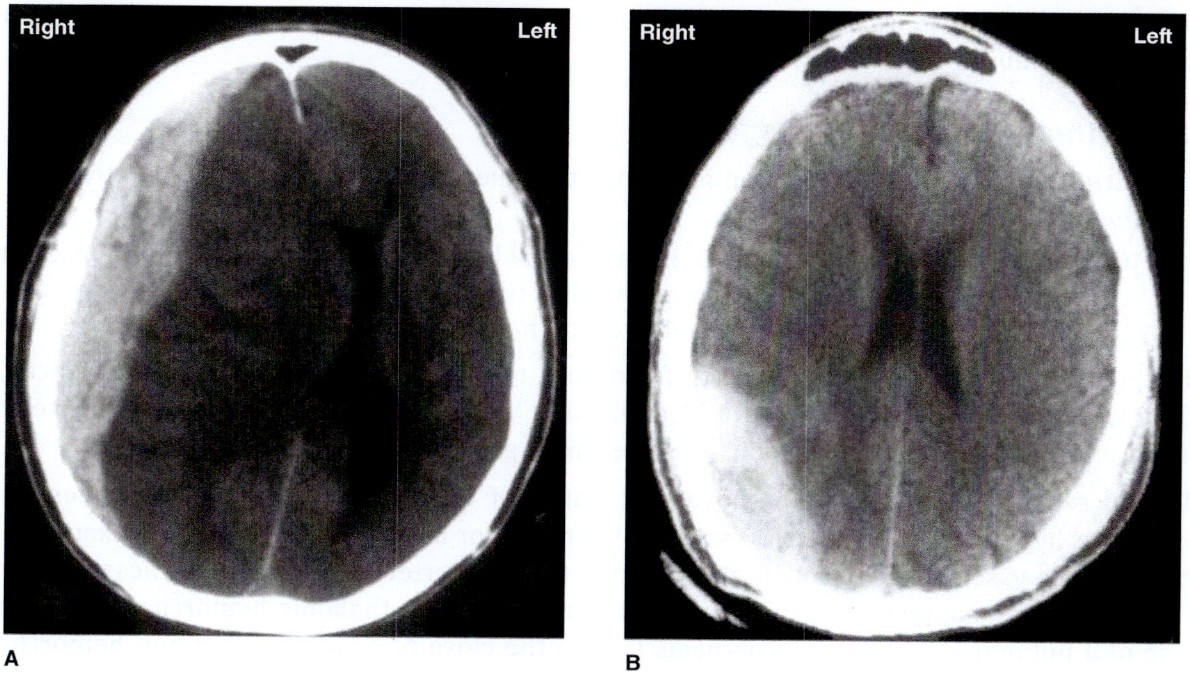

Figure 2.6. (A) Subdural hematoma. Unenhanced CT scan showing a large, high-density crescentic mass over the right cerebral hemisphere, with shift of the lateral ventricles across the midline. (B) Epidural hematoma. Unenhanced CT scan showing a large, high-density lens-shaped mass in the right parietooccipital region. Fracture of the occipital bone was seen on bone windows.

Source: https://dl.mehrsys.ir/pdf-books/Clinical%20Neurology%209%20Edition%20(www.myuptodate.com).pdf.

2.3.1.2. Epidural Hematoma

Usually, a lateral skull fracture coupled with head trauma that tears the middle meningeal artery and vein causes an epidural hematoma. Initial loss of consciousness may or may not occur in patients. Before the onset of a coma, there is frequently a lucid period of several hours during which headache, vomiting, obtundation, seizures, and focal neurologic signs can appear. A CT scan and MRI are used to make the diagnosis (Figure 2.6), which traditionally reveals a mass that resembles a radiodense biconvex lens that is compressing the cerebral hemisphere. To avoid a catastrophic outcome, the hematoma must be surgically removed as soon as possible.

2.3.1.3. Cerebral Contusion

A cerebral contusion is brain bruising that occurs as a result of a head injury. This injury can lead to temporary unconsciousness, but the patient typically recovers. Sweling around the bruised area can cause changes in consciousness levels, as well as the development of seizures and neurological symptoms in a specific area of the body. It is important to monitor patients closely for any worsening of neurological symptoms due to increasing swelling and potential herniation.

A lumbar puncture is needless and could be harmful. The preferred diagnostic techniques are MRIs and CT scans. Surgical intervention is rarely necessary for cerebral contusions, unlike subdural and epidural hematomas.

2.3.1.4. Intracerebral Hemorrhage

- **Etiology:** Chronic hypertension is the most frequent cause of nontraumatic intracerebral hemorrhage.
- **Clinical Findings:** The majority of intracerebral hemorrhage happens when the patient is conscious. Transient prodromal symptoms, like transient ischemic attacks (TIAs) frequently linked to cerebral infarction, do not precede hemorrhage.

Frequent headaches range in intensity from mild to severe. If a headache is experienced, it could be widespread or restricted to the bleeding site. Vomiting and nausea are typical. Over the course of minutes to hours, altered consciousness may gradually lead to stupor or coma.

During examination, even in the advanced stages of transtentorial herniation, patients are almost always hypertensive (blood pressure 170/90 mm Hg or higher). The funduscopic examination typically reveals vascular alterations linked to long-term hypertension. Nuchal stiffness is typical. Gaze deviation may happen, either downward and medially in a thalamic hemorrhage or toward the side of a putaminal or lobar hemorrhage. Due to the close proximity of common hemorrhage sites, like the thalamus and basal ganglia, to the internal capsule, which transmits descending motor fibers from the cerebral cortex, hemiparesis is a common condition.

About 10% of cases result in seizures, which are frequently focal. Deficits in the nervous system do not change on their own.

- **Investigative Studies:** The diagnosis is confirmed by an MRI or CT brain scan without contrast that reveals intraparenchymal blood.
- Treatment
  - **Blood Pressure**: Systolic blood pressure should be reduced to 140 mm Hg or less to limit hematoma expansion, but excessive blood pressure reduction should be avoided, as it may compromise blood flow in brain tissue adjacent to the hemorrhage.
  - **Cerebral Edema**: The mass effect of intracerebral hemorrhage is typically compounded by progressive cerebral edema, which becomes evident at approximately 24 hours and maximal within 5 to 6 days. Cerebral edema may be treated with mannitol or intravenous hypertonic saline (Table 2.6), but this is usually only useful as a temporizing measure prior to surgery, when indicated, and alone rarely alters the eventual outcome.

3. **Surgical treatment**: Evacuation of the clot may be appropriate in cases (approximately 10%) in which hemorrhage is located superficially in the cerebral hemisphere and produces a mass effect. However, most hemorrhages are deep within the brain and less accessible to surgery.

- **Prognosis:** About 25% of patients who suffer an intracerebral hemorrhage pass away within 72 hours, which is a high rate of early mortality. However, as the clot heals over a few weeks to months, those who survive could experience surprisingly minor deficits.

2.3.1.5. Brain Abscess

A brain abscess is a rare condition that makes up only 2% of intracranial masses.

- **Etiology:** Blood-borne metastasis from distant systemic infection (especially pulmonary infection), direct extension from parameningeal sites (otitis, cranial osteomyelitis, sinusitis), an unknown source, infection associated with recent or distant head trauma or craniotomy, and infection associated with cyanotic congenital heart disease are the common conditions predisposing to brain abscess, roughly in order of frequency.

Table 2.6. Drug Therapy for Cerebral Edema

Drug	Dose	Route	Indications and Comments
Glucocorticoids			
Dexamethasone	10-100 mg, then 4 mg 4 times daily	Intravenous or orally	Dexamethasone preferred for lowest mineralocorticoid effect. Antacid treatment indicated. Effective for edema associated with brain tumor or abscess; not indicated for intracerebral hemorrhage or infarction.
Prednisone	60 mg, then 25 mg 4 times daily	Orally	
Methylprednisolone	60 mg, then 25 mg 4 times daily	Intravenous or orally	
Hydrocortisone	300 mg, then 130 mg 4 times daily	Intravenous or orally	
Osmotic diuretic agents			
Mannitol	1.5-2 g/kg over 30 min–1 h	20% intravenous solution	Effective acutely. Major dehydrating effect on normal tissue; osmotic effect short-lived, and more than two intravenous doses rarely effective. Hypertonic saline has both osmotic and vasoregulatory effects.
Hypertonic saline	3% continuous infusion or 23.4% or 29.2% by 20 mL bolus	Intravenously	Continuous infusion of 3% hypertonic saline to target a serum sodium of 145-155 mEq/L; boluses of hypertonic saline may be more effective than other osmotic agents.

Source: https://dl.mehrsys.ir/pdf-books/Clinical%20Neurology%209%20Edition%20(www.myuptodate.com).pdf.

Gram-negative anaerobes like Prevotella, Fusobacterium, and Bacterioides, as well as aerobic, anaerobic, and microaerophilic streptococci, are the most prevalent pathogenic agents. Less frequent are Proteus, Staphylococcus aureus, and other gram-negative bacilli. There are also Actinomyces, Nocardia, and Candida. In most cases, abscesses contain multiple organisms.

- **Clinical Findings:** In a conscious patient, the course is that of an expanding mass lesion, typically manifesting as focal neurologic deficits and headaches. A coma rarely lasts for hours, but it can happen over days. Table 2.7 lists common presenting signs and symptoms. It is noteworthy that in 40% of patients, the temperature is normal, and in 20% of cases, the peripheral white blood cell count is below 10,000/μL. These are common correlates of infection that may not be present.
- **Investigative Studies:** A mass lesion with a contrast-enhanced rim on an MRI or CT scan, or an avascular mass on an angiography, strongly supports the diagnosis. Upon examination, the CSF shows that in 75% of patients, the opening pressure is greater than 200 mm water;

in approximately 60% of patients, the protein level is elevated (45–500 mg/dL) and there is pleocytosis of 25 to 500 or more white cells/μL, depending on how close the abscess is to the ventricular surface and how much it has been encapsulated. The majority of CSF cultures are negative. If a brain abscess is suspected, lumbar puncture should not be done because patients may experience marked clinical deterioration after the procedure.

Table 2.7. Brain Abscesses: Presenting Features in 123 Cases

Fever	58%
Headache	55%
Disturbed consciousness	48%
Hemiparesis	48%
Nausea, vomiting	32%
Nuchal rigidity	29%
Dysarthria	20%
Seizures	19%
Sepsis	17%
Visual disturbances	15%

Source: Modified from Lu CH, Chang WN, Lin YC, et al. Bacterial brain abscess: microbiological features, epidemiological trends and outcomes. Q J Med. 2002;95:501–509.

- Treatment: Antibiotics alone or in conjunction with surgical drainage are two possible treatments for pyogenic brain abscesses. When there is a large mass effect or the abscess is close to the ventricular surface, surgical therapy should be seriously considered because there is a risk of catastrophic rupture into the ventricular system.

  For multiple, early, or surgically inaccessible abscesses, medical treatment alone is recommended. It is recommended to use broad-spectrum antibiotic coverage if the causative organism is unknown. In North America, ceftriaxone 2 g every 12 hours in addition to metronidazole is the first-line recommendation. Certain countries still use penicillin G 3 to 4 million units intravenously every 4 hours and metronidazole 7 to 5 mg/kg intravenously or orally every 6 hours. Add 3 g of oxacillin or nafcillin intravenously every 6 hours if staphylococcal infection is suspected. Vancomycin 1 g every 12 hours adjusted to serum levels is the first line of treatment for many centers due to the rising prevalence of methicillin-resistant staphylococcal infections. It is advised that trauma patients receive cefcillin in addition to either cefotaxime or ceftriaxone to treat aerobic gram-negative bacteria and staphylococci. Glucocorticoids (Table 2.6) have the potential to lessen surrounding abscess edema. Clinical examination and repeated CT or MRI scans should be used to evaluate how the patient is responding to medical treatment. In order to determine the organisms present in an abscess, needle aspiration is recommended for patients receiving medical treatment who do not improve.

2.3.1.6. Stroke (Cerebral Infarction)

Since bilateral hemispheric lesions are necessary for consciousness to be lost, an embolic or thrombotic occlusion of one carotid artery does not directly cause coma. On the other hand, cerebral edema following a massive hemispheric infarction may result in transtentorial herniation or compression of the contralateral hemisphere, both of which may result in coma. Within 48 to 72 hours of the infarction, edema reaches its peak and can lead to stupor and coma as well as the progression of the initial neurologic deficit. An MRI or CT scan rules out cerebral hemorrhage.

There is no obvious benefit to treating cerebral edema linked to stroke with corticosteroids and dehydrating agents.

2.3.2. Brain Tumor

- ***Clinical Findings:*** Comas are uncommon presentations of primary or metastatic brain tumors, though they can happen when there is a hemorrhage within the tumor or when seizures are caused by the tumor. More often than not, a headache, focal neurologic deficits, and altered consciousness precede the coma, which sets in late in the clinical course of the brain tumor. In 25% of cases, papilledema is a sign on presentation.
- **Investigative Studies:** An MRI or CT scan of the head should be performed if a brain tumor is suspected. A biopsy may be necessary to ascertain the nature of the tumor based solely on its imaging appearance. Because lung carcinoma is the most common cause of intracranial metastasis and because other tumors that metastasize to the brain typically involve the lungs first, a chest X-ray or CT scan is helpful.
- **Treatment:** Corticosteroids (Table 2.6) are frequently remarkably effective in reducing tumor-associated vasogenic brain edema from leaking capillaries and improving related neurologic deficits, in contrast to their lack of therapeutic effect on edema resulting from cerebral ischemia. Depending on the location and type of lesion, specific tumor treatment methods include radiotherapy, chemotherapy, and excision.

2.4. Subtentorial Structural Lesions

2.4.1. Basilar Artery Thrombosis or Embolic Occlusion

- **Clinical Findings:** These comparatively common vascular syndromes block blood supply to the brainstem reticular activating system, which results in coma. The majority of patients are middle-aged or older, and they frequently have a history of TIAs, hypertension, or atherosclerotic vascular disease. Typically, embolic occlusion affects the top of the basilar artery, while thrombosis affects its middle section. Almost all patients arrive with some form of altered consciousness, and half are unconscious when they do. Neurologic focal signs are evident right away.

  Differentiating between midsized fixed pupils with midbrain involvement and pinpoint pupils with pontine lesions, the abnormalities in pupil function depend on the location of the lesion. During head or cold-water caloric testing, it is common for the eyes to deviate vertically, and horizontal eye movements may be absent or asymmetrical. If conjugate eye deviation is seen, it points toward the hemiparesis rather than the side of the lesion. There may be intact or impaired vertical eye movements. There may be symmetric or asymmetric symptoms, including hyperreflexia, hemiparesis, and Babinski responses. The CSF is free of blood.
- **Treatment and Prognosis:** Anticoagulation is the standard treatment for progressive subtotal basilar artery thrombosis, even though there isn't much proof that it works. If recurrent cardiac emboli are the cause, anticoagulation lowers their frequency. Specialized centers are now using intravascular clot retrieval, also known as endovascular therapy. The degree of brainstem injury directly affects the prognosis.

2.4.2. Pontine Hemorrhage

Just about 6% of hypertensive intracerebral hemorrhages occur at the pontine hemorrhage site, although this type of hemorrhage almost exclusively affects patients with high blood pressure. The defining feature of this syndrome is the abrupt, "apoplectic" onset of coma. Many of the findings seen in basilar artery infarction are visible on physical examination, but transient ischemic episodes do not precede the condition. Specific pupils, loss of horizontal eye movements, and ocular bobbing—spontaneous, brisk, periodic, mostly conjugate, downward eye movements with a slower return to the primary position—are characteristics that are particularly suggestive of pontine involvement. Most patients who survive for longer than a few hours experience hyperthermia, which is defined as a temperature elevation of 39.5°C (103°F) or higher. A CT scan or MRI is used to make the diagnosis. Although there is obvious blood and increased pressure in the CSF, a lumbar puncture is not recommended. There's no cure that works.

2.4.3. Cerebellar Hemorrhage or Infarction

Cerebellar hemorrhage or infarction can manifest clinically as a sudden onset of coma that rapidly progresses to death, or as a syndrome that begins with headache, dizziness, vomiting, and inability to stand and progresses over hours or even days to coma. Since acute deterioration can happen suddenly, it's important to monitor patients closely and start treating them as soon as possible. An MRI or CT scan verifies the diagnosis.

With the right surgical care, patients who are lethargic or even stuporous after surgery may recover with little to no residual deficits and retain their full mental capacity. Surgical decompression may also result in a dramatic reduction of symptoms. Nonetheless, there is little chance of a useful survival if the patient is profoundly unconscious.

2.4.4. Posterior Fossa Subdural and Epidural Hematomas

These extremely rare lesions are important to identify because they are treatable and have similar clinical pictures. Usually, occipital trauma occurs hours to many weeks before brainstem involvement begins. Physical signs of extra-axial (extrinsic) compression of the brainstem include progressive obtundation, nystagmus, vertigo, and ataxia. In more persistent cases, there may be papilledema and nuchal rigidity. A fracture line that crosses the transverse or sigmoid sinus is frequently visible on skull CT scans. The traumatic tearing of these vessels is the cause of the hematoma. Analyzing the CSF is not beneficial. Decompression surgery is the mode of treatment.

2.5. Diffuse Encephalopathies

2.5.1. Meningitis and Encephali

Meningitis and encephalitis are often accompanied by fever and headache, and they can present as an acute confused state or coma. Meningeal irritation symptoms are also commonly observed in meningitis and should be carefully sought after to enable prompt lumbar puncture, diagnosis, and treatment. These symptoms include flexion of the knee during passive neck flexion, flexion of the neck or contralateral knee during passive elevation of the extended straight leg, and resistance of the neck to full forward flexion. Meningeal signs may not be present in cases of deeply unconscious or immunocompromised patients, meningitis that occurs at the oldest ages, or encephalitis without meningeal involvement. Typically, a neurologic examination reveals symmetric findings; however, certain infections, like herpes simplex encephalitis or bacterial meningitis complicated by vasculitis, can show focal features. It is not recommended to postpone a CSF examination to get a CT scan if there are indications of meningeal irritation.

2.5.2. Subarachnoid Hemorrhage

The symptoms of subarachnoid hemorrhage, headache, and facial pain usually start out abruptly and include headache, which is usually, but not always, severe. At the onset, consciousness is often lost, either temporarily or permanently. At this point, decerebrate posturing or, very infrequently, seizures, may happen. Prominent focal neurologic signs are rare, except in cases of oculomotor (III) or abducens (VI) nerve palsies; bilateral extensor plantar responses are common. Meningeal irritation and meningeal signs are caused by subarachnoid blood. Acute hemorrhages resulting from abruptly elevated intracranial pressure or the more common superficial subhyaloid hemorrhages can both be seen upon examination of the optic fundi. Blood is seen in the subarachnoid space on the CT brain scan, and the CSF is bloody.

2.5.3. Hypoglycemia

- **Etiology:** Hypoglycemic encephalopathy and coma typically occur due to insulin overdose, with other possible causes including alcoholism, severe liver disease, oral hypoglycemic medications, insulin-secreting tumors (insulinoma), and large retroperitoneal tumors.
- **Clinical Findings:** Patients may be alerted to hypoglycemia by symptoms of sympathetic nervous system hyperactivity, such as tachycardia, sweating, and anxiety, which manifest as blood glucose levels drop. Patients with diabetic autonomic neuropathy, however, may not experience these prodromal symptoms. Seizures, delirium, stupor, coma, and focal neurologic signs that may alternate sides are among the neurologic findings associated with hypoglycemia. Progressive loss of body heat is frequent.
- **Investigative Studies:** Blood glucose levels and symptoms are not exactly correlated; therefore, a level of 30 mg/dL may be linked to delirium in one patient, hemiparesis with preserved consciousness in another, or coma in a third. It has been documented that blood glucose levels between 2 and 28, 8 and 59, and 9 and 60 mg/dL can cause coma, stupor, and confusion, respectively.
- **Treatment:** It is possible to prevent hypoglycemia-induced permanent brain damage if glucose is quickly given intravenously, orally, or through a nasogastric tube. Every patient presenting with altered consciousness (acute confusional state, coma, or psychosis) should have blood drawn for a subsequent glucose determination and receive 50 mL of 50% dextrose intravenously right away because hypoglycemia is so easily treated and delaying treatment can have tragic consequences. This makes blood analysis possible without postponing treatment.
- **Prognosis:** The amount of time hypoglycemia will persist before causing irreversible brain damage varies. Hypoglycemic coma can be tolerated for 60 to 90 minutes, but if recovery is to be expected, glucose must be given within 15 minutes of the patient reaching the stage of flaccidity with hyporeflexia. Full recovery should happen seconds after intravenous glucose administration and 10 to 30 minutes after nasogastric glucose administration, assuming no irreversible brain damage has occurred. While full recovery usually

happens quickly, it can occasionally take several days or even hours to fully recover. Any residual symptoms or indicators point to either an additional neuropathologic process or irreversible brain damage caused by hypoglycemia.

2.5.4. Global Cerebral Ischemia

Encephalopathy and coma are the results of global cerebral ischemia, and they typically follow cardiac arrest. Rapid pupil dilation and tonic, frequently opisthotonic, posturing with a few tonic-clonic movements resembling seizures may be present. Urinary incontinence is widespread.

Recovery starts at the brainstem level with the restoration of reflex eye movements and pupillary function if cerebral perfusion is quickly restored. After that, purposeful movements take the place of reflex motor activity (flexor or extensor posturing), and consciousness returns.

The prognosis is based on how quickly brain function returns. Patients with a poor prognosis are those who do not regain consciousness within 4 days or who do not exhibit pupillary reactivity within 1 day.

Meaningful recovery is essentially precluded in adults whose brainstem function (unreactive pupils) is persistently impaired after cardiac function returns. If recovery is not complete, higher-order cognitive functions may not return, and wakefulness—the opening of the eyes during sleep–wake cycles—will take over. A persistent vegetative state is the term used to describe the state in which these patients are conscious but not awake. Global ischemia is the most common cause, though other significant brain insults like trauma, bihemispheric stroke, or subarachnoid hemorrhage may also result in this kind of outcome. Prognosis has improved with the introduction of therapeutic hypothermia for patients in a coma following cardiac arrest resuscitation; however, this has necessitated a reevaluation of prognostic indicators. The prognosis is now clinically assessed 72 hours following rewarming, or 96 hours following arrest. While motor responsiveness, which is predictive of a normothermic anoxia patient's prognosis, is unclear in patients receiving hypothermia treatment, loss of pupillary light reflex is still a serious prognostic indicator. In certain centers, prognostication is based on a combination of brainstem signs, EEG findings, and somatosensory-stimulated potential study results.

2.5.5. Drug Intoxication

- **Sedative Drugs:** In many series, sedative drug overdose—of which barbiturates and benzodiazepines are the archetypal drugs—is the most common cause of coma.

  A period of intoxication characterized by prominent nystagmus in all gaze directions, dysarthria, and ataxia precedes the coma. A brief neurologic examination shortly after the loss of consciousness may indicate a structural lesion affecting motor pathways, accompanied by hyperreflexia, extensor plantar responses, ankle clonus, and (in rare cases) decerebrate or decorticate posturing. Nonetheless, the absence of eye movements during doll's head or cold-water calorie testing, combined with preserved pupillary reactivity, is a defining characteristic of sedative-hypnotic overdose. Pupil reactivity can occasionally be compromised by barbiturates or other sedative drug concentrations high enough to cause severe hypotension, respiratory depression, and the need for pressors and ventilator support. This can lead to pupils that are 2 to 3 mm in diameter and nonreactive to light. Hypothermia and bullous skin eruptions are additional signs of barbiturate-induced coma.

Full recovery with support for cardiopulmonary function will occur even though the electroencephalogram (EEG) may be flat and, in the event of an overdose with long-acting barbiturates, may remain isoelectric for a full day or longer. Supportive care should be administered with an emphasis on preserving appropriate circulation and ventilation. Barbiturates can be dialyzed; however, patients receiving more conservative care have lower rates of morbidity and death when using shorter-acting barbiturates. Flumazenil, a benzodiazepine-receptor antagonist, can be used to reverse sedative drug intoxication in some cases. However, in patients with mixed overdose, it can cause status epilepticus by exposing tricyclic antidepressant-induced seizures. Flumazenil should only be administered intravenously up to a maximum dose of 1 mg.

- **Ethanol:** The symptoms of an ethanol overdose are comparable to those of a sedative drug overdose, but they are less likely to include nystagmus during wakefulness, early lateral eye movement impairment, and coma progression. Tachycardia, hypotension, and hypothermia are all evident, along with peripheral vasodilation. Blood ethanol levels between 250 and 300 mg/dL are normally associated with stupor, while levels between 300 and 400 mg/dL are associated with coma. However, alcoholic patients who have grown tolerant to the drug may tolerate much higher levels and still be awake and seemingly sober.
- **Opioids:** Pupilary constriction, which can also result from organophosphate poisoning, miotic eye drops, pontine hemorrhage, and Argyll Robertson pupils, is a hallmark of an opioid overdose. Rapid pupillary dilation and awakening following intravenous injection of 0.4–1.2 mg of the opioid antagonist naloxone are indicative of opioid intoxication. In most cases, naloxone works for one to four hours. Therefore, repeated doses might be required, particularly in cases where long-acting opioids like methadone have caused intoxication.

2.5.6. Hepatic Encephalopathy

- **Clinical Findings:** Patients with severe liver disease, particularly those with portacaval shunting, may experience hepatic encephalopathy that progresses to coma. Jaundice is not a requirement. An acute insult, particularly a gastrointestinal hemorrhage, can cause coma. The pathogenesis may be aided by colonic bacteria's ammonia production. Increased levels of endogenous benzodiazepine receptor agonists in the brain may lead to an increase in inhibitory γ-aminobutyric acid-mediated neurotransmission, which in turn may cause neuronal depression. Similar to other metabolic encephalopathies, delirium or somnolence are the patient's initial symptoms. Asterixis might be particularly noticeable. There have been reports of alternating hemiparesis, decorticate or decerebrate posturing, and frequently elevated muscle tone and hyperreflexia. Seizures that are focal or generalized do happen occasionally.
- **Investigative Studies:** The almost constant presence of respiratory alkalosis due to hyperventilation is

a useful diagnostic clue; however, serum bicarbonate levels rarely decrease below 16 mEq/L. Although the CSF is typically normal, patients with serum bilirubin levels higher than 4 to 6 mg/dL may see a yellow appearance (xanthochromic). The elevated CSF glutamine concentration confirms the diagnosis. Although it can happen with values as low as 35 mg/dL, coma is typically linked to concentrations over 50 mg/dL. Reducing protein intake to less than 20 g/d, controlling gastrointestinal bleeding or systemic infection, and lowering intracolonic pH with lactulose (30 mg orally 2–3 times per day or titrated to produce 2–4 bowel movements daily) are the treatment strategies for hepatic encephalopathy. During the first 48 hours of lactulose treatment, abdominal cramps may happen. Neomycin 6 g/d, taken orally in three or four divided doses, has the potential to decrease the production of ammonia by colonic bacteria.

2.5.7. Hyperosmolar States

The hyperosmolar state, most commonly linked to nonketotic hyperglycemia, frequently manifests as coma with focal seizures.

2.5.8. Hyponatremia

In cases where serum sodium levels drop below 120 mEq/L, particularly when the drop occurs quickly, hyponatremia may result in neurologic symptoms. Seizures and delirium are frequent initial symptoms.

2.5.9. Hypothermia

A patient cannot go into a coma if their temperature is below 26°C (79°F). However, mild hypothermia (>32°C [90°F]) does not result in a coma. Hypoglycemia, sedative drug intoxication, Wernicke encephalopathy, and hypothyroidism (myxedema) are among the conditions that can cause coma in cases of hypothermia. When a structural brain lesion results in an acute coma outside or in another unheated area, exposure can also cause hypothermia. For this reason, the lesion should not be ruled out in the differential diagnosis of coma with hypothermia.

Upon physical examination, the patient appears noticeably cold to the touch, though it's possible that they aren't shivering—shivering stops at temperatures below 32.5°C (90.5%F). A neurologic examination reveals diffusely elevated muscle tone and an unresponsiveness to pain in the patient. Pupillary responses could be slow or nonexistent.

Prolonged PR, QRS, and QT intervals, bradycardia, and the distinctive J-point elevation (Osborn waves) can all be seen on the ECG. In the absence of myocardial infarction, serum creatine kinase may be elevated, and elevated serum amylase levels are typical. Temperature-related errors in arterial blood gas measurements and pH will result in reported values of falsely high PCO2 and PO2 as well as falsely low pH.

The goal of treatment is to return the body temperature to normal while also addressing the underlying illness causing the hypothermia. While there is debate over the best way to reheat food and how quickly, using blankets in a warm room to passively reheat food is a quick and easy remedy. When rewarming, ventricular fibrillation might happen. Warming causes vasodilation, which can result in hypotension, so intravenous fluids might be necessary.

Most hypothermic patients recover without experiencing any neurological aftereffects. There is no direct relationship between recorded temperature and survival, except for myxedema. The underlying disease process that causes hypothermia or ventricular fibrillation, to which the human myocardium becomes particularly susceptible at temperatures below 30°C (86°F), is the cause of death when it happens. The maximum temperature at which myocardial sensitivity can occur is below 21 to 24°C (70–75°F).

2.5.10. Hyperthermia

Coma develops when body temperature rises above 42 to 43°C (107.6–109.4°F), as the brain's metabolic activity is unable to keep up with the increased energy demands. Exposure to high ambient temperatures is the most frequent cause of hyperthermia (heat stroke). Additional causes include anticholinergic medications, hypothalamic damage, delirium tremens, status epilepticus, and idiosyncratic reactions to halogenated inhalational anesthetics (malignant hyperthermia) or antipsychotic drugs (neuroleptic malignant syndrome). The centrally mediated temperature elevations in patients who survive pontine hemorrhage for longer than a few hours range from 38.5 to 42.8°C (101.3–109°F).

In hyperthermia, reactive pupils, a diffuse increase in muscle tone, and coma are found on the neurologic examination.

The patient's body temperature is immediately brought down to 39°C (102.2°F) with the use of an electric fan or cooling blanket, as well as ice packs and alcohol. It is important to avoid becoming overly dehydrated because cooling causes vasoconstriction in patients with volume expansion, which can lead to pulmonary edema.

2.5.11. Seizure or Prolonged Postictal State

Coma differential diagnosis should always take status epilepticus into account. Motor activity can be limited to the repetitive motions of one side of the face or one limb. Even though these indications of seizure activity may be subtle, one should not ignore them because status epilepticus needs to be treated right away.

2.5.12. Other Diffuse Encephalopathies

Multifocal conditions such as disseminated intravascular coagulopathy, sepsis, pancreatitis, vasculitis, thrombotic thrombocytopenic purpura, fat emboli, hypertensive encephalopathy, and diffuse micrometastases are uncommon causes of coma that manifest as metabolic coma.

2.6. Differential Diagnosis

Several neurological and psychiatric conditions can be mistaken for comas.

2.6.1. Psychogenic Unresponsiveness

Psychogenic unresponsiveness is an exclusionary diagnosis that ought to be made only in the presence of strong supporting data. It could be an indication of malingering, somatoform disorders (conversion disorder or somatization disorder), or catatonic schizophrenia.

During the general physical examination, no abnormalities are found. The neurologic examination typically shows decreased muscle tone, normal reflexes, and a normal response to plantar stimulation. Pupils are usually 2 to 3 mm in diameter and respond well to light. Lateral eye movements on doll's head testing may not always be present due to visual fixation. Slow conjugate roving eye movements of metabolic coma cannot be mimicked and are not compatible with a diagnosis of psychogenic unresponsiveness. In addition, the slow, often asymmetric eye closure observed in comatose patients cannot be voluntarily reproduced. Patients with psychogenic unresponsiveness often show some voluntary muscle tone in the eyelids during passive eye opening. Irrigation of the tympanic membrane with cold water is a helpful test, as brisk nystagmus is seen in conscious patients, while coma patients do not exhibit this response. EEG findings in psychogenic unresponsiveness are similar to those of a normal awake person.

2.6.2. Persistent Vegetative State

Cerebral hypoxia, global cerebral ischemia, head trauma, and bilateral hemispheric strokes can all cause comatose patients to regain wakefulness but not awareness (Figure 2.7). This is referred to as a persistent vegetative state if it lasts for at least one month. In addition to having intact brainstem and autonomic function, these patients differ from those in comas in that they exhibit spontaneous eye opening and sleep-wake cycles. They do not, however, understand or speak language, and they do not respond to stimuli with intention. This might continue for years. It is uncommon to regain consciousness from nontraumatic causes beyond three months, and it is even less common to recover from traumatic causes beyond twelve months. It's possible that a portion of these patients exhibit minimal but distinct signs of environmental awareness, a condition known as minimally conscious. There have been reports of late responsiveness recovery with significant residual disability.

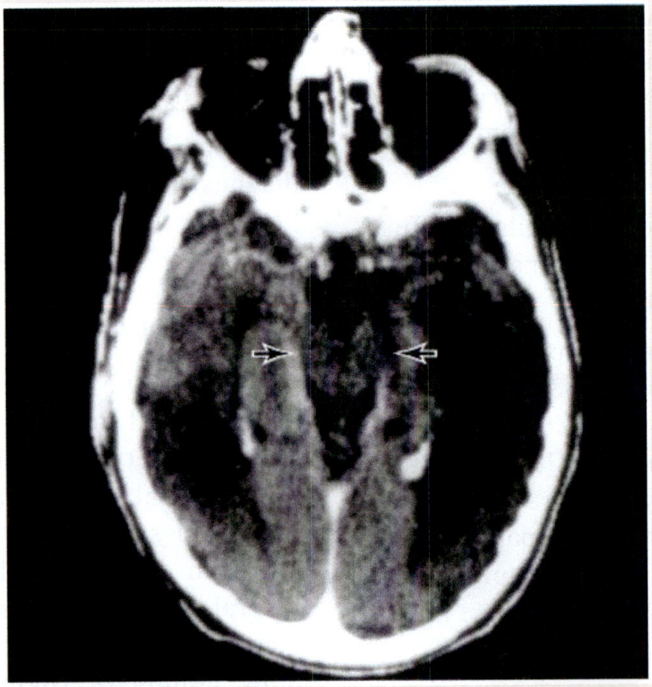

Figure 2.7. CT brain scan (contrast-enhanced) of a patient with bilateral middle cerebral artery infarcts who is in a persistent vegetative state. The reticular activating system in the intact midbrain (arrows) allows wakefulness, but the bihemispheric lesions preclude awareness.

Source: https://dl.mehrsys.ir/pdf-books/Clinical%20Neurology%209%20Edition%20(www.myuptodate.com).pdf.

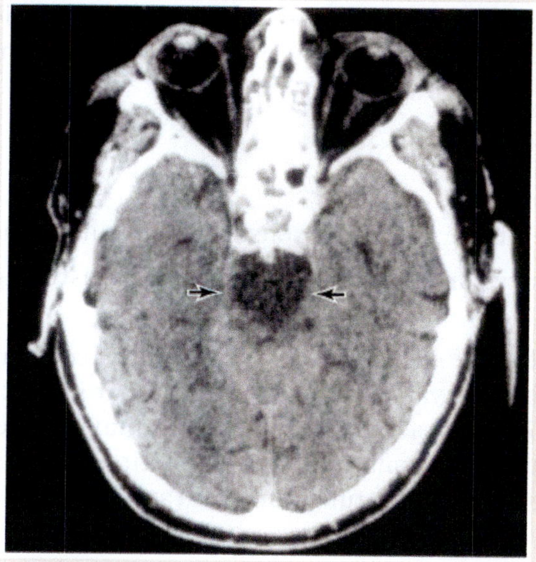

Figure 2.8. A CT brain scan (contrast-enhanced) of a man with basilar artery occlusion who exhibits the "locked-in" syndrome. The pontine infarction (arrows) is below the level of the reticular activating system, allowing wakefulness, but the bilateral descending motor tracts have been transected.

Source: https://dl.mehrsys.ir/pdf-books/Clinical%20Neurology%209%20Edition%20(www.myuptodate.com).pdf.

2.6.3. Locked-In Syndrome

Functional transection of the brainstem below this level—by pontine infarction (Figure 2.8), hemorrhage, central pontine myelinolysis, tumor, or encephalitis—can interrupt descending neural pathways to produce an akinetic and mute state, with preserved consciousness, because the portion of the reticular formation responsible for consciousness lies above the level of the midpons. Despite appearing comatose, these patients are awake and conscious despite being quadriplegic and mute. Flexor spasms or decerebrate posturing could be observed. When voluntary eye opening, vertical eye movements, ocular convergence, or a combination of these volitional midbrain-mediated movements are preserved, the diagnosis can be made. Any patient who appears to be in a comatose state should be instructed to make certain movements during the examination, such as "open your eyes," "look up," "look down," and "look at the tip of your nose.." The EEG is in the normal range. The degree of the brainstem lesion and the underlying cause influence the outcome, which varies. When a vascular disturbance is the cause, mortality from pneumonia is typically 70%, whereas in nonvascular cases, it is approximately 40%. Over the course of several weeks to months, survivors may fully or partially recover.

2.7. Brain Death

Here is a summary of the current criteria for determining brain death that were created by the President's Commission for the Study of Ethical Problems in Medicine and Biomedical and Behavioral

Research in 1981. A diagnosis of brain death requires the irreversible loss of all brain function. When diagnosing brain death in children under the age of five, care must be taken.

2.7.1. Cessation of Brain Function

- Unresponsiveness
  - The patient must be unresponsive to sensory input, including speech and pain.
  - The presence of seizures or decorticate/decerebrate posturing is incompatible with brain death.
- **Absent Brainstem Reflexes:** There are no pupillary, corneal, oropharyngeal responses, and doll's head and cold-water caloric testing fail to elicit eye movements. After the patient's PCO_2 is allowed to rise to 60 mm Hg for maximal ventilatory stimulation, there are no more respiratory responses, and oxygenation is maintained by providing 100% oxygen through an endotracheal tube cannula (apnea test).

2.7.2. Irreversibility of Brain Dysfunction

The coma's cause needs to be identified, sufficient to account for the clinical picture, and irreversible. It is necessary to rule out sedative drug intoxication, shock, hypothermia (<32°C [90°F]), neuromuscular blockade, and hypothermia because these conditions can cause a clinical picture that mimics brain death but may still allow for neurologic recovery.

2.7.3. Persistence of Brain Dysfunction

The criteria for brain death described in the preceding section must persist for an appropriate length of time, as follows:

1. Six hours with a confirmatory isoelectric (flat) EEG, performed according to the technical standards of the American Electroencephalographic Society.
2. Twelve hours without a confirmatory isoelectric EEG.
3. Twenty-four hours for anoxic brain injury without a confirmatory isoelectric EEG.

A Closer Look

Brain Stem Stroke

Brain stem strokes can have complex symptoms and can be hard to diagnose. A person may have vertigo, dizziness and severe imbalance without the hallmark of most strokes — weakness on one side of the body. Vertigo dizziness symptoms or imbalance usually occur together; dizziness alone is not a sign of stroke. A brain stem stroke can also cause double vision, slurred speech and decreased consciousness.

Only a half-inch in diameter, the brain stem controls all basic activities of the central nervous system: consciousness, blood pressure and breathing. All motor control for the body flows through it. Brain stem strokes can impair any or all these functions. More severe brain stem strokes can cause locked-in syndrome, a condition in which survivors can move only their eyes.

If a stroke in the brain stem results from a clot, the faster blood flow can be restored, the better the chances for recovery.

Like all strokes, brain stem strokes produce a wide spectrum of deficits and recovery. Whether a survivor has minor or severe deficits depends on the location of the stroke within the brain stem, the extent of injury and how quickly treatment is provided.

Risk factors for brain stem stroke are the same as for strokes in other areas of the brain: high blood pressure, diabetes, heart disease, atrial fibrillation and smoking. Similarly, brain stem strokes can be caused by a clot or a hemorrhage. Rare causes include injury to an artery due to sudden head or neck movements.

Recovery is possible. Because brain stem strokes don't usually affect language ability, the patient is often able to participate more fully in rehabilitation. Double vision and vertigo usually resolve after several weeks of recovery in mild to moderate brain stem strokes.

Summary

- Comas may arise from a blow to the head during a traumatic event, from an infection, from complications of diabetes, or from low oxygen levels.
- A sudden onset of coma suggests a vascular origin, especially a brainstem stroke or subarachnoid hemorrhage.
- Palpation of the head may demonstrate a depressed skull fracture or swelling of soft tissues at the site of trauma.
- Strong pressure is applied to the sternum, nail beds, or supraorbital ridge in order to evaluate the motor response to pain.
- A coma caused by diffuse encephalopathies, also known as metabolic comas, encompass not only metabolic conditions like hypoglycemia and drug intoxication but also other diffuse brain disorders like meningitis, subarachnoid hemorrhage, and seizures.
- A cerebral contusion is brain bruising that occurs as a result of a head injury. This injury can lead to temporary unconsciousness, but the patient typically recovers.
- Comas are uncommon presentations of primary or metastatic brain tumors, though they can happen when there is a hemorrhage within the tumor or when seizures are caused by the tumor.
- Meningeal irritation symptoms are also commonly observed in meningitis and should be carefully sought after to enable prompt lumbar puncture, diagnosis, and treatment.
- Encephalopathy and coma are the results of global cerebral ischemia, and they typically follow cardiac arrest.

References

1. Becker, D. A., Balcer, L. J., & Galetta, S. L. (2012). The neurological complications of nutritional deficiency following bariatric surgery. *Journal of Obesity, 2012*, 608534.
2. Bernat, J. L. (2006). Chronic disorders of consciousness. *The Lancet, 367*, 1181–1192.
3. Bernat, J. L. (2010). Current controversies in states of chronic unconsciousness. *Neurology, 75*(18 Suppl 1), S33–S38.
4. Braun, M., Schmidt, W. U., Möckel, M., Römer, M., Ploner, C. J., & Lindner, T. (2016). Coma of unknown origin in the emergency department: implementation of an in-house management routine. *Scandinavian Journal of Trauma, Resuscitation and Emergency Medicine, 24*, 61.
5. Donnino, M. W., Vega, J., Miller, J., & Walsh, M. (2007). Myths and misconceptions of Wernicke's encephalopathy: what every emergency physician should know. *Annals of Emergency Medicine, 50*(6), 715–721.
6. Edlow, J. A., Rabinstein, A., Traub, S. J., & Wijdicks, E. F. (2014). Diagnosis of reversible causes of coma. *The Lancet, 384*(9959), 2064–2076.
7. Forsberg, S., Höjer, J., & Ludwigs, U. (2012). Prognosis in patients presenting with non-traumatic coma. *Journal of Emergency Medicine, 42*(3), 249–253.
8. Giacino, J. T., Fins, J. J., Laureys, S., & Schiff, N. D. (2014). Disorders of consciousness after acquired brain injury: the state of the science. *Nature Reviews Neurology, 10*, 99–114.

9. Green, S. M. (2011). Cheerio, laddie! Bidding farewell to the Glasgow Coma Scale. *Annals of Emergency Medicine, 58*(5), 427–430.
10. Hoffman, R. S., & Goldfrank, L. R. (1995). The poisoned patient with altered consciousness. Controversies in the use of a 'coma cocktail.' *JAMA, 274*(7), 562–569.
11. Huff, J. S., Stevens, R. D., Weingart, S. D., & Smith, W. S. (2012). Emergency neurological life support: approach to the patient with coma. *Neurocritical Care, 17*(Suppl 1), S54–S59.
12. Maramattom, B. V., & Wijdicks, E. F. (2005). Uncal herniation. *Archives of Neurology, 62*(12), 1932–1935.
13. Mattle, H. P., Arnold, M., Lindsberg, P. J., Schonewille, W. J., & Schroth, G. (2011). Basilar artery occlusion. *The Lancet Neurology, 10*(11), 1002–1014.
14. Posner, J. B., Saper, C. B., Schiff, N. D., & Plum, F. (2007). Plum and Posner's Diagnosis of Stupor and Coma (4th ed.). Oxford University Press.
15. Ropper, A. H. (2012). Hyperosmolar therapy for raised intracranial pressure. *New England Journal of Medicine, 367*(8), 746–752.
16. Samuels, M. A. (1993). The evaluation of comatose patients. *Hospital Practice, 28*(3), 165–182.
17. Schmidt, W. U., Ploner, C. J., Lutz, M., Möckel, M., Lindner, T., & Braun, M. (2019). Causes of brain dysfunction in acute coma: a cohort study of 1027 patients in the emergency department. *Scandinavian Journal of Trauma, Resuscitation and Emergency Medicine, 27*(1), 101.
18. Smith, E., & Delargy, M. (2005). Locked-in syndrome. *BMJ, 330*(7488), 406–409.
19. Stead, L. G., Wijdicks, E. F., Bhagra, A., Kashyap, R., Bellolio, M. F., Nash, D. L., Enduri, S., Schears, R., & William, B. (2009). Validation of a new coma scale, the FOUR score, in the emergency department. *Neurocritical Care, 10*(1), 50–54.
20. Sternbach, G. L. (2000). The Glasgow coma scale. *Journal of Emergency Medicine, 19*(1), 67–71.
21. Stevens, R. D., Huff, J. S., Duckworth, J., Papangelou, A., Weingart, S. D., & Smith, W. S. (2012). Emergency neurological life support: intracranial hypertension and herniation. *Neurocritical Care, 17*(Suppl 1), S60–S65.
22. Stevens, R. D., Shoykhet, M., & Cadena, R. (2015). Emergency Neurological Life Support: Intracranial Hypertension and Herniation. *Neurocritical Care, 23*(Suppl 2), S76–S82.
23. Teasdale, G., & Jennett, B. (1974). Assessment of coma and impaired consciousness. A practical scale. *The Lancet, 2*(7872), 81–84.
24. Wijdicks, E. F., Bamlet, W. R., Maramattom, B. V., Manno, E. M., & McClelland, R. L. (2005). Validation of a new coma scale: The FOUR score. *Annals of Neurology, 58*(4), 585–593.
25. Wijdicks, E. F. M. (2019). C. Miller Fisher and the Comatose Patient. *Neurocritical Care, 30*(1), 1–4.
26. Young, G. B., & Wijdicks, E. F. M. (Eds.). (2008). Disorders of Consciousness. *Handbook of Clinical Neurology,* Vol 90. Elsevier.

Chapter

3

APOPTOSIS IMPLICATION IN NEURODEGENERATIVE DISORDERS

Contents

Introduction

Apoptotic cell death has been shown to occur in several human neurodegenerative disorders and animal models of human disease during the course of the illness. In addition to being a hallmark of neurodegeneration, programmed cell death of neurons, glial cells, and other nervous system components is also a common occurrence of healthy fetal and postnatal development. The studies on development and neurodegeneration in *C. elegans.* provide the most elegant illustration of this. It makes sense to assume that the capacity of the nervous system to remove cells gracefully and on purpose during development might reappear in the event of injury, neurodegenerative illness, or aberrant aging. However, it is important to consider whether the timing and quantity of cells involved in a particular mode of cell death in each model or neurodegenerative disease are sufficient to regard apoptotic cell death as a crucial component of the disease process. We will focus on Batten disease, which is the "gold standard" of neurodegenerative disorders where the gene defect directly affects apoptotic mechanisms.

Orientation and Directional Terms

Term	Definition	Illustration
Apoptosis	Apoptosis is the process of programmed cell death. It is used during early development to eliminate unwanted cells; for example, those between the fingers of a developing hand.	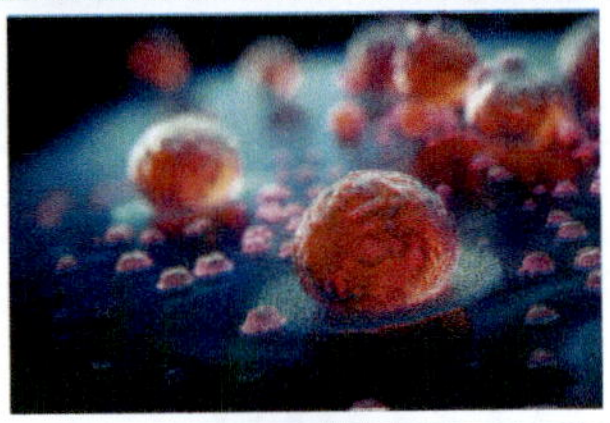
Neuraxis	The neuraxis is the long axis of the central nervous system. It refers to the direction in which the central nervous system lies.	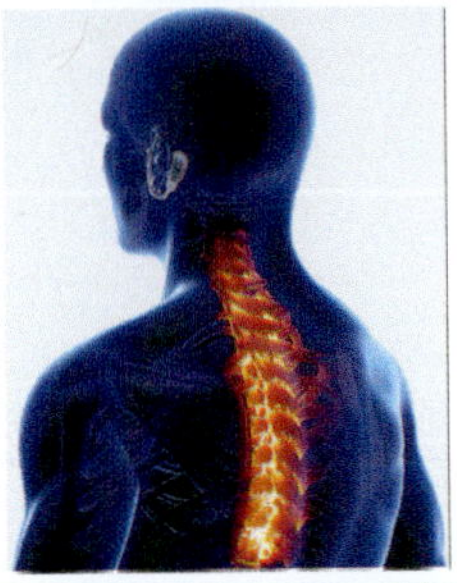
Neocortex	The neocortex comprises the largest part of the cerebral cortex and makes up approximately half the volume of the human brain.	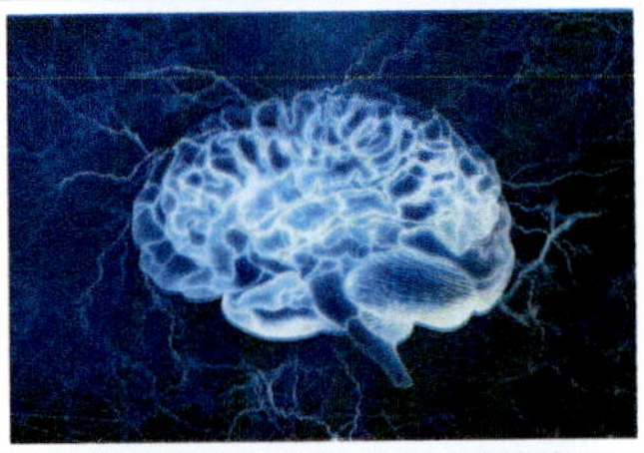
Neuronal ceroid lipofuscinoses	The neuronal ceroid lipofuscinoses (NCLs) are a group of rare and fatal diseases of the nervous system that typically begin in childhood.	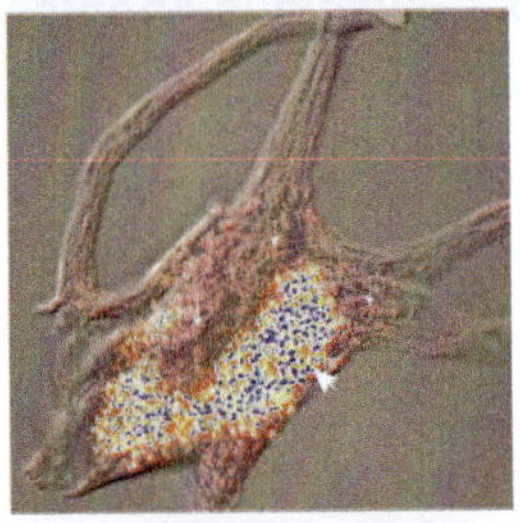
Retinitis pigmentosa	Retinitis pigmentosa is a rare, inherited degenerative eye disease that causes severe vision impairment considered legally blind.	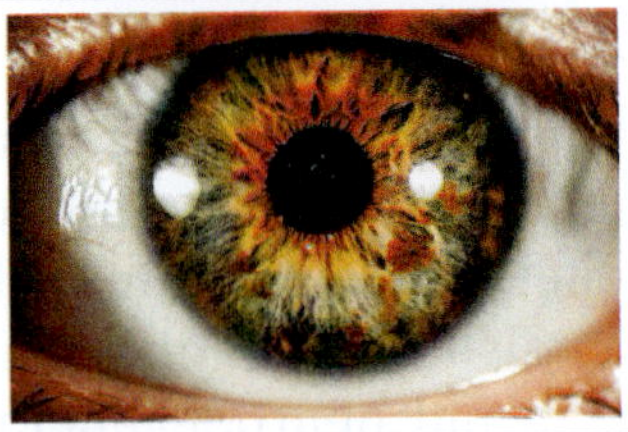

3.1. Cell Death in Normal Development and Aging

3.1.1. Spinal Cord

A great deal of research has been done on the developing spinal cord and its relationships with targets of innervation, particularly striated muscle, as well as inducing structures like the notochord. It is now evident that development involves programmed cell death, which can lead to the eventual loss of up to 50% of certain cell classes, including neurons. Throughout the later stages of spinal cord development, programmed cell death persists from the very beginning. The discovery that early spinal motoneurons' apoptotic death may be governed by intrinsic programs or local factors inside the spinal cord is intriguing. Later stages of motoneuron apoptotic death, however, may be dominated by trophic factors related to interactions and target muscle innervation. Apoptosis is therefore heterogeneous in mechanism, even within this specific region of the neuraxis and for this particular discrete group of cells. Furthermore, apoptotic cell death affects peripheral nerves, interneurons intrinsic to the spinal cord, glial cell elements in the spinal cord, and projection neurons innervating skeletal muscle and sensory neurons of the dorsal root ganglia.

3.1.2. Midbrain, Forebrain, Retina

Significant cell death is also a characteristic of neuraxis development at higher levels. This is well known for the cerebellum, whose development in rodents can be studied postnatally, and for the visual pathway, which can be studied in animals with late eye opening with ease. The occurrence of distinct periods of apoptotic activity and apoptosis in both neuronal and glial populations is an intriguing finding in these systems. These processes are probably related to the rate of neurogenesis, the formation of postmitotic neurons' neural connections, and the interactions between neurons and glia. This brief stage of apoptosis ends when these pathways and systems begin to function. Even though additional gliogenesis, myelination, and changes in axonal connectivity take place, apoptosis is evidently only a significant factor in the early stages of the nervous system's development under normal conditions.

Low background rates of apoptosis in the adult nervous system are of uncertain significance, but they should not be disregarded as important biological factors in animals with long lifespans because they occur at low steady rates over time. This might be especially true for cells that are stem cell populations that remain in the subventricular zone or that are poised midway through differentiation. Similarly, low levels of apoptotic cell death within specific neuronal subsets may eventually indicate a significant attrition. For instance, according to neuropeptide content, subclasses of GABAergic inhibitory neurons typically make up 1 to 5% of all neurons, and in most forebrain regions, these subclasses account for 20 to 30% of all neurons. These or comparable neuronal subsets may experience significant cell loss via apoptosis, which may not be readily apparent using standard histological techniques.

3.1.3. Cerebral Cortex: Example of Cortical Subplate

A temporary area in the growing cerebral cortex that integrates the cortical plate's basic level of organization is known as the cortical subplate. This region lies beneath the main cortical plate and is home to neurons that are generated early in the development of the neocortex. Subplate neurons participate in crucial cell-cell interactions with migrating neurons as well as with incoming afferent and efferent projections. They also form connections with neurons in layer I. This structure is especially noticeable in the brains of humans and primates. Its disappearance during development serves as an example of another apoptotic principle: earlier, developmentally active phylogenetic patterns of organization are removed in favor of more complex patterns. Thus, with subsequent neurogenesis, the primitive developmental pattern of cerebral cortical organization and activity is altered.

There is evidence of neuronal loss even though some of these neurons are diluted in the marked expansion of the cerebral cortical mantle. Local circuit neurons in layer I experience glial reaction to eliminate the cell and its processes, especially those in the cortical subplate. Additionally, the remodeling and loss of long axonal projections of other systems coincide with this timing. Up to 50% of the neuronal projections from the retina to the posterior visual structures in the visual system are lost. Both the transient subplate neurons and projection neurons have been significantly lost in other areas of the cerebral cortex. There is a noticeable amount of microglial activity in the deep white matter beneath the cortex at this stage of development. This brings up an additional concern regarding the occurrence of apoptosis and cell death during development: the response of the glia to the extensive cell death. An early and important interaction between immune-competent cells and dying neurons and glial cells is represented by the recruitment and activation of microglia. In certain instances, these early interactions may modify the adult nervous system's subsequent cellular and immune response to cell death.

3.1.4. Hippocampus

With its highly ordered geometry and significance for memory and cognition, the hippocampus is a crucial region to take into account when discussing apoptotic cell death. Numerous studies imply that even after development, the hippocampal tissue may be susceptible to apoptotic cell death. Specifically, several studies have shown the effects of the hypothalamic-pituitary axis and adrenal steroids on hippocampal neurons. In hippocampal granule cell neurons, the most direct model—adrenectomy with loss of corticosteroid levels—causes a substantial amount of cell death through apoptosis. Because of the way that the dentate gyrus and the granule cells that make it up are organized, the granule cell losses are likely to occur gradually and with little to no behavioral impact. The important clinical issue is that significantly low levels of apoptotic cell death could occur with gradual denervation over time.

This raises two questions:

(1) why would these neurons be particularly sensitive to systemic factors and subject to apoptotic cell death?, and

(2) would low rates of apoptotic cell death in such nervous system structures eventually serve as a priming event or portal into neurodegenerative disorders? Although this process may not be very noticeable to the patient, it still represents a significant pathological event for the disease.

3.1.5. Deafferentation

For many classes of neurons, deafferentation of adult or mature neurons can undoubtedly be a cause of apoptosis. The response of the nervous system to two common aging events—the denervation of a neuron from its target cells or tissue and the activation of immune-competent glial cells from systemic factors or acquired illness—is a significant factor in neurodegenerative illness. It is abundantly evident from the first example that many neurons rely on trophic factors from their innervated targets for both their biological program and moment-to-moment sustenance. Therefore, failing to innervate a target tissue during development is one of the factors that may result in apoptotic cell death (e.g., motoneurons' striated muscle), the inability to successfully sustain innervation once it has been attained (e.g., competition, atrophy from lack of use), harm or compromise to the integrity of that relationship (e.g., axonal damage), and/or the target's decreased ability to produce trophic factors. Depending on the connectivity, redundancy of connections, and age of the nervous system of a given class of neurons, the significance of the loss of trophic factors for adult neurons varies.

The aforementioned neuronal reliance on its connections is directly impacted by glial response and glial cell immunocompetence. For instance, at the spinal cord level, there is an instant reaction and proliferation of satellite glial cells surrounding the motoneuron cell body when an axon experiences reversible crush injury.

Positively, these activated glial cells could aid in severing the afferent connections to that particular cell and take part in the neuron's recuperation process (also known as chromatolysis or the neuron's retrograde cell reaction). However, these cells may serve as a substrate for harmful genetic factors that lead to neurodegenerative illness because they are immunocompetent. For instance, discrete injury to peripheral nerve trunks may occur before amyotrophic lateral sclerosis (ALS), also known as motor neuron disease.

ALS may "begin" at this level in the spinal cord before progressing to other levels. The general rule is that glial cells respond to any damage done to neurons or their processes both at the site of the injury and at the parent neuronal cell body. Thus, it is necessary to link the idea that glial cells are also involved in the outcome from the earliest time points of injury with the consideration of deafferentation and loss of trophic factors or their influence.

3.2. Apoptotic Cell Death in Early Onset Neurodegenerative Disorders

3.2.1. Necrosis–Apoptosis Continuum

The challenge of accurately identifying apoptosis in human tissues has cast doubt on the role of apoptotic cell death in neurodegenerative disorders. The techniques that must be used are anatomical techniques that use TUNEL (terminal deoxynucleotidyl dUTP nick end labeling) staining, morphological analysis, ultrastructural study, and biochemical techniques that identify endonucleosomal DNA cleavage and the distinctive laddering of DNA fragments. Apoptosis as a disease process in many illnesses is further complicated in the nervous system by factors such as the timing of the disease's onset, the pace of apoptosis during the disease's course, and the possibility of restriction to a single cell class in a complex tissue with multiple cell classes. Furthermore, the possible triggers (e.g., cell necrosis and apoptosis in the same tissue can be caused by ischemia, excitotoxic injury, toxic injury to mitochondria, and the ensuing process of active tissue injury. This raises the question of how to evaluate cell death across a possible continuum that stretches from necrotic, or unintentional, cell death to apoptotic, or deliberate cell death.

It is evident from experimental research that examining the function of apoptosis in a particular disease may be significantly influenced by other secondary factors. Individuals who pass away later in their illness have perimortem morbidity from dehydration and sepsis, among other illnesses. The levels of apoptosis found during postmortem examination can be influenced by the degree of hypoxia and rate of decline during the dying process, as well as the status of the hypothalamic-pituitary-adrenal axis and the effect of steroid levels. This presents a unique challenge for research involving humans, as nearly all brain samples are collected after death, often at a later stage of the neurodegenerative disease.

Determining the role of apoptotic cell death for a particular neurodegenerative disease is a real problem, since common environmental assaults on the nervous system, along with the intricate process of cell injury and glial response, can produce both apoptotic and necrotic cell death. For illnesses where a genetic defect in a gene directly related to the apoptotic cell response occurs, the strongest argument can be made (e.g., Batten disease). It should come as no surprise that a significant genetic influence on apoptosis is linked to early disease onset. Defects in genes that affect a cell's response to injury or cellular defenses like free radical-absorbing enzymes, or genes that have been demonstrated to affect apoptosis in vitro, are present in many other neurodegenerative diseases. A number of these illnesses have devastating midlife late onsets of illness. One way to look at these diseases is as secondary genetic relationships to apoptosis. Apoptosis can, however, also be caused by environmental stimuli in a host that is genetically neutral or "normal.." Two typical instances are toxic injury and ischemia. For instance, delayed neuronal death via apoptosis can be caused by carbon monoxide poisoning and most likely other mitochondrial toxins. Such environmental damage may combine with hereditary elements to cause neurodegenerative illness in later life. Thus, a secondary or environmental relationship to apoptosis can be used to characterize another category of neurodegenerative disease. Table 3.1 shows the representation of these three categories.

Table 3.1. Apoptosis and Neurodegenerative Disease

Neurodegenerative Disease	Biomarkers of Apoptosis	Neurons Affected	Clinical Features
Alzheimer's disease	Caspase-3 activation; reduced expressions of B-cell lymphoma 2 (Bcl-2); DNA fragmentation identified via terminal deoxynucleotidyl transferase dUTP nick end labeling (TUNEL) assay; BCL2 Associated X (BAX) overexpression	Loss of synapses and neurons in certain subcortical areas and cerebral cortex	Behavioral abnormalities; increased memory loss and confusion
Parkinson's disease	Activations of caspase-3, -8, and -9; decreased level of Bcl-2 expression; BAX overexpression; DNA fragmentation identified via TUNEL assay	Dopaminergic neurons of the substantia nigra pars compacta	Bradykinesia; postural instability, resting tremor; rigidity; gait impairment

Huntington's disease	Activations of caspase-3, -8, and -9; decreased level of Bcl-2 expression; BAX overexpression; DNA fragmentation identified via TUNEL assay	Affected regions include the temporal lobe, frontal lobe, and striatum (globus pallidus, putamen, and caudate nucleus); loss of medium spiny neurons	Various psychiatric disturbances; cognitive deficits; chorea
Amyotrophic lateral sclerosis	Activation of caspase-9; decreased level of Bcl-2 expression; BAX overexpression; DNA fragmentation identified via TUNEL assay	Motor neurons of the brain stem, cortex, and spinal cord	Speech problems; spasticity; muscle weakness or stiffness; muscular paralysis; muscular atrophy

Source: Dailah HG. Potential of Therapeutic Small Molecules in Apoptosis Regulation in the Treatment of Neurodegenerative Diseases: An Updated Review. *Molecules*. 2022; 27(21):7207. https://doi.org/10.3390/molecules27217207.

3.2.2. Batten Disease

Often known as neuronal ceroid lipofuscinosis, Batten disease is an eponymic term for a family of autosomal recessive or seemingly sporadic neurodegenerative disorders. The juvenile form is most commonly affected. These progressive disorders are characterized by a neuropathology that includes massive neuronal death and, in the majority of subtypes, the death of retinal photoreceptors, which leads to blindness. As a result, they signify a debilitating syndrome characterized by a decline in motor and cognitive abilities, milestone loss, visual loss, and seizures. Their descriptive name refers to inclusions that occur in the involved cells and that turn autofluorescent to represent deposits of lipofuscin. Numerous inclusions, such as granular osmiphilic deposits, curvilinear profiles, and fingerprint-like bodies, can be seen through ultrastructural analysis. The following conditions are also arranged according to the age at which they manifest: adult Kuf's disease, Batten disease, late infantile neuronal ceroid lipofuscinosis (LINCL), juvenile neuronal ceroid lipofuscinosis (JNCL), and infantile neuronal ceroid lipofuscinosis (INCL). It's interesting to note that there were no abnormalities in the gene encoding this protein to go along with the accumulation of subunit 9 of the mitochondrial ATPase synthase complex in lysosomes of the last three forms, along with a corresponding change in subunit 9 (nuclear coded) mRNA and protein expression.

Histological evidence showing that apoptotic cell death is the hallmark of cell death in Batten disease has led to recent progress in our understanding of these disorders. Furthermore, upregulation of Bcl-2 and ceramide levels has been observed in other neurochemical studies, suggesting a close connection to the control of apoptosis. The identification of the cloned and sequenced responsible gene, CLN3, on chromosome 16 has furthered the findings that associate apoptosis with juvenile NCL or Batten disease. The 438-amino acid protein product of this gene is active in a novel antiapoptotic pathway, according to recent research. The CLN3 peptide appears to mediate its antiapoptotic effect by reducing ceramide levels, as it modulates both endogenous and vincristine-stimulated levels of ceramide. The deletions linked to the human disease appear to cause a loss of function in the CLN3 gene. This program of apoptosis could also be connected to the lysosomal peptidase gene defect in LINCL, which is encoded on chromosome 11. A mutation in the chromosome 1 CLN1 gene (palmitoyl protein thioesterase) causes infantile neuronal ceroid lipofuscinosis; the connection to apoptotic mechanisms is unknown.

3.2.3. Spinal Muscular Atrophy

In spinal muscular atrophy (SMA), the prominent apoptosis of spinal motor neurons that takes place during normal development and results in the normal complement of motor neurons persists unabatedly. There are various forms of sickle cell disease (SMA). The most prevalent form is SMA I, which usually strikes young infants and results in death before the age of two. SMA II is a milder form with a slightly shorter lifespan. SMA III begins late in the first decade and has an almost normal lifespan. SMA I is caused by deletions in the chromosome 5 neuronal apoptosis inhibitor protein (NAIP) gene. There are additional copies of the NAIP gene, some of which have been truncated and may have some biological activity. The ability of lingering copies of the NAIP gene to make up for the loss of the full-length form may therefore be represented by the various forms of SMA, which vary in severity and age of onset. The similarity of the NAIP gene to a viral gene that prevents apoptosis is intriguing.

Another gene known as the survival motor neuron gene (SMN) has been linked to additional instances of spinal muscular atrophy in the same region of chromosome 5. These two genes suggest that active genetic mechanisms that are antiapoptotic are also necessary for the absence of apoptosis in the mature nervous system. The tissues that are at risk contain the necessary proteins.

3.2.4. Retinal Degeneration

Genes responsible for apoptotic cell death and photoreceptor loss in retinal degeneration have been thoroughly examined in both human and animal models of the condition. The genes in question cause the loss of photoreceptors, which leads to retinitis pigmentosa in the early to midlife stages. This condition has severe consequences, including blindness. During this process, additional pro- and antiapoptotic genes as well as related ones are activated. Defective genes that are directly involved in signal transduction include rhodopsin. It appears that the faulty proteins cause altered G-protein-related signaling, which tips the scales in favor of apoptotic cell death. This imbalance can also be impacted by environmental factors like light flux, ischemia, or retinal detachment because it involves signaling mechanisms for the physiological transduction of vision. As a result, in experimental models, changing the amount of light and wavelength that reach the retinal tissue that is at risk can start the process of apoptotic cell death.

Spinal muscular atrophy, previously discussed, is a theme that is repeated in retinal degeneration. In fact, the survival of individual cells within the mature nervous system depends on maintaining appropriate interactions with other cells and components of the intricate biological system. Therefore, the same mechanisms that result in the exit of mature components that are regrettably no longer in excess can also cause the graceful and planned death of excess cells and connections during the nervous system's development.

The apoptotic pathway may be activated as a result of aberrant G-protein system signaling and balance. Retinal degeneration is a disorder that is one step removed from spinal muscular atrophy, where mutations in antiapoptotic genes cause loss of function and directly involve the apoptotic pathway. Instead, alteration in normal signaling pathways is "interpreted" by the cell as a sign of physiological failure and triggers the genetic program for cell removal.

3.2.5. Triplet Repeat Disorders

A variety of illnesses known as triplet repeat expansion disorders cause specific subsets of nervous system cells to undergo apoptosis. These conditions include dentatorubral pallidoluysian atrophy (DRPLA), Huntington's disease, Machado-Joseph disease, and spinocerebellar ataxia type I (SCA-1). The theme that unites them is the acquisition of aberrant function via the expansion of a CAG repeat, which causes the polyglutamine hinge region of that specific protein to lengthen. This causes neurodegeneration in early to midlife in the caudate-putamen and cerebral cortex (Huntington's disease), spinocerebellar tracts (Machado-Joseph disease), cerebellum, red nucleus, and pallidoluysian nuclei (DRPLA), depending on the specific gene and its tissue and cellular distribution. The idea that abnormal gain of function is the primary mechanism shared by all of the aforementioned disorders is supported by genetic animal models and cell culture models for these diseases. Depending on the length of repeat and expression level, the involved gene product, its distribution, and the stochastic risk of an adverse protein-protein interaction may all contribute to the disease's specificity.

The capacity of the polyglutamine region to aggregate over a length of more than 35 amino acids is the mechanism of injury, which can then impact intracellular metabolism and function through aberrant protein–protein interactions. Glyceraldehyde-6-phosphate dehydrogenase (GAPDH), a crucial enzyme in glycolysis, is one enzyme that is impacted. Apoptosis is also linked to posttranslational modification of GAPDH, which is thought to affect intermediate metabolism. With disastrous consequences for the nervous system, these effects lead to an apparent stochastic increase in the likelihood that specific sets of neurons will depart through apoptotic cell death. It's interesting to note that, although this process is anatomically rather specific and is caused by apoptotic cell death, there may be difficulty in proving this at every stage of the illness. Therefore, apoptotic cell death in the caudate-putamen can be easily observed at certain early stages of the disease, while apoptotic figures become relatively rare at the very end stages (where few neurons remain).

3.3. Role of Mitochondria in Apoptosis

Apoptosis, also known as programmed cell death, is an evolutionary conserved mechanism that uses a sophisticated signaling network to eliminate cells. Cell removal is crucial for a number of processes, including development, organ homeostasis, and the removal of autoreactive lymphocytes, cancerous, damaged, or infected cells.

Generally speaking, two categories of stimuli cause apoptosis: i.e., physiological and stress-related factors. Surface receptors like TNF or CD95 are examples of physiological stimuli; UV light, radiation, bacterial and viral infections, etc., are examples of stress stimuli. While many physiological stimuli cause death through surface receptors, the exact mechanism by which stress-induced apoptosis begins is not well understood, although it appears to involve mitochondria very early in the intracellular signaling cascade.

3.3.1. Receptor-Induced Apoptosis

Apoptosis is triggered by CD95 (Figure 3.1) by the acid sphingomyelinase moving from an intracellular compartment onto the surface of the cell membrane. The small, discrete domains that make up the cell membrane are primarily made of cholesterol and sphingolipids. These tiny domains separate from the phospholipids in the cell membrane due to homo- and heterotypic interactions between sphingolipids and cholesterol, which make these domains less fluid than the other portions of the membrane.

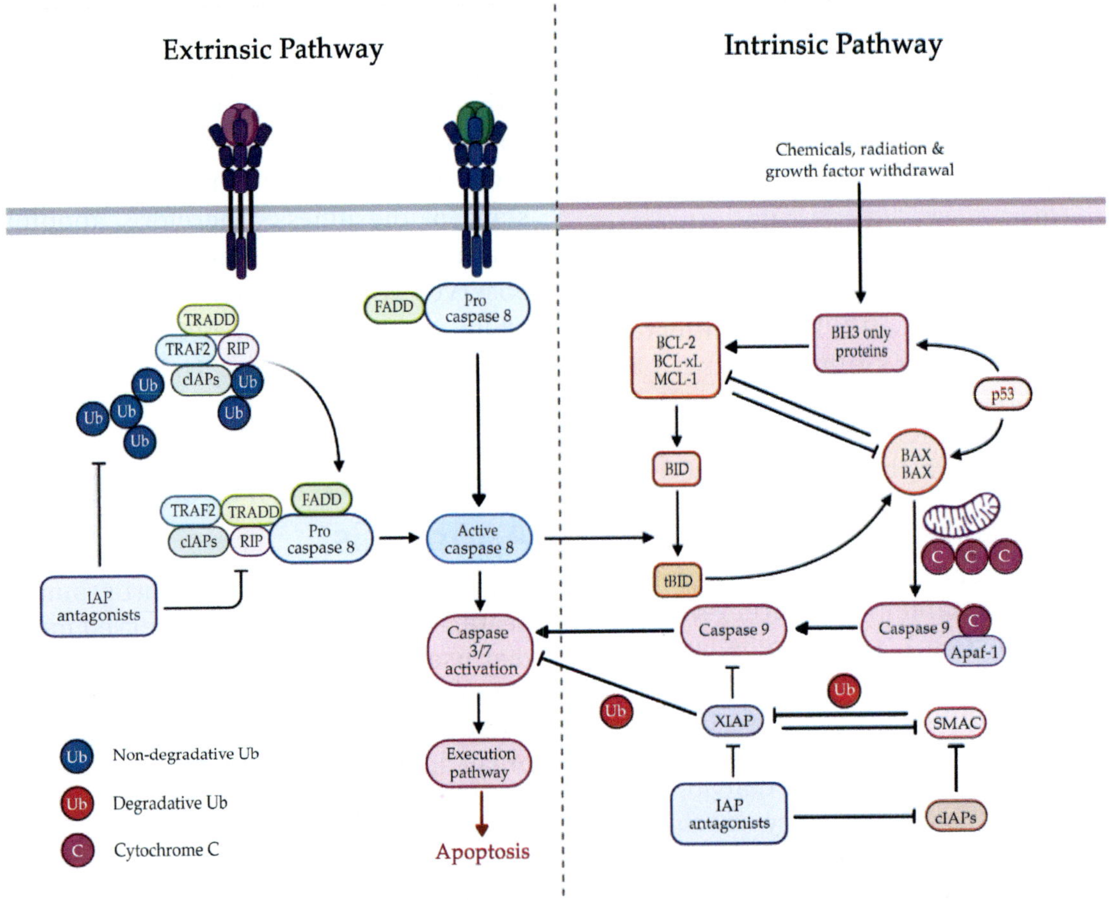

Figure 3.1. Pathways leading to apoptosis. Apoptosis initiated by receptor molecules or by intracellular or extracellular stress merges at the level of mitochondria. Key molecules integrating apoptotic stimuli to mitochondria seem to be Bcl-2-like proteins. The release of pro-apoptotic molecules from mitochondria triggers apoptosis.

Source: Singh V, Khurana A, Navik U, Allawadhi P, Bharani KK, Weiskirchen R. Apoptosis and Pharmacological Therapies for Targeting Thereof for Cancer Therapeutics. *Sci.*, 2022; 4(2):15. https://doi.org/10.3390/sci4020015.

These domains, also referred to as rafts, are changed by ceramide that is released by acid sphingomyelinase. Ceramide causes a fusion of numerous small raft domains to form a large platform that functions to cluster CD95, an event necessary for the start of particular CD95 signaling. An adapter protein called Fas-associated death domain (FADD), which binds to the protease caspase 8, is effectively recruited by clustered CD95. A family of cysteine proteases known as caspases selectively cleaves substrates after aspartate residues. They begin life as inactive pro-enzymes and undergo restricted proteolysis to transform into catalytically active proteases. Through Bcl-2-like proteins and other unidentified mechanisms, caspase 8 transmits the apoptotic signal from CD95 to mitochondria or directly to other caspases, specifically caspase 3. By cleaving numerous intracellular proteins, such as enzymes involved in genome function, regulators of cell-cycle progression, and structural proteins of the nucleus and cytoskeleton, this caspase facilitates the execution of apoptosis. These proteins cleave to produce morphological changes suggestive of apoptosis, such as e.g., fragmentation of DNA and membrane blebbing.

3.3.2. Stress-Induced Apoptosis

On the other hand, very little is understood about how stress-induced apoptosis begins (Figure 3.1). Apoptosis appears to be triggered at or right upstream of mitochondria by a variety of stressors. Furthermore, during stress-induced apoptosis, Bcl-2-like proteins appear to play a key role in the transfer of the apoptotic signal to mitochondria. Bcl-2 family proteins are characterized by their pro-apoptotic or pro-survival characteristics, respectively, and by the quantity of Bcl-2 homology domains (BH1–4). The pro-survival group consists of A1/Bfl-1, Mcl-1, Boo/Diva, Bcl-2, Bcl-xL, and Bcl-w. Certain proteins encoded by viruses, such as. g. Similar to Bcl-2, E1B19K and BHRF1 also inhibit apoptosis. Pro-apoptotic proteins include Bak, Bok, Bax, and a subset of Bcl-2-like proteins called BH3-only proteins, which only have BH3 domains, Bid, Noxa, Puma, Bim, Bmf, and Bad. It has been demonstrated that the 'multidomain' pro-apoptotic members, Bax or Bak, are essential for the induction of mitochondrial dysfunction during apoptosis, even though it is unclear how Bcl-2-like proteins cause apoptosis. The association of Bcl-2 and Bcl-xL with Bax or BH-3-only molecules, which sequesters the pro-apoptotic proteins and thereby blocks apoptosis, is one of the mechanisms that appear to regulate Bcl-2-like proteins. The regulation of Bcl-2-like proteins appears to involve similar mechanisms, as evidenced by their association with 14–3-3 proteins, their interaction with dynein, their binding of Bmf to the actin cytoskeleton, and their binding of phosphorylated Bad to lipid rafts. Furthermore, it has been demonstrated that the activity of Bcl-2-like proteins is regulated by phosphorylation/dephosphorylation events mediated by a protein kinase B/Akt (PKB/Akt) signaling pathway.

It appears that distinct apoptotic stimuli attract distinct sets of Bcl-2-like proteins. For example, TNF and CD95 cause Bid to cleave and become active. Bax undergoes a conformational shift and oligomerization caused by Active Bid, which ultimately leads to the insertion of Bax into the outer mitochondrial membrane. On the other hand, the absence of growth factors causes Bad to be dephosphorylated and undergo limited proteolysis, which triggers apoptosis. When staurosporine or etoposide induce apoptosis, Bax is cleaved at its N-terminus, producing an 18 kDa fragment that encourages cell death.

3.3.3. Activation of the Devil – Release of Pro-Apoptotic Factors from Mitochondria

Numerous signals that promote cell death gather at the mitochondria, causing a change in the permeability of the mitochondrial membrane, allowing the release of various proteins into the cytoplasm. This release is a critical event in the process of mitochondria-mediated apoptosis. This suggests that mitochondria act as gatekeepers, capturing pro-apoptotic proteins and preventing their function in the cytosol. The release of these proteins in the cytosol ultimately leads to apoptosis. The proteins released during apoptosis from mitochondria include cytochrome c, caspase 9, Smac/DIABLO, AIF, HtrA2, and endonuclease G.

A notable increase in both the outer and, to some extent, the inner mitochondrial membrane permeability is what triggers the release of these proteins. Below is a discussion of the permeability change's molecular specifics. AIF, HtrA2, and endonuclease G appear to play a specific role in apoptosis, whereas cytochrome c, caspase 9, and Smac/DIABLO appear to be involved in nearly all forms of mitochondria-induced apoptosis (Figure 3.2).

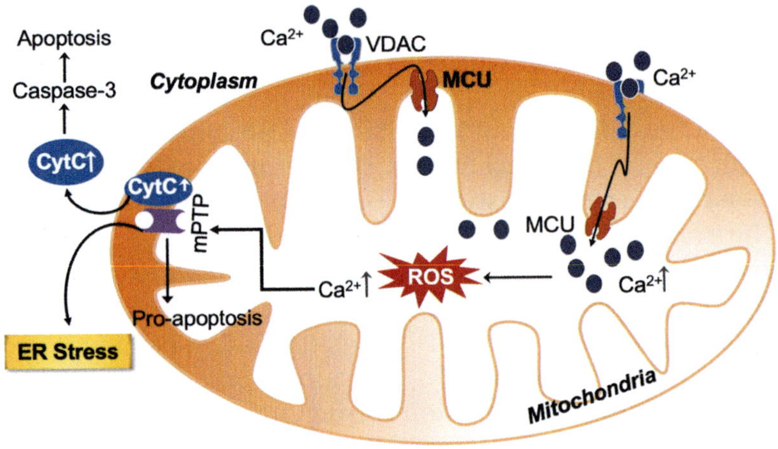

Figure 3.2. Role of mitochondria in apoptosis. Mitochondria release several pro-apoptotic factors upon induction of apoptosis. These factors are either directly triggering apoptosis by associating with cytosolic factors to form the apoptosome or they neutralize cytosolic proteins that inhibit apoptosis. Finally, some mitochondrial, pro-apoptotic proteins translocate into the nucleus to induce DNA fragmentation.

Source: Arumugam MK, Gopal T, Kalari Kandy RR, Boopathy LK, Perumal SK, Ganesan M, Rasineni K, Donohue TM Jr., Osna NA, Kharbanda KK. Mitochondrial Dysfunction-Associated Mechanisms in the Development of Chronic Liver Diseases. *Biology*. 2023; 12(10):1311. https://doi.org/10.3390/biology12101311.

3.3.3.1. Cytochrome C

The first apoptogenic intermembrane protein found to be released from mitochondria during apoptosis was cytochrome c. Xiaodong Wang and associates demonstrated using a cell-free system that cytochrome c is necessary for the proteolytic activation of procaspase-3. Furthermore, apoptosis is the outcome of cytochrome c microinjection. After being released from mitochondria, cytochrome c forms a high molecular weight caspase-activating complex known as the "apoptosome" with the help of cytosolic procaspase-9, dATP, and "apoptotis protease-activator factor 1" (Apaf-1). After the apoptosome is put together, it processes and activates procaspase-9, the initiator caspase, which then proteolytically activates procaspase-3 and procaspase-7, the executioner caspases. Then, a proteolytic cascade is started, in which procaspase-2, -6, -8, and -10 are activated by caspase-3, leading to a feedback amplification of the apoptotic signal. By producing a different proteolytic p10 caspase-9 fragment without the amino-terminal XIAP-interacting motif and avoiding caspase inhibition, caspase-3 can further enhance the proteolytic processing of caspase-9. The apoptosome's three-dimensional structure was recently discovered, and it shows a structure that resembles a wheel and has sevenfold symmetry.

The initial activation of procaspase-9 differs fundamentally from other procaspases in that it requires Apaf-1 and dATP. Apaf-1 is a cytosolic protein with three distinct regions: a nucleotide-binding domain, a C-terminal domain with multiple WD-40 repeats, and an N-terminal caspase-recruitment domain (CARD). The CARD domain of Apaf-1 functions as a docking region for procaspase-9 recruitment, but it is typically hidden until cytochrome c and dATP activate Apaf-1. Apaf-1 has a weak affinity for dATP, but when cytochrome c is bound, both molecules' affinity increases noticeably. Many different proteins contain WD-40 repeats, which are motifs for protein–protein interactions. It has been demonstrated that cytochrome c binding requires the WD-40 motif of Apaf-1. Mutational substitution analysis has indirectly demonstrated that Apaf-1 is completely encircled by cytochrome c at the time of binding. In contrast, only the lysine-rich interphase linked to heme binding is involved in the interaction of cytochrome c with its partners in the electron transfer pathway. However, the dual roles of cytochrome c in oxidative phosphorylation and apoptosome formation can be separated, as demonstrated by *Saccharomyces cerevisiae*, a yeast that lacks the ability for cytochrome c to activate Apaf-1 in a system devoid of cells.

Genetic studies in mice have confirmed the significance of cytochrome c, Apaf-1, and caspase-9 for the execution of apoptosis through the targeted disruption of the corresponding genes, resulting in the embryonic or perinatal death of the homozygous knockout-animals. These null-mice embryonic stem cells and fibroblasts exhibit abnormalities in response to a range of apoptotic stimuli, and none of the knockout cells showed procaspase-9 activation. The fact that the phenotypes of Apaf-1 and caspase-9 knockout mice are remarkably similar has proven that these proteins function in the same pathway. Midgestation is when cytochrome c deficient mice pass away in the womb. Contrary to AIF, cytochrome c is not required for cavitation, as evidenced by the ability of cytochrome c knockout embryos to develop differentiated tissues derived from the three germ layers, despite their severe phenotype and developmental delay.

3.3.3.2. Apoptosis Inducing Factor (AIF)

It was discovered that the 57 kDa flavoprotein AIF found in the mitochondria of mammals shares similarities with oxidoreductases found in plants, bacteria, and fungi. Bearing both nuclear and mitochondrial signal sequences, AIF is normally restricted to the intermembrane space of the mitochondria. However, in response to apoptogenic stimuli, it translocates to the nucleus, causing peripheral chromatin condensation and large-scale (approximately 50 kb) DNA fragmentation, but not oligonucleosomal DNA laddering. In addition to its nuclear effects, overexpression of AIF causes other features of apoptotic cell death, including the exposure of phosphatidylserine on the plasma membrane and the dissipation of the mitochondrial transmembrane potential. Since oxidoreductase activity is not necessary for its apoptogenic function and it lacks intrinsic nuclease activity, the molecular mechanism by which it carries out its cytotoxic activity is still unknown. Still, none of these AIF effects are countered by the broad-spectrum caspase inhibitor zVAD-fmk. According to recent research, heat-shock protein Hsp 70 can bind to and inhibit AIF, which helps to explain some of Hsp70's cytoprotective qualities. AIF is released along with cytochrome c and other proapoptotic mitochondrial factors, so it's unclear what role it plays in the apoptotic process, even though it appears to mediate apoptotic functions in a caspase-independent manner. Furthermore, it was demonstrated that embryonic stem cells from animals lacking in AIF were susceptible to the majority of common inducers of genuine apoptosis, including staurosporine, etoposide, and UV radiation. They do not, however, perish after growth factor deprivation. However, mice lacking AIF display a phenotype that is clearly linked to cell death, as embryoid bodies derived from AIF−/−ES cells do not form the amniotic cavity, which is typically triggered by the death of the central core of ectodermal cells. This phenomenon is thought to represent the initial wave of programmed cell death, which is necessary for healthy morphogenesis. It's unclear if the observed phenotype results from AIF's oxidoreductase function or its loss of cytotoxic property. Apaf-1−/− and caspase-9−/− ES cells demonstrated that AIF-dependent cell death could be genetically separated from Apaf-1 and caspase-9 expression, suggesting that AIF functions independently of the cytochrome c/Apaf-1/caspase-9 apoptosome. Given that plants and fungi have homologs for AIF, an ancestral route independent of caspase may be involved in AIF's function in cell death.

3.3.3.3. Smac/DIABLO

The inhibitor of apoptosis protein XIAP, which binds and sequesters activated caspase-3 generated within the apoptosome, was found to be present in the Apaf-1/cytochrome c apoptosome complex. Additionally, Alnemri and associates showed how XIAP interacts with caspase-9 within the apoptosome complex. After Procaspase-9 is first processed at Asp315, the small subunit's linker region produces an aminoterminal recognition motif that binds to the BIR3 domain of XIAP. On the other hand, processed caspase-3 interacts with XIAP's BIR2 domain. Through these interactions with caspase-9 and -3, XIAP can effectively block caspases that have been activated, thereby stopping the proteolytic cascade. The protective effect of XIAP may be overcome if the proapoptotic stimulus is strong enough or persistent enough to cause the progressive generation of activated caspases and the competition of mitochondrial proteins that block XIAP activity.

Smac/DIABLO, a 29 kDa mitochondrial protein that matures to a 23 kDa protein and translocates to the cytosol in response to an apoptotic trigger, is one of these mitochondrial XIAP antagonists. Smac/DIABLO has been demonstrated to bind additional IAP proteins, such as c-IAP1, c-IAP2, survivin, and baculoviral Op-IAP, in addition to its interaction with XIAP. Similar to caspase-9, the BIR3 domain of XIAP is bound by a recognition motif found at the amino-terminus of mature Smac/DIABLO. The BIR2-domain of XIAP and the same aminoterminal sequence of Smac/DIABLO combine to form a stable complex that permits competition with the XIAP-dependent inhibition of caspase-3 and -7. It's interesting to note that the aminoterminal residues of caspase-9 and Smac/DIABLO that interact with the BIR3 domain of XIAP have a lot in common with the cytosolic proteins Hid, Grim, and Reaper from Drosophila, which inhibit DIAP-1 and -2 and encourage apoptosis in the fly. Recently, Sickle, a different Drosophila cell death protein, was identified. It binds to IAPs via a related motif and counteracts their anti-apoptotic action. It is amazing that proteins with no additional homology, like caspase-9, Smac/DIABLO, and Omi/HtrA2 in mammals, and Sickle, Grim, Hid, and Reaper in Drosophila, share this aminoterminal IAP-binding motif. The same motif is used in entirely different protein contexts: proapoptotic mechanisms like Grim, Hid, Reaper, Sickle, Smac/DIABLO, and Omi/HtrA2 block IAPs, while caspase-9 uses it as an anti-apoptotic mechanism to recruit IAPs. This suggests a strict co-evolution of pro- and anti-apoptotic mechanisms. Smac/DIABLO has an additional mechanism for apoptosis induction that is not dependent on its IAP-binding domain. This can be seen in the proapoptotic activity of Smac β, a Smac/DIABLO splice variant that cannot bind IAPs or have a mitochondrial-targeting sequence. Moreover, overexpression of a shortened Smac/DIABLO mutant, which is devoid of the complete IAP-interacting domain, increases apoptosis to the same degree as Smac/DIABLO and Smac β, indicating that Smac/DIABLO may have a different proapoptotic mechanism that works better. This IAP-independent activity and its underlying mechanism are presently unknown. It is still unknown if Smac/DIABLO is a necessary component of the apoptotic process or merely a misdirected mitochondrial protein, however, the first theory is supported by the presence of the IAP binding motif. Mice deficient in Smac/DIABLO, however, remain fully viable and exhibit no abnormalities. Different kinds of Smac/DIABLO-deficient primary cells react appropriately to a variety of apoptotic cues. These findings point to either the existence of redundant factors—likely Omi/HtrA2—that compensate for the loss of Smac/DIABLO or the possibility that Smac/DIABLO plays no universally important role in apoptosis during development.

3.3.3.4. Omi/HtrA2

Another mitochondrial factor, the serine protease Omi, also referred to as HtrA2, is functionally similar to Smac/DIABLO. This protease is released from the mitochondrial intermembrane space upon apoptosis induction by anti-Fas, TRAIL, staurosporin, and UV radiation. It then interacts with cytosolic IAP proteins through a similar IAP binding motif as previously mentioned. It was proposed that Omi/HtrA2, a 49 kDa serine protease homologous to the bacterial DegP/HtrA protein, is involved in pathways leading to cellular stress responses. A mitochondrial localization signal was discovered using computational models, and its presence in mitochondria was verified using Omi/HtrA2 specific antibodies, despite the signal's original definition as being localized to either the nucleus or the endoplasmic reticulum. An aminoterminal presequence is broken during mitochondrial transport, allowing Omi/HtrA2 to mature into a 37 kDa protein that is released into the cytosol in response to an apoptotic trigger. It is unknown if Omi/HtrA2 is cleaved by another mitochondrial protease or if autocatalytic cleavage occurs for proper processing. The "conserved" tetrapeptide motif, which is necessary for IAP interaction, is exposed by the free amino-terminus of processed mature Omi/HtrA2. While Smac/DIABLO preferentially binds the BIR3 domain, Omi/HtrA2 interacts with both the BIR2 and BIR3 domains of XIAP, albeit with a greater affinity for the BIR2 domain. This selectivity implies that through inhibiting XIAP, Omi/HtrA2 may preferentially promote caspase-3 activation as opposed to caspase-9 activation.

While both Omi/HtrA2 and Smac/DIABLO appear to target XIAP after being released into the cytosol, their patterns of distribution diverge significantly. Using Northern blot analysis of mRNA, it was possible to determine the abundance of Smac/DIABLO in the heart, liver, kidney, and testis. No expression of Smac/DIABLO was found in the skeletal muscle, lung, thymus, or brain. On the other hand, Omi/HtrA2 mRNA is widely expressed, just like XIAP. This implies that in some cell types, Omi/HtrA2 and Smac/DIABLO may have redundant functions. In addition to its ability to interact with IAP, Omi/HtrA2's serine protease catalytic domain also functions as an inducer or accelerator of cell death. Independent of caspase activation or IAP interaction, cell death is induced by overexpressing the mature protein in the cytoplasm without its mitochondrial presequence. This cytotoxic activity requires the catalytic domain. Omi/HtrA2 possesses a carboxyterminal PDZ domain in addition to its catalytic domain and amino-terminal mitochondrial presequence. The proteins disc large tumor suppressor, postsynaptic density protein, and Zo-1 tight junction protein are the acronym for PDZ domains, which were first identified in these domains. It has been discovered that PDZ domains are involved in a range of protein–protein interactions, such as the formation of multimeric complexes that can start signal transduction at particular subcellular locations, especially at the cell surface. The MAGUK (membrane-associated guanylate kinase) protein class, which is generally linked to cell junctions or other specialized sites on the plasma membrane, is one set of proteins that is indicative of the presence of such PDZ modules.

The proteins CARD11 and CARD14, belonging to the MAGUK family, were found to interact with Bcl-10 and activate NF-κB signaling pathways. Omi/HtrA2, through its PDZ domain, binds Mxi2, a variant of p38 stress-activated kinase, although the purpose of this interaction remains unclear. The exact physiological targets of Omi/HtrA2 in cell death processes are still unidentified and require further examination. Recent findings have unveiled the trimeric structure of Omi/HtrA2, essential for its protease activity and functionality. The protein forms a pyramid-shaped structure, with IAP-binding sequences at the top and PDZ domains at the base. Mutant forms of monomeric Omi/HtrA2 are inactive, emphasizing the importance of trimerization for its function. Surprisingly, the IAP-binding motif appears to be unnecessary for its cell-killing capabilities, while the PDZ domain seems to regulate its protease activity. It is suggested that Omi/HtrA2 may interact with death receptors like TNFR and Fas in a trimeric state and contribute to apoptosis activation through its proteolytic effects in the DISC complex.

The evolutionarily conserved protease Omi/HtrA2 has a bacterial ortholog called the *E. coli* DegP/HtrA endoprotease, which is required for osmotic, thermo-, and oxidative tolerance in bacteria. Bacterial HtrA acts as a chaperone at normal temperature and as a protease at high temperature. These prokaryotic roles might imply that Omi/HtrA2 is a multipurpose protein that has cytotoxic properties when released into the cytosol and protective properties within mitochondria. Nevertheless, the exact role of Omi/HtrA2 in caspase-dependent and caspase-independent cell death is still unknown and might only be discovered through "knockin" transgenic studies employing mutant versions of HtrA2/Omi devoid of one of the functional domains.

3.3.3.5. Endonuclease G

Endonuclease G and the C homolog cps-6. elegans, which are 30 kDa proteins, have a mitochondrial localization signal that is eliminated upon importation into the intermembrane space of the mitochondria. Endonuclease G was first discovered to be a protein involved in mitochondrial DNA replication, but more recently, research has shown that it is also involved in nuclear DNA breakdown in the cell nucleus after being released from mitochondria during apoptosis induced by TNF, agonistic anti-Fas antibodies, and UV radiation. Numerous DNAses have been linked to the degradation of apoptotic DNA. The most well-studied enzyme is the caspase-activated DNAse CAD/DFF40, which together with its inhibitor and chaperone, ICAD/DFF45, forms an inactive heterodimer. ICAD is broken down by caspase-3 during apoptosis induction, releasing active CAD that can break down nuclear DNA. ICAD is not the only DNAse linked to apoptosis, though, as evidenced by the phenotypic normality of transgenic or ICAD-deficient mice that nevertheless exhibit residual DNA fragmentation. Thus, after TNF treatment or UV light induces apoptosis, it is plausible that endonuclease G is the cause of the nuclear DNA degradation seen in the embryonic fibroblasts from these mice.

During apoptosis, DNA breaks down into two main stages: first, high molecular weight fragments (around 50 kb) that match the size of chromatin loop domains are generated, and second, oligonucleosomal fragments (also known as "DNA laddering") are formed. High molecular weight DNA cleavage and early chromatin condensation can occur without CAD/DFF40, but oligonucleosomal fragmentation and final chromatin condensation require it. Although endonuclease G-dependent DNA "laddering" was demonstrated by Wang and colleagues, we were only able to witness higher-order DNA degradation in isolated nuclei. The high concentration of endonuclease G needed to cause DNA degradation in vitro in comparison to CAD/DFF40 (100 times more endonuclease G is required than CAD) raises more questions about the role of endonuclease G in apoptosis. Endonuclease G most likely needs additional nucleases or cofactors to function properly. It was demonstrated that exonucleases and DNAse I aid the capacity of endonuclease G to produce DNA cleavage products, indicating that these processes cooperate in vivo to guarantee effective DNA degradation in apoptotic cells. It was demonstrated that AIF and endonuclease G-induced DNA degradation are independent of caspase activation, in contrast to CAD/DFF40. However, endonuclease G is a self-nuclease, whereas AIF is not. It's also feasible that both proteins depend on one another for complete function rather than acting independently. When caspase activation is restricted or compromised, as may be the case during viral infection, both proteins may guarantee nuclear degradation. or they might be the cause of the DNA degradation that occurs in plants, fungi, and protozoa but is not dependent on caspase.

3.4. Apoptosis in Alzheimer's, Parkinson's, and Motor Neuron Disease

3.4.1. Modeling Chronic Neurodegenerative Diseases

Modeling the different stages of the disease is a problem in chronic neurodegenerative disease, which usually manifests in mid- to late-life and lasts for five to twenty-five years until death. The majority of data regarding AD and other related chronic neurodegenerative disorders comes from postmortem examinations conducted at the very end of the disease, when several other factors, most notably the dying process, have already taken place. As a result, a lot of data on apoptosis in AD has been acquired, primarily from the disease's endpoints. Modeling the onset of AD pathology is critical, especially the likely preclinical pathology present even at a very young age in individuals at genetic and/or environmental risk. The development of in vitro and in vivo models of AD pathology in animals or human-derived tissue, as well as the creation of genetic models of AD—especially in light of the identification of specific genes for AD—are the solutions to these issues.

3.4.2. Evidence for Apoptosis in AD

The work of Cotman and others, which showed the anatomical and biochemical characteristics of apoptotic cell death in AD brain tissue, is the source of very strong evidence for apoptotic cell death in the AD brain. This includes correlation with apoptosis-related markers like Bcl-2, Bax, c-Jun, Fos, and others, as well as the display of TUNEL-positive staining. While there has been little published ultrastructural evidence for apoptosis, there has been a fair amount of agreement among various workers.

3.4.3. Role of AD Genes: Presenilins, Amyloid Precursor Polypeptide, Apolipoprotein E

The finding that most, if not all, of the genes linked to AD affected cellular apoptosis supports the idea that AD is caused by apoptotic cell death. Not surprisingly, presenilin 1 (chromosome 12), presenilin 2 (chromosome 1), and amyloid precursor polypeptide (APP) on chromosome 21 are the three genes implicated in early onset, autosomal dominant AD. It is unclear, nevertheless, whether these gene products are directly linked to the apoptotic pathway, in contrast to the unambiguous case of Batten disease. Rather, mutations in these three AD genes modify the course of cell injury and repair in a way that triggers apoptotic pathways by affecting membrane events, free radical production, and protein trafficking.

Potentiating oxidative damage, making the cell more susceptible to trophic factor deficiency, changing rough endoplasmic reticulum protein trafficking, modifying APP metabolism, and influencing signal transduction—particularly G-protein related signal transduction—are some of the mechanisms that have been proposed to start apoptotic programs. There's a compelling argument for a shared mechanism involving G-protein signaling that causes apoptosis in AD without necessarily entailing extracellular AB deposition events. Nevertheless, there is also proof of heightened oxidative damage in AD associated with intra- and extracellular protein–protein interactions, specifically with presenilin, oxidative priming events, and APP and its fragments interacting to make the cell more susceptible to apoptosis. Therefore, there are currently many possible ways in which presenilin or APP mutations can cause apoptotic cell death. Interestingly, though, in the genetic animal models based on these mutations, there isn't much evidence to date for neuronal degeneration or even apoptotic cell death. It's crucial to remember that the majority of AD cases occur in late life and have normal presenilin and APP gene expression. More "humanization" of the rodent with human APOE, tau, and other AD-related gene products might be required.

In the most common late-onset cases of Alzheimer's Disease, the APOE gene, which is associated with increased risk, interacts with normal presenilin 1 and 2 as well as APP genes. While there is no evidence for increased cell death with the APOE allele 4, there is evidence from in vitro studies suggesting that APOE and APP interactions can lead to heightened oxidative damage.

3.4.4. Evidence for Apoptosis in Parkinson's Disease

Traditionally, Parkinson's disease (PD) has been viewed as primarily an environmental disorder with established etiologies, such as exposure to MPTP toxin, carbon monoxide, postencephalitic related exposure, manganese exposure, and other possible chemical exposures involving damage to mitochondrial complex I enzymes. However, the majority of cases are idiopathic and lack a clear etiology, though it is evident that some cases have a genetic component. An oxidative stress theory for the pathogenesis of Parkinson's disease (PD) and an emphasis on apoptosis as a potential mechanism of cell loss have resulted from the understanding that Parkinson's disease (PD) is related to progressive dopaminergic cell loss in the substantia nigra, with symptomatology typically appearing at 80 to 90% cell depletion and the evidence linking Parkinsonism to environmental exposures.

The primary cell population at risk of Parkinson's disease, the dopaminergic neurons of the substantia nigra, has been shown to undergo apoptosis in both animal models and human material. There has been "mixed" evidence supporting both classical cellular apoptosis and a possible variant of apoptotic cell death in certain experimental models of Parkinson's disease. It is important to note that dopaminergic neurons do die in the presence of some degree of cellular inflammation and microglial response in both human disease and experimental animals. This suggests that the demise of certain dopaminergic neurons could occur quite quickly and follow the path of unintentional or necrotic cell death, accompanied by inflammation. There is probably a continuum between necrotic and apoptotic cell death, and the amount of each will probably depend on when and how much of the environmental stressor or toxin occurs.

The potential involvement of exogenous L-DOPA, which is used in therapy as neurotoxins, and endogenous L-DOPA, which is produced by the remaining dopaminergic neurons, in Parkinson's disease is another concern. Several studies have shown that L-DOPA can cause cell culture to undergo apoptosis. To make up for the loss of neurons during the illness, L-DOPA synthesis and release are increased in dopaminergic neurons that have survived. This could potentially lead to secondary injury. Toxins that impact complex I in mitochondria, calcium stress, aging-related conditions, or inherited mtDNA defects have also been proposed as entry points for dopaminergic neurons to undergo apoptosis. The targets of protective therapy may be the apoptotic or mitochondrial pathways of cell damage and demise.

3.4.5. Evidence for Apoptosis in Motor Neuron Disease (ALS) and Related Disorders

Apoptotic cell death has been identified as a major pathogenetic mechanism in motor neuron disease, also known as amyotrophic lateral sclerosis, or Lou Gehrig's disease. Progressive loss of both upper and lower motor neurons causes severe disability and, in the end, death in ALS. Similar to AD and Parkinson's disease, there have been suggestions of environmental and genetic factors. Apoptotic motor neuron cell death has been linked to immunological assault and the breakdown of cellular defense mechanisms against oxidative stress.

Given that the mutation results in the conversion of an antioxidant defense enzyme into a proapoptotic gene, the identification of Cu, Zn-superoxide dismutase mutations as the causative agent for certain cases of familial ALS has provided compelling evidence for the involvement of apoptosis. Furthermore, NAIP mutations have been linked to additional uncommon cases of familial ALS. This shows that ALS may be very similar to late-onset AD and Parkinson's disease in that 25–50% of familial cases may be caused by many specific gene defects or allelic effects that have been identified. These genes probably interact with environmental factors to determine the onset and nature of illness. Many of the remaining cases might be caused by a combination of stronger and more detrimental environmental or aging-related events with multiple genetic factors. It is crucial to understand that the majority of ALS cases—95%—are sporadic, and that the genes that have been found to date only contribute to a small percentage of familial ALS cases.

Since apoptotic cell death may be the primary mechanism of motor neuron loss in other neurodegenerative diseases, understanding the pathophysiology of ALS is crucial. The potential for both necrotic and apoptotic cell death, with possibly all intermediates, depending on the timing and extent of injury, is the concern raised for excitoxic injury to the nervous system. There is strong evidence that excitotoxicity is a mode of cell injury in ALS.

Changes in the extracellular glutamate buffering during cellular responses to injury may cause damage to neurons and initiate apoptosis. Changes in glutamate transporters, for instance, may occur with aging or from prior cellular damage. Therefore, ALS and other motor neuron disorders represent an example of apoptotic cell injury that is influenced by both environmental and genetic factors.

Furthermore, it has been proposed that some of these defects result from faulty RNA splicing in cases of spinal muscular atrophy caused by mutations in the SMN gene. This gene might produce an enzyme that splices RNA. Age-related neurodegenerative diseases may share a common mechanism: abnormal RNA splicing.

3.4.6. Role of ALS Genes: Copper, Zinc Superoxide Dismutase Mutations

About 15 to 25% of cases of familial ALS are caused by a mutation in Cu, Zn-SOD that results in an enzyme that is proapoptotic but still has enzymatic activity. Aggregation, akin to triplet repeat diseases, disruption of other intracellular functions, or efficient sequestration of activity in an ineffective location are some possible mechanisms.

Another possibility is that these proteins aggregate and are lost from the intracellular copper stores, which leaves other copper proteins and cuproenzymes with insufficient copper charging.

3.4.7. Evidence for Apoptosis in Toxic Environmental Exposures

Many toxic environmental exposures that can harm the nervous system are probably the cause of apoptotic cell death. Two well-known instances are subacute carbon monoxide poisoning and organic mercury or cadmium poisoning, which happened during the Minimata disease outbreak in Japan. Both types of exposures have the potential to cause long-term and chronic damage to the nervous system, leading to delayed neuronal degeneration syndromes in both human cases and in vitro models. It is likely that many environmental exposures, especially those that are subacute and sublethal with less tissue injury and necrotic cell death, result in apoptotic cell death of photoreceptor cells since well-studied experimental models of physical, ischemic, and toxic injury to the retina result in this type of cell death. Such exposures to the environment (e.g., ischemic stroke, head trauma, low estrogen levels) are all plausible candidates for playing a role in the development of neurodegenerative diseases in people with a higher genetic risk.

3.4.8. Minocycline

A tetracycline of the second generation with exceptional neuroprotective qualities is minocycline. Minocycline was tested in experimental models of cerebral ischemia because it prevents the inducible form of nitric oxide synthetase from producing nitric oxide. Minocycline dramatically lessened the degree of tissue damage and neurologic dysfunction caused by ischemia. Minocycline inhibited ischemia-induced up-regulation of nitric oxide synthase, caspase 1, and reactive microgliosis in addition to providing neuroprotection. Additionally, in mouse models of multiple sclerosis, Parkinson's disease, brain damage, Huntington's disease, and ALS, minocycline has been shown to provide neuroprotection. Minocycline works primarily by directly inhibiting the release of cytochrome c; secondarily, it blocks subsequent cell-death-related processes, particularly the activation of caspase 3. It's unclear if minocycline directly inhibits reactive microgliosis or nitric oxide synthase synthesis, or if it does so through a secondary mechanism that comes after cytochrome c release inhibition. Minocycline is orally bioavailable, crosses the blood–brain barrier-crossing, and is safe for humans. Clinical trials involving patients with ALS and Huntington's disease are being conducted to assess it.

3.5. Contagious Apoptosis ("The Kindergarten Effect")

The dynamics of cell death in nearby cells can be influenced by the process of cell death in one cell. Neighboring cells suffer from factors produced by dying and post-dying cells. Similar triggering factors that impact a dying cell are also experienced by nearby cells. For instance, a neuron in an ischemic environment during a stroke initiates the cascade of cell death and releases interleukin-1β, TNF-α, and free radicals, all of which contribute to the cell's own demise. Neighboring neurons that have been similarly exposed to ischemia are impacted by these diffusible factors. Neurons that may not have perished from the ischemic insult alone succumb to a combination of exposure to a sublethal ischemic environment and the diffusible toxic factors produced by their dying neighbors because there is a gradient of ischemia.

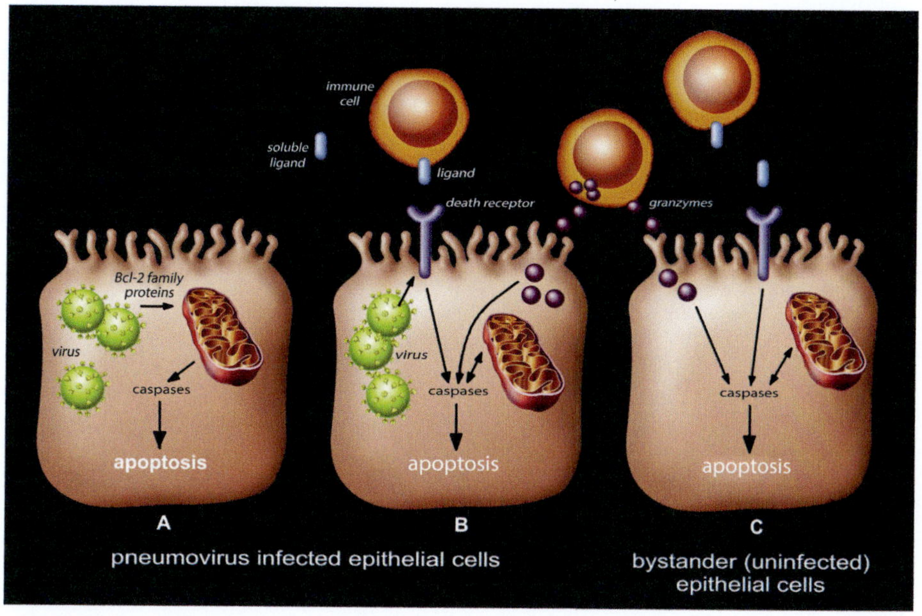

Figure 3.3. Contagious apoptosis and cell dysfunction.

Source: Van den Berg E, Van Woensel JBM, Bem RA. Apoptosis in Pneumovirus Infection. *Viruses*. 2013; 5(1):406–422. https://doi.org/10.3390/v5010406.

Neurodegenerative diseases that are chronic also exhibit this phenomenon. For instance, in ALS caused by a mutant SOD1 protein, a single motor neuron triggers the cell-death cascade. Proapoptotic factors are released by the dying neuron as it moves through the cascade and affects nearby cells. These factors may also cause the neighboring cells to initiate the cell-death cascade, as they share the same genetic predisposition (Figure 3.3). This idea is significant from a therapeutic perspective because an apoptosis inhibitor will likely prevent the production of the diffusible toxic factors that could start a cell-death cascade in a nearby cell in addition to slowing the process of cell death in that specific cell.

A Closer Look

Cerebral Cortex,

The cerebral cortex, also known as the cerebral mantle, is the outer layer of neural tissue of the cerebrum of the brain in humans and other mammals. The six-layered neocortex makes up approximately 90% of the cortex, with the allocortex making up the remainder. The cortex is separated into two cortices by the longitudinal fissure that divides the cerebrum into the left and right cerebral hemispheres. The two hemispheres are joined beneath the cortex by the corpus callosum. The cerebral cortex is the largest site of neural integration in the central nervous system. It plays a key role in attention, perception, awareness, thought, memory, language, and consciousness. The cerebral cortex is part of the brain responsible for cognition.

In most mammals, apart from small mammals that have small brains, the cerebral cortex is folded, providing a greater surface area in the confined volume of the cranium. Apart from minimizing the brain and cranial volume, cortical folding is crucial for the brain circuitry and its functional organization. In mammals with small brains, there is no folding and the cortex is smooth.

A fold or ridge in the cortex is termed a gyrus (plural gyri) and a groove is termed a sulcus (plural sulci). These surface convolutions appear during fetal development and continue to mature after birth through the process of gyrification. In the human brain the majority of the cerebral cortex is not visible from the outside but buried in the sulci. The major sulci and gyri mark the divisions of the cerebrum into the lobes of the brain. The four major lobes are the frontal, parietal, occipital and temporal lobes. Other lobes are the limbic lobe, and the insular cortex often referred to as the *insular lobe*.

There are between 14 and 16 billion neurons in the human cerebral cortex. These are organized into horizontal cortical layers, and radially into cortical columns and minicolumns. Cortical areas have specific functions such as movement in the motor cortex, and sight in the visual cortex. The motor cortex is primarily located in the precentral gyrus, and the visual cortex is located in the occipital lobe.

Summary

- Apoptotic cell death has been shown to occur in several human neurodegenerative disorders and animal models of human disease during the course of the illness.
- A temporary area in the growing cerebral cortex that integrates the cortical plate's basic level of organization is known as the cortical subplate.
- The aforementioned neuronal reliance on its connections is directly impacted by glial response and glial cell immunocompetence.
- Batten disease is an eponymic term for a family of autosomal recessive or seemingly sporadic neurodegenerative disorders.
- In spinal muscular atrophy (SMA), the prominent apoptosis of spinal motor neurons that takes place during normal development and results in the normal complement of motor neurons persists unabatedly.
- Apoptosis, also known as programmed cell death, is an evolutionary conserved mechanism that uses a sophisticated signaling network to eliminate cells.
- Modeling the different stages of the disease is a problem in chronic neurodegenerative disease, which usually manifests in mid- to late-life and lasts for five to twenty-five years until death.
- Traditionally, Parkinson's disease (PD) has been viewed as primarily an environmental disorder with established etiologies, such as exposure to MPTP toxin, carbon monoxide, postencephalitic related exposure, manganese exposure, and other possible chemical exposures involving damage to mitochondrial complex I enzymes.

References

1. Bender, A., Krishnan, K. J., Morris, C. M., Taylor, G. A., Reeve, A. K., Perry, R. H., et al. (2006). High levels of mitochondrial DNA deletions in substantia nigra neurons in aging and Parkinson's disease. *Nature Genetics, 38*, 515.
2. Bratton, S. B., Walker, G., Srinivasula, S. M., Sun, X. M., Butterworth, M., Alnemri, E. S., & Cohen, G. M. (2001). Recruitment, activation and retention of caspases-9 and -3 by Apaf-1 apoptosome and associated XIAP complexes. *The EMBO Journal, 20*, 998–1009.
3. Dolle, C., Flones, I., Nido, G. S., Miletic, H., Osuagwu, N., Kristoffersen, S., et al. (2016). Defective mitochondrial DNA homeostasis in the substantia nigra in Parkinson's disease. *Nature Communications, 7*, 13548.
4. Du, C., Fang, M., Li, Y., Li, L., & Wang, X. (2000). Smac, a mitochondrial protein that promotes cytochrome c-dependent caspase activation by eliminating IAP inhibition. *Cell, 102*, 33–42.
5. Gao, G., & Dou, Q. P. (2000). N-terminal cleavage of Bax by calpain generates a potent proapoptotic 18-kDa fragment that promotes Bcl-2-independent cytochrome C release and apoptotic cell death. *Journal of Cellular Biochemistry, 80*, 53–72.
6. Grassmé, H., Jekle, A., Riehle, A., Schwarz, H., Berger, J., Sandhoff, K., Kolesnick, R., & Gulbins, E. (2001). CD95 signaling via ceramide rich membrane rafts. *Journal of Biological Chemistry, 276*, 20589–20596.

7. Kanduc, D., Mittelman, A., Serpico, R., et al. (2002). Cell death: apoptosis versus necrosis. *International Journal of Oncology, 21*, 165–170.

8. Kim, B. C., Mamura, M., Choi, K. S., Calabretta, B., & Kim, S. J. (2002). Transforming growth factor beta 1 induces apoptosis through cleavage of BAD in a Smad3-dependent mechanism in FaO hepatoma cells. *Molecular and Cellular Biology, 22*, 1369–1378.

9. Kuhn, H. G., Palmer, T. D., & Fuchs, E. (2001). Adult neurogenesis: a compensatory mechanism for neuronal damage. *European Archives of Psychiatry and Clinical Neuroscience*, 251, 152–158.

10. Lassus, P., Opitz-Araya, X., & Lazebnik, Y. (2002). Requirement for caspase-2 in stress-induced apoptosis before mitochondrial permeabilization. *Science, 297*, 1352–1354.

11. Murphy, K. M., Streips, U. N., & Lock, R. B. (2000). Bcl-2 inhibits a Fas-induced conformational change in the Bax N-terminus and Bax mitochondrial translocation. *Journal of Biological Chemistry, 275*, 17225–17228.

12. Rossi, F., & Cattaneo, E. (2002). Neural stem cell therapy for neurological diseases: dreams and reality. *Nature Reviews Neuroscience, 3*, 401–409.

13. Widlak, P., Li, L. Y., Wang, X., & Garrard, W. T. (2001). Action of recombinant human apoptotic endonuclease G on naked DNA and chromatin substrates. Cooperation with exonuclease and DNase I. *Journal of Biological Chemistry, 276*, 48404–48409.

Chapter

DISORDERS OF EQUILIBRIUM

4

Contents

Introduction

Balance disorders, commonly referred to as disorders of equilibrium, are a broad category of conditions that impair the body's capacity to sustain stability and orientation in space. To coordinate movements and maintain balance, the equilibrium system depends on sensory data from the vestibular system, proprioception, and visual input. Numerous equilibrium disorders can result from compromised or improperly processed sensory inputs. Vertigo, a common disorder marked by a spinning or dizzy feeling, is one example. Meniere's disease and benign paroxysmal positional vertigo (BPPV), among other inner ear disorders, as well as vestibular neuritis or migraines, can also be the cause of this.

Other disorders of equilibrium include oscillopsia, in which objects seem to bounce or oscillate, and disequilibrium, which results in a feeling of unsteadiness or imbalance. These disorders may be caused by problems with the central nervous system, anomalies in the inner ear, adverse drug reactions, or neurological disorders such as Parkinson's disease.

A disturbance of equilibrium can have a major influence on day-to-day functioning; it can cause falls, make it difficult to walk, and lower quality of life. Finding the diagnosis usually entails a thorough assessment of the patient's symptoms, medical history, and results from specialized tests like vestibular function testing. Depending on the underlying cause of the condition, treatment options may involve medications, lifestyle changes, vestibular rehabilitation exercises, or surgical interventions.

Orientation and Directional Terms

Term	Definition	Illustration
Nonvertiginous dizziness	Non-vertiginous dizziness is a term that describes a range of sensations that are different from vertigo, which is the feeling of spinning or rotation while still.	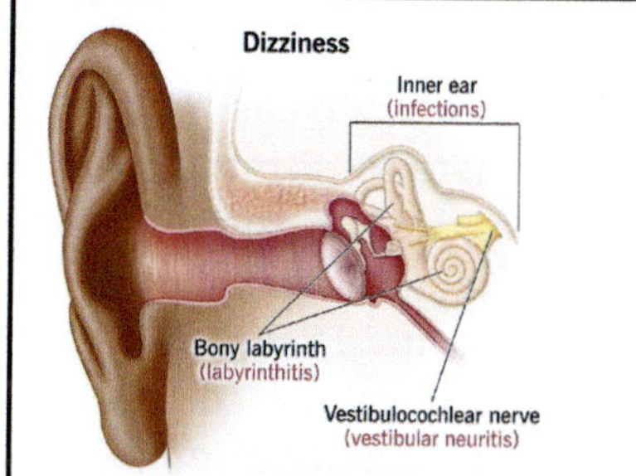
Nystagmus	Nystagmus is a vision condition in which the eyes make repetitive, uncontrolled movements.	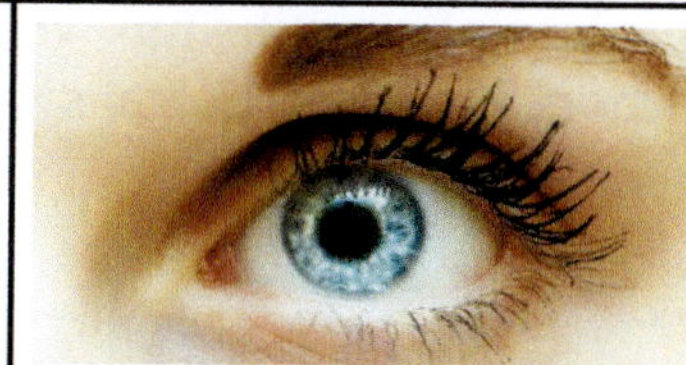
Antagonist muscle	An agonist muscle is a muscle that contracts to provide the main force to move or rotate a bone through its joint. An antagonist muscle is a muscle that produces the opposite action of an agonist.	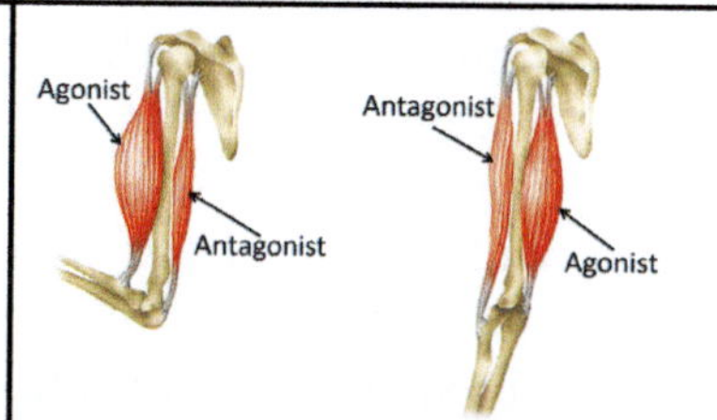
Hemiataxia	Hemiataxia is a type of ataxia that affects only one side of the body. Ataxia is caused by damage to the cerebellum, the part of the brain that controls voluntary movement.	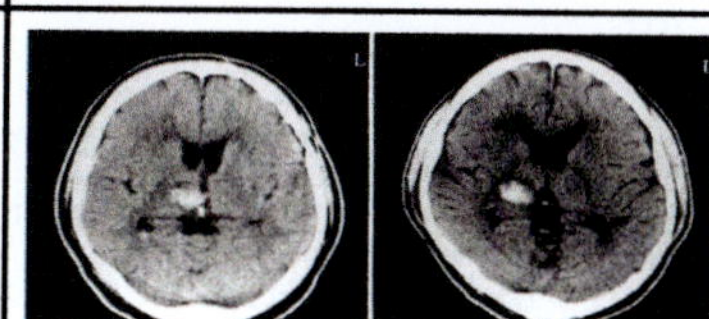
Medial lemnisci	The medial lemniscus, also known as Reil's band or Reil's ribbon, is a bundle of myelinated axons in the brainstem that carries sensory information from the medulla oblongata to the thalamus.	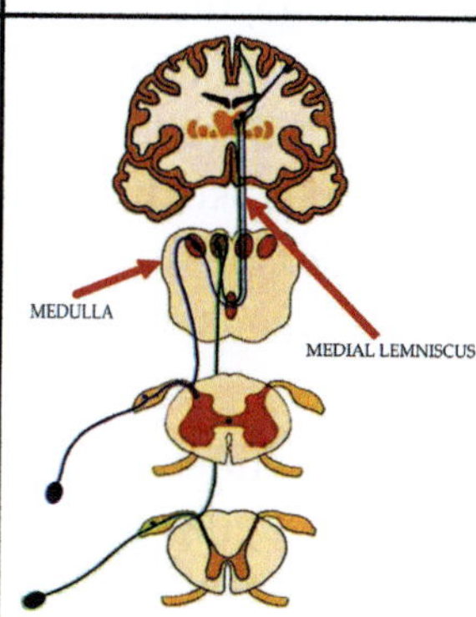

4.1. Equilibrium Approach to Diagnosis

The capacity to keep the body and its components oriented in respect to the surrounding environment is known as equilibrium. It depends on constant somatosensory input that is integrated into the brainstem and cerebellum, including visual, labyrinthine, and proprioceptive input. Diseases affecting the cerebellum, peripheral or central vestibular pathways, or proprioceptive sensory pathways can cause disorders of equilibrium. Vertigo or ataxia are the most common clinical symptoms of these disorders.

4.1.1. Vertigo

The illusion of movement in the body or surroundings is known as vertigo. Other symptoms like nausea, vomiting, oscillopsia (a visual illusion of moving back and forth), impulsion (a feeling that the body is being thrown or pulled in space), or gait ataxia may also be present.

It's important to differentiate between vertigo and nonvertiginous dizziness, which comprises feelings of lightheadedness, faintness, or giddiness that aren't connected to an illusion of movement. Unlike vertigo, these symptoms—which can result in loss of consciousness—are caused by situations that deprive the brain of blood, oxygen, or glucose (such as excessive vagal stimulation, orthostatic hypotension, cardiac arrhythmia, myocardial ischemia, hypoxia, or hypoglycemia).

The initial stage of the differential diagnosis for vertigo involves identifying the pathologic process and localizing it to either the central or peripheral vestibular pathways (Figure 4.1). Peripheral and central causes of vertigo can be distinguished from one another using specific features of the condition, such as the existence of any related abnormalities (Table 4.1).

- **Peripheral Vertigo:** The vestibular division of the vestibulocochlear (VIII) nerve or the inner ear labyrinth are both impacted by peripheral vestibular lesions. Compared to vertigo of central origin, vertigo originating from peripheral lesions is typically more sporadic, lasts shorter periods of time, and causes greater distress (see the following section). Peripheral vertigo is always accompanied by nystagmus, a rhythmic oscillation of the eyes that is typically unidirectional rather than vertical. Additional symptoms of the inner ear or vestibulocochlear (VIII) nerve dysfunction, such as hearing loss and tinnitus (the delusional perception of sound, such as ringing in the ears), are frequently caused by peripheral lesions.
- **Central Vertigo:** Rarely, a cerebral cortical lesion can cause vertigo, such as when it manifests as a symptom of complex partial seizures. Instead, lesions affecting the brainstem vestibular nuclei or their connections are typically the cause of vertigo of central nervous system origin.

Nystagmus can be present in conjunction with or separate from central vertigo; if it is, it can be vertical, unidirectional, or multidirectional, and it can have different characteristics in each eye. Nystagmus caused by upgaze or downgaze is not always in the vertical plane; vertical nystagmus is the oscillation in a vertical plane. Intrinsic brainstem or cerebellar signs, such as motor or sensory deficits, hyperreflexia, extensor plantar responses, dysarthria, or limb ataxia, may coexist with vertigo resulting from central lesions.

4.1.2. Ataxia

Incoordination or clumsiness in movement that is not caused by weak muscles is known as ataxia. Vestibular, cerebellar, or sensory (proprioceptive) disorders may be the cause. Ataxia can impact the trunk, stance, gait, individual limbs, speech (causing dysarthria), eyes, and other body parts (Table 4.2).

4.1.2.1. Vestibular Ataxia

Vestibular ataxia can be caused by the same central and peripheral lesions that result in central or peripheral vertigo (refer to the section above). Nystagmus is a common occurrence, usually affecting one eye, and is most noticeable when looking away from the side of vestibular involvement. Vestibular ataxia does not include dysarthria. Vestibular ataxia is a gravity-dependent condition in which the patient's limb coordination is not evident until they try to stand or walk.

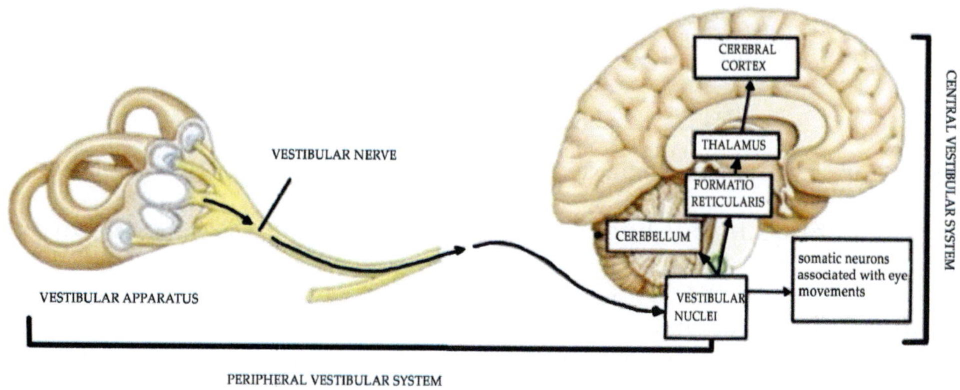

Figure 4.1. Peripheral and central vestibular pathways. The vestibular nerve terminates in the vestibular nucleus in the brainstem and midline cerebellar structures that project to the vestibular nucleus. From here, bilateral pathways in the medial longitudinal fasciculus ascend to the abducens (VI) and oculomotor (III) nuclei and descend to the spinal cord (vestibulospinal tracts).

Source: Balkan, E. (2023). Initial approach to patients with balance disorders. IntechOpen. doi: 10.5772/intechopen.111837.

4.1.2.2. Cerebellar Ataxia

Lesions affecting the cerebellum or its afferent or efferent connections in the pons, spinal cord, red nucleus, or cerebellar peduncles can result in cerebellar ataxia (Figure 4.2).

Unilateral frontal disease can sometimes mimic a disorder of the contralateral cerebellar hemisphere due to the crossed connection between the frontal cerebral cortex and the cerebellum. The rate, rhythm, amplitude, and force of voluntary movements can all be abnormal in cerebellar ataxia patients.

- **Hypotonia:** Hypotonia, or low muscle tone, is frequently linked to cerebellar ataxia and causes poor posture maintenance. The examiner can easily move the limbs with a small amount of force, and they show greater range of excursion when shaken. There may be a comparable increase in the range of arm swing when walking. Tendon reflexes have a pendular quality, which means that after the reflex is elicited, the limb may oscillate multiple times. The antagonist muscle does not check the movement when muscles are contracted against resistance that is later removed, and compensatory muscular relaxation does not happen quickly. The limb moves backward as a result of this.

Table 4.1. Characteristics of Peripheral and Central Vertigo

	Peripheral	Central
Vertigo	Often intermittent; severe	Often constant; usually less severe
Nystagmus	Always present; unidirectional, never vertical	May be absent; uni- or bidirectional, may be vertical
Hearing loss or tinnitus	Often present	Rarely present
Intrinsic brainstem or cerebellar signs[1]	Absent	Typically present

[1]Motor or sensory deficits, hyperreflexia, extensor plantar responses, dysarthria, or limb ataxia.

Source: https://dl.mehrsys.ir/pdf-books/Clinical%20Neurology%209%20Edition%20(www.myuptodate.com).pdf.

- **Incoordination:** Cerebellar ataxia is linked to voluntary movement incoordination in addition to hypotonia. Simple movements have slower rates of acceleration and deceleration and have a delayed onset. There is a jerky appearance due to variations in the force, amplitude, rhythm, and rate of movement. Clinical signs include terminal intention tremor as the limb approaches the target and terminal dysmetria, or "overshoot" when the limb is pointed at a target. Rather than being one fluid motor act, more complicated movements can be broken down into a series of smaller movements (asynergia). The most severely affected movements are those that involve quick direction changes or higher levels of physiological complexity, like walking.
- **Eye Movement Abnormalities:** Ocular abnormalities are a common result of cerebellar disease due to the cerebellum's prominent role in controlling eye movements. These include gaze paresis, abnormal saccadic and pursuit movements, and nystagmus and associated ocular oscillations.
- **Anatomic Basis of Clinical Signs:** The somatotopic organization of the motor, sensory, visual, and auditory connections in different anatomic regions of the cerebellum (Figure 4.3) corresponds to their functional differences (Figure 4.4).
  - **Midline Lesions:** The middle zone of the cerebellum— the vermis and flocculonodular lobe and their associated subcortical (fastigial) nuclei—is involved in the control of axial functions, including eye movements, head and trunk posture, stance, and gait. Midline cerebellar disease results in a clinical syndrome characterized by nystagmus and other disorders of ocular motility, dysarthria, oscillation of the head and trunk (titubation), instability of stance, and gait ataxia (Table 4.3). Selective involvement of the superior cerebellar vermis, as in alcoholic cerebellar degeneration, produces exclusively or primarily gait ataxia, as predicted by the somatotopic map of the cerebellum (Figure 4.4).

- **Hemispheric Lesions**: The lateral cerebellum (cerebellar hemispheres) helps coordinate movements and maintain tone in the ipsilateral limbs. The hemispheres also regulate ipsilateral gaze. Disorders affecting one cerebellar hemisphere cause ipsilateral hemiataxia and limb hypotonia as well as nystagmus and transient ipsilateral gaze paresis (inability to look voluntarily toward the affected side). Involvement of the medial (paravermian) portion of either cerebellar hemisphere can also produce dysarthria.

Table 4.2. Characteristics of Vestibular, Cerebellar, and Sensory Ataxia

	Vestibular	Cerebellar	Sensory
Vertigo	Present	May be present	Absent
Nystagmus	Present	Often present	Absent
Dysarthria	Absent	May be present	Absent
Limb ataxia	Absent	Usually present (one limb, unilateral, legs only, or all limbs)	Present (typically legs)
Stance	May be able to stand with feet together; typically worse with eyes closed	Unable to stand with feet together and eyes either open or closed	Often able to stand with feet together and eyes open but not with eyes closed (Romberg sign)
Vibration and position sense	Normal	Normal	Impaired
Ankle reflexes	Normal	Normal	Depressed or absent

Source: https://dl.mehrsys.ir/pdf-books/Clinical%20Neurology%209%20Edition%20(www.myuptodate.com).pdf.

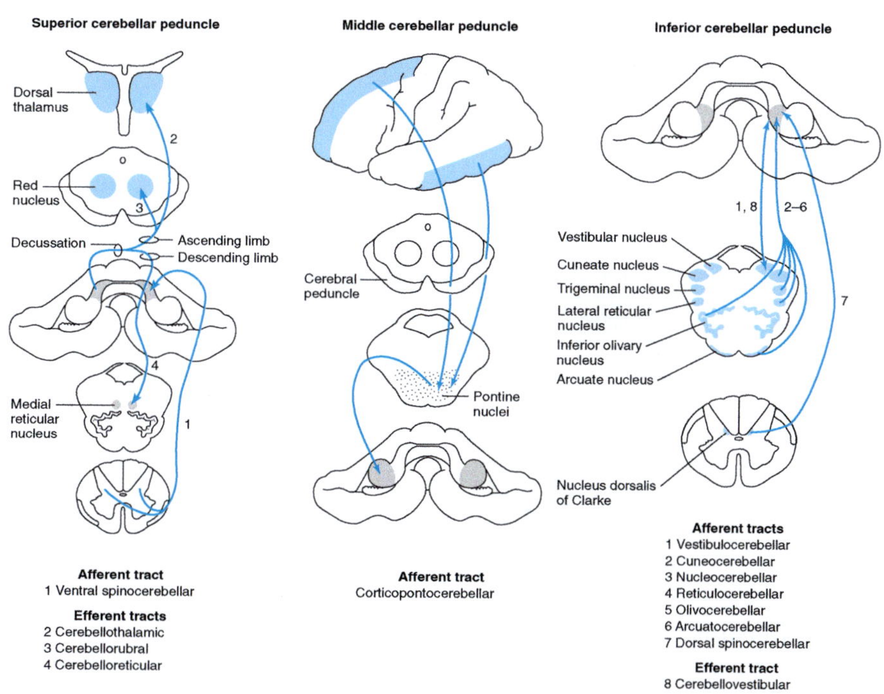

Figure 4.2. Cerebellar connections in the superior, middle, and inferior cerebellar peduncles.

Source: https://neupsykey.com/wp-content/uploads/2017/01/f0190-01.jpg.

3. **Diffuse Disease:** Many cerebellar disorders—typically toxic, metabolic, and degenerative conditions—affect the cerebellum diffusely. The clinical picture in such states combines the features of midline and bilateral hemisphere disease.

4.1.2.3. Sensory Ataxia

Disorders affecting the proprioceptive pathways in the medial lemnisci, posterior columns of the spinal cord, sensory roots, or peripheral sensory nerves can cause sensory ataxia. Seldom do parietal lobe and thalamic lesions cause contralateral sensory hemiataxia.

Kinesthesis, or the sensation of joint position and movement, is a result of unencapsulated nerve endings in joint capsules, ligaments, muscles, and the periosteum as well as pacinian corpuscles. Primary afferent neurons with heavily myelinated A fibers enter the spinal cord's dorsal horn and ascend in the posterior columns uncrossed to transmit these sensations (Figure 4.5). The fasciculus gracilis, which is situated medially, transmits proprioceptive information from the legs, while the fasciculus cuneatus, which is situated more laterally, transmits information from the arms. These tracts form synapses with second-order sensory neurons in the nucleus cuneatus and nucleus gracilis of the lower medulla. In the contralateral medial lemniscus, the second-order neurons ascend after decussating as internal arcuate fibers. Third-order sensory neurons in the ventral posterior nucleus of the thalamus, where they end, project to the parietal cortex.

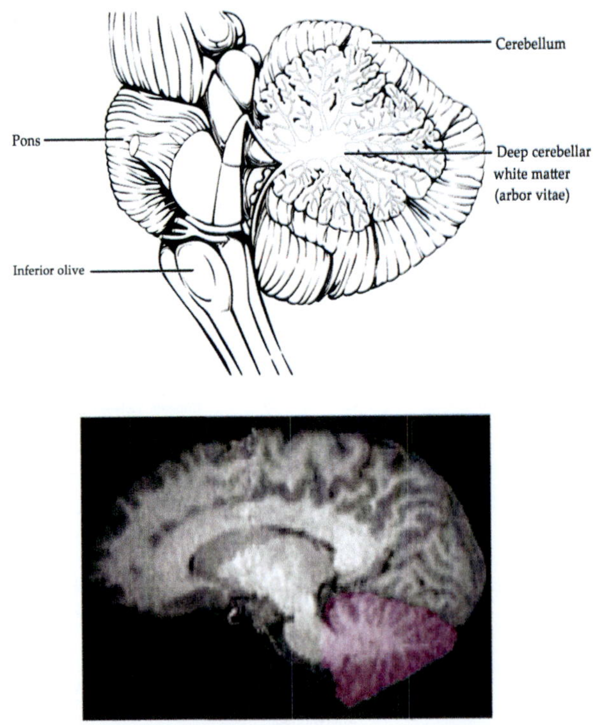

Figure 4.3. Anatomic divisions of the cerebellum in midsagittal view.

Source: https://courses.lumenlearning.com/atd-herkimer-biologyofaging/chapter/the-central-nervous-system/.

Sensory ataxia resulting from polyneuropathy or lesions in the posterior column usually affects the gait and legs symmetrically, with the arms either not affected at all or only slightly affected. Upon examination, it is found that the affected limbs have poor joint position feeling, and vibration sense is frequently compromised. The absence of vertigo, nystagmus, and dysarthria is typical.

4.1.3. History

4.1.3.1. Symptoms and Signs

- **Vertigo:** It's important to distinguish between presyncopal or dizziness and true vertigo. Most people who experience vertigo describe it as spinning, rotating, or moving; however, if the patient gives a vague description, it is important to specifically ask them if they feel as though they are moving.

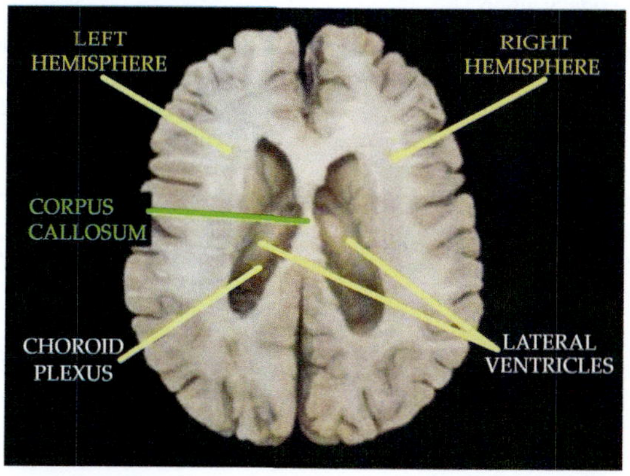

Figure 4.4. Functional organization of the cerebellum. The view is similar to that in Figure 4.3B but is of a monkey rather than a human cerebellum. The three cerebellar homunculi represent areas to which proprioceptive and tactile stimuli project, and the stripes represent areas to which auditory and visual stimuli project.

Source: https://courses.lumenlearning.com/child/chapter/brain-development-2/.

The conditions that give rise to symptoms could also be useful in the diagnostic process. Head position changes are a common cause of vertigo. On the other hand, symptoms that arise from extended recumbency and can be promptly alleviated by sitting or lying down are indicative of orthostatic hypotension. Though it is rarely connected to actual vertigo, orthostatic hypotension and other cerebral hypoperfusion states can also cause loss of consciousness.

Vertigo symptoms could be useful in locating the location of the causing lesion. A problem with the peripheral vestibular apparatus (labyrinth or vestibulocochlear [VIII] nerve) is strongly suggested by hearing loss or tinnitus. A central (brainstem) lesion is likely indicated by dysarthria, dysphagia, diplopia, focal weakness, or sensory loss affecting the face or limbs.

- **Ataxia:** While ataxia accompanied by tingling or numbness in the legs is typical in patients with sensory ataxia, ataxia accompanied by vertigo may indicate a vestibular disorder. Patients with sensory ataxia may report that by watching their feet when they walk, using a cane or a companion's arm for support, their balance is improved. This is because proprioceptive deficits may be partially compensated for by other sensory cues. Because of this, they might be less stable in the dark and find it harder to go down stairs than to climb them.

Table 4.3. Clinical Patterns of Cerebellar Ataxia

Pattern of Involvement	Signs	Causes
Midline	Nystagmus, dysarthria, head and trunk titubation, gait ataxia	Tumor, multiple sclerosis
Superior vermis	Gait ataxia	Wernicke encephalopathy, alcoholic cerebellar degeneration, tumor, multiple sclerosis
Cerebellar hemisphere	Nystagmus, ipsilateral gaze paresis, dysarthria, ipsilateral hypotonia, ipsilateral limb ataxia, gait ataxia, falling to side of lesion	Infarction, hemorrhage, tumor, multiple sclerosis
Pancerebellar	Nystagmus, bilateral gaze paresis, dysarthria, bilateral hypotonia, bilateral limb ataxia, gait ataxia	Sedative drug intoxication, hypothyroidism, autosomal dominant spinocerebellar ataxias, paraneoplastic cerebellar degeneration, Wilson disease, infectious and parainfectious encephalomyelitis, Creutzfeldt-Jakob disease, multiple sclerosis

Source: https://dl.mehrsys.ir/pdf-books/Clinical%20Neurology%209%20Edition%20(www.myuptodate.com).pdf.

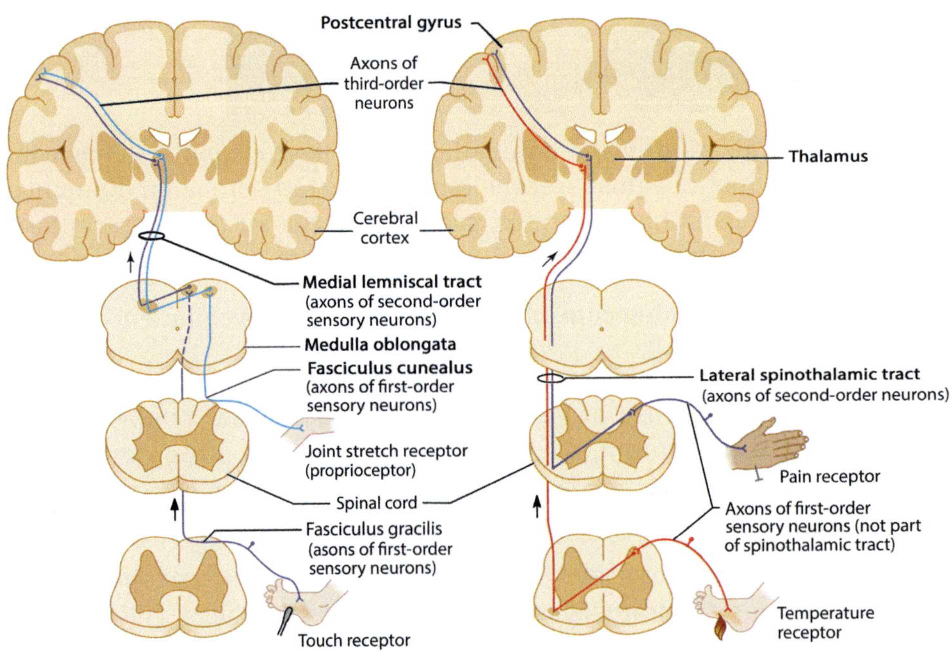

Figure 4.5. Pathways mediating proprioception (left, light blue) and other somatic sensory modalities (left and right).

Source: Used with permission from Fox SI. Human Physiology. 10th ed. Boston, MA: McGraw-Hill; 2008.

4.1.3.2. Onset and Time Course

The cause of an equilibrium disturbance may be ascertained with the aid of the mode of onset and time course.

- **Sudden:** Infarcts and hemorrhages in the brainstem or cerebellum (e.g., lateral medullary syndrome, cerebellar hemorrhage or infarction) cause sudden onset of disequilibrium.
- **Episodic:** Acute episodic disequilibrium may indicate benign positional vertigo, vestibular migraine, Ménière disease, or transient ischemic attacks in the basilar artery distribution. Transient ischemic attack-induced disorientation is typically accompanied by deficits in the cerebral nerves, neurologic symptoms in the limbs, or both. Vertigo, tinnitus, and progressive hearing loss are frequently linked to Ménière disease.
- **Chronic and Progressive:** The most likely cause of a chronic, progressive disequilibrium that develops over weeks to months is a toxic or nutritional disorder (nitrous oxide exposure, vitamin B12 or vitamin E deficiency, etc. An inherited spinocerebellar degeneration exhibits a characteristic of evolution over months to years.

4.1.3.3. Medical History

Examining the medical history closely is necessary to look for conditions that affect the cerebellum (hypothyroidism, paraneoplastic syndromes, tumors) or sensory pathways (syphilis, vitamin B12 deficiency), as well as medications that affect these areas (ethanol, sedatives, phenytoin, aminoglycoside antibiotics, quinine, salicylates).

4.1.3.4. Family History

Cerebellar ataxia that is progressive and chronic may be caused by a hereditary degenerative disease. These conditions include Wilson disease, Friedreich ataxia, ataxia-telangiectasia, and spinocerebellar degenerations.

4.1.4. General Physical Examination

Several features of the general physical examination may provide clues to the underlying disorder.

1. Orthostatic hypotension is associated with tabes dorsalis, polyneuropathies, and spinocerebellar degenerations.
2. The skin may show oculocutaneous telangiectasia (ataxia-telangiectasia), or it may be dry, with brittle hair (hypothyroidism) or have a lemon-yellow coloration (vitamin B12 deficiency).
3. Pigmented corneal (Kayser-Fleischer) rings are seen in Wilson disease.
4. Skeletal abnormalities include kyphoscoliosis in Friedreich ataxia, hypertrophic or hyperextensible joints in tabes dorsalis, and pes cavus in certain hereditary neuropathies. Abnormalities at the craniocervical junction may be associated with Arnold-Chiari malformation or other congenital anomalies involving the posterior fossa.

4.1.5. Neurologic Examination

1. **Mental Status Examination:** An acute confusional state accompanied by ataxia may indicate Wernicke encephalopathy, ethanol or sedative drug intoxication. Wilson disease, Creutzfeldt-Jakob disease, hypothyroidism, paraneoplastic syndromes, and certain spinocerebellar degenerations are among the conditions that cause dementia with cerebellar ataxia. A vitamin B12 deficiency or

syphilitic taboparesis may be the cause of dementia with sensory ataxia. Cerebellar ataxia and amnesia are linked to long-term alcohol abuse.

2. **Stance and Gait:** It is possible to differentiate between vestibular, cerebellar, and sensory ataxia by observing stance and gait. Any patient suffering from ataxia will have a wide-based, unsteady gait that is frequently accompanied by reeling or lurching motions.

i. **Stance:** The ataxic patient asked to stand with the feet together may be reluctant or unable to do so. With urging, the patient may gradually move the feet closer together but will leave some space between them.

a. Patients with sensory ataxia and some with vestibular ataxia may be able to stand with the feet together, using vision to compensate for the loss of proprioceptive or labyrinthine input. This is demonstrated when the patient closes the eyes, eliminating visual cues, leading to markedly increased unsteadiness or falling (Romberg sign). With a vestibular lesion, the tendency is to fall toward the side of the lesion.

b. Patients with cerebellar ataxia cannot compensate for their deficit using visual input and are unstable on their feet whether the eyes are open or closed.

ii. **Gait:** The gait in cerebellar ataxia is wide-based, often with a staggering quality that can suggest drunkenness. Oscillation of the head or trunk (titubation) may be present. With a unilateral cerebellar hemisphere lesion, there is a tendency to deviate toward the side of the lesion when the patient tries to walk in a straight line or circle, or marches in place with eyes closed. Tandem (heel-to-toe) gait, which requires walking with an exaggerated narrow base, is always impaired in cerebellar ataxia.

a. In sensory ataxia, the gait is also wide-based and tandem gait is poor. In addition, the feet are typically lifted high off the ground and slapped down heavily (steppage gait) to enhance proprioceptive input. Stability may be dramatically improved by letting the patient use a cane or lightly rest a hand on the examiner's arm for support. If the patient attempts to walk in the dark or with eyes closed, gait is much more impaired.

b. Gait ataxia may also be a manifestation of conversion disorder or malingering. The most helpful observation in identifying factitious gait ataxia is that such patients may exhibit wildly reeling or lurching movements from which they can recover without falling, whereas recovery from such awkward positions actually requires excellent equilibrium.

3. **Cranial Nerves:** Vestibular disease is usually associated with abnormalities of extraocular (III, IV, and VI) and vestibulocochlear (VIII) nerve function, which frequently coexist with cerebellar lesions.

i. Eye Movements

a. The eyes are examined in the primary position of gaze (looking directly forward) to detect misalignment in the horizontal or vertical plane.

b. The patient is asked to turn the eyes in each of the cardinal directions of gaze to detect ocular nerve palsy or gaze paresis (inability to move the two eyes coordinately in any of the cardinal directions of gaze).

c. Nystagmus—an involuntary oscillation of the eyes—is characterized in terms of the positions of gaze in which it occurs (gaze-evoked nystagmus), its amplitude, and the direction of its fast phase. Pendular nystagmus, usually due to visual impairment beginning in infancy, has the same velocity in both directions, whereas jerk nystagmus has fast (vestibular-induced) and slow (cortical) phases. The direction of jerk nystagmus is defined by the direction of the fast component.

d. Fast voluntary eye movements (saccades) are elicited by having the patient rapidly shift gaze between targets in different regions of the visual field. Slow voluntary eye movements (pursuits) are assessed by having the patient track a slowly moving target such as the examiner's finger.

e. Peripheral vestibular disorders produce unidirectional horizontal jerk nystagmus that is maximal on gaze away from the involved side.

f. Central vestibular disorders can cause unidirectional or bidirectional horizontal nystagmus, vertical nystagmus, or gaze paresis.

g. Cerebellar lesions are associated with a wide range of ocular abnormalities, including gaze paresis, defective saccades or pursuits, nystagmus in any or all directions, and ocular dysmetria (overshoot of visual targets during saccadic eye movement).

ii. **Hearing:** Otoscopic inspection of the auditory canals and tympanic membranes, evaluation of auditory acuity in each ear, and Weber and Rinne tests using a 256-Hz tuning fork should all be part of a preliminary vestibulocochlear (VIII) nerve examination.

a. In the Weber test, unilateral sensorineural hearing loss (from lesions of the cochlea or vestibulocochlear nerve) causes the patient to perceive the sound produced by a vibrating tuning fork placed at the vertex of the skull as coming from the normal ear. With a conductive (external or middle ear) disorder, sound is localized to the abnormal ear.

b. The Rinne test may also distinguish between sensorineural and conductive defects in the affected ear. Air conduction (tested by holding the vibrating tuning fork next to the external auditory canal) normally produces a louder sound than bone conduction (tested by placing the base of the tuning fork over the mastoid bone). This also occurs with sensorineural hearing loss due to vestibulocochlear nerve lesions but is reversed in conductive hearing loss.

Table 4.4. Assessment of Hearing Loss

	Weber Test	Rinne Test
Normal	Sound perceived as coming from midline	Air conduction > bone conduction
Sensorineural hearing loss	Sound perceived as coming from normal ear	Air conduction > bone conduction
Conductive hearing loss	Sound perceived as coming from affected ear	Bone conduction > air conduction on affected side

Source: https://dl.mehrsys.ir/pdf-books/Clinical%20Neurology%209%20Edition%20(www.myuptodate.com).pdf.

iii. **Positional Vertigo Testing:** When a patient says that shifting positions causes dizziness, one can try to replicate the situation that causes it by performing the Nylen-Bárány or Dix-Hallpike maneuver. The head descends quickly to a position 30 degrees below horizontal. The head and eyes are turned to the right, then the left, and this process is repeated. The patient is asked to record the beginning, intensity, and end of vertigo, and their eyes are checked for nystagmus (Figure 4.6).

Positional nystagmus and vertigo are frequent symptoms of benign positional vertigo and are typically linked to peripheral vestibular lesions. Severe distress, a lag of few seconds between assuming the position and the onset of vertigo and nystagmus, a tendency for the response to remit spontaneously (fatigue) while maintaining the position, and attenuation of the response (habituation) as the offending position is repeatedly assumed are typical characteristics of this. In addition, central vestibular disease can cause positional vertigo.

iv. **Caloric Testing:** Calorimetric testing can identify vestibuloocular pathway disorders. A thorough otoscopic examination should come before beginning any calorie testing, and it should not be done if the tympanic membrane is perforated. The lateral semicircular canal, which is superficially located, is brought into an upright position by placing the patient supine with their head elevated 30 degrees. At least five minutes pass between tests as each ear canal is individually irrigated for 40 seconds with either warm (~44°C) or cold (~33°C) water. Generally speaking, warm water causes less pain than cold water.

a. In the normal, awake patient, cold-water caloric stimulation produces nystagmus with the slow phase toward and the fast phase away from the irrigated ear. Warm water irrigation produces the opposite response.

b. In patients with unilateral labyrinthine, vestibulocochlear (VIII) nerve, or vestibular nuclear dysfunction, irrigation of the affected side fails to cause nystagmus or elicits nystagmus that is later in onset or briefer in duration than on the normal side.

v. **Other Cranial Nerves:** When papilledema and disequilibrium coexist, it may indicate an intracranial mass lesion that is raising intracranial pressure. This lesion typically occurs in the posterior fossa. Multiple sclerosis, neurosyphilis, and vitamin B12 deficiency can all cause optic atrophy. Cerebellopontine angle tumors may appear with a depressed corneal reflex or facial palsy ipsilateral to the lesion (as well as ataxia). Diseases of the lower brainstem cause hoarseness, dysphagia, and weakness of the tongue or palate.

A

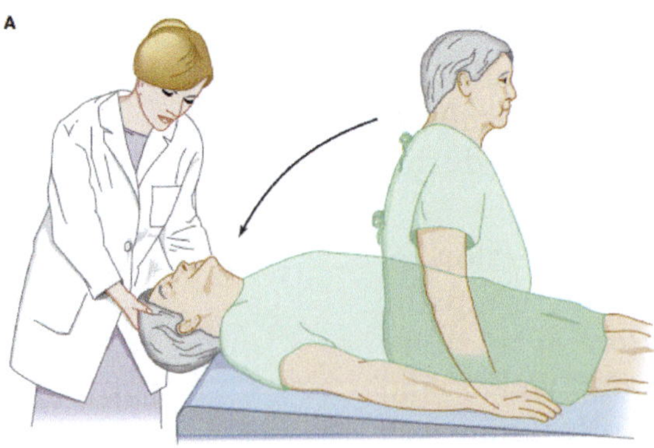

Source: https://neupsykey.com/wp-content/uploads/2017/01/f0196-01.jpg.

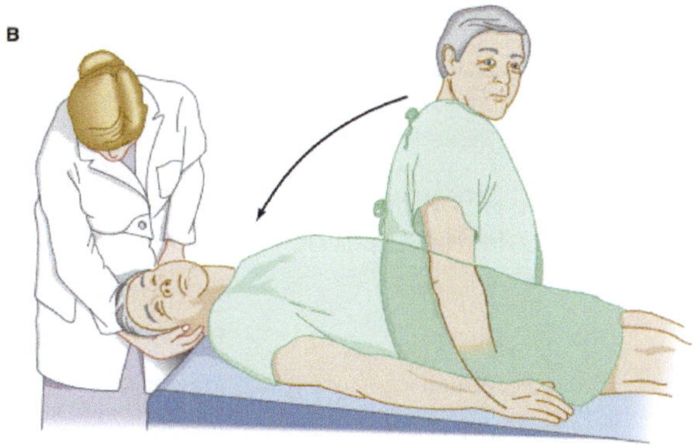

Figure 4.6. Test for positional vertigo and nystagmus. The patient is seated on a table with the head and eyes directed forward (A) and is then quickly lowered to a supine position with the head over the table edge, 45 degrees below horizontal. The patient's eyes are then observed for nystagmus, and the patient is asked to report any vertigo. The test is repeated with the patient's head and eyes turned 45 degrees to the right (B), and again with the head and eyes turned 45 degrees to the left (not shown).

Source: https://neupsykey.com/wp-content/uploads/2017/01/f0196–02.jpg.

Table 4.5. Characteristics of Positional Nystagmus

Feature	Peripheral Lesion	Central Lesion
Vertigo	Severe	Mild
Latency	2-40 s	No
Fatigability	Yes	No
Habituation	Yes	No

Source: https://dl.mehrsys.ir/pdf-books/Clinical%20Neurology%209%20Edition%20(www.myuptodate.com).pdf.

4. **Motor System:** An assessment of motor function in a patient presenting with an imbalance should reveal the type and degree of ataxia as well as any associated involvement of pyramidal, extrapyramidal, or lower motor neurons that may indicate a possible cause. Table 4.6 summarizes the clinical characteristics that aid in differentiating cerebellar disease from illnesses affecting these other motor systems.

Table 4.6. Clinical Features Distinguishing Cerebellar from Other Motor Systems Disorders

	Cerebellar	Upper Motor Neuron	Lower Motor Neuron	Extrapyramidal
Strength	Normal	Decreased	Decreased	Normal
Tone	Decreased	Increased (spastic)[1]	Normal	Increased (rigid)[1] or decreased
Tendon reflexes	Normal	Increased[1]	Decreased[1]	Normal
Plantar responses	Flexor	Extensor[1]	Flexor	Flexor
Atrophy	Absent	Absent	Present[1] or absent	Absent
Fasciculations	Absent	Absent	Present[1] or absent	Absent
Tremor	Intention tremor[1] or absent	Absent	Absent	Resting tremor[1] or absent
Chorea or athetosis	Absent	Absent	Absent	Present[1] or absent
Akinesia	Absent	Absent	Absent	Present[1] or absent
Ataxia	Present[1]	Absent	Absent	Absent

[1] Most helpful diagnostic features.

Source: https://dl.mehrsys.ir/pdf-books/Clinical%20Neurology%209%20Edition%20(www.myuptodate.com).pdf.

i. Muscle Tone

a. Hypotonia is characteristic of cerebellar disorders; with unilateral cerebellar hemispheric lesions, the ipsilateral limbs are hypotonic.

b. Extrapyramidal hypertonia (rigidity) may occur in disorders that affect both the cerebellum and basal ganglia (e.g., Wilson disease, acquired hepatocerebral degeneration, Creutzfeldt-Jakob disease, and some spinocerebellar ataxias).

c. Ataxia with spasticity may be seen in conditions that affect both the cerebellum and upper motor neuron pathways (e.g., multiple sclerosis, posterior fossa tumors or congenital anomalies, vertebrobasilar infarction, some spinocerebellar ataxias, Friedreich ataxia, neurosyphilis, Creutzfeldt-Jakob disease, and vitamin B12 deficiency).

ii. Coordination

a. Truncal stability is assessed by examining gait (discussed earlier) and by observing the seated, unsupported patient. In addition to gait ataxia, patients with midline or pancerebellar disease may show oscillation of the head or trunk (titubation) and truncal ataxia while seated, causing a tendency to fall over when they sit.

b. Movement of the patient's arm is observed as his or her finger tracks back and forth between his or her own nose or chin and the examiner's finger. With mild cerebellar ataxia, an intentional tremor characteristically appears near the beginning and end of each such movement, and the patient may overshoot the target.

c. When the patient is asked to raise the arms rapidly to a given height—or when the extended and outstretched arms are displaced by a sudden force—there may be an overshoot (rebound). Impaired ability to check the force of muscle contractions can also be demonstrated by having the patient flex the arm at the elbow against resistance, and then suddenly removing the resistance. If the limb is ataxic, continued contraction without resistance may cause the hand to strike the patient, whose head should be turned to the side to avoid being hit in the face.

d. Ataxia of the legs is demonstrated by the supine patient's inability to run the heel of the foot smoothly up and down the opposite shin.

e. Ataxia of any limb is reflected by irregularity in the rate, rhythm, amplitude, and force of rapid successive tapping movements.

iii. Weakness

a. Pure vestibular, cerebellar, or sensory disorders do not cause weakness, but weakness may occur in disorders that also affect motor pathways.

b. Distal weakness can be caused by disorders that also produce sensory ataxia, such as polyneuropathies and Friedreich ataxia.

c. Paraparesis may be superimposed on ataxia in vitamin B12 deficiency, multiple sclerosis, foramen magnum lesions, or spinal cord tumors.

d. Ataxic quadriparesis, hemiataxia with contralateral hemiparesis, or ataxic hemiparesis suggests a brainstem lesion.

iv. Abnormal Involuntary Movements

a. Titubation and intention tremors are common in cerebellar disorders. Other abnormal movements can occur with diseases that affect both the cerebellum and other brain structures.

b. Asterixis may occur in hepatic encephalopathy, other acute metabolic encephalopathies, or acquired hepatocerebral degeneration.

c. Myoclonus occurs in the same conditions as asterixis and is a prominent manifestation of Creutzfeldt-Jakob disease.

d. Chorea may accompany cerebellar signs in Wilson disease, acquired hepatocerebral degeneration, or ataxia-telangiectasia.

5. **Sensory System**

i. **Joint Position Sense:** Joint position sense is always compromised in the legs and may be compromised in the arms in cases of sensory ataxia. In order to determine the upper limit of any deficit in each limb, joint position sense is tested by asking the patient to detect passive movement of the joints, starting distally and moving proximally. Nearly any displacement should be detectable with normal joint position sense. Another way to show abnormal position sense is to have the patient place one limb in a certain way and then, with their eyes closed, place the other limb in the same spot.

ii. Vibration Sense

A common feature of sensory ataxia is also impaired vibration sense. The patient is asked to feel if a tuning fork with a frequency of 128 Hz vibrates on a bony prominence. The upper limit of the deficit in each limb is ascertained by testing progressively more proximal sites. The examiner's ability to detect vibration in the hand holding the tuning fork is compared to the patient's threshold for vibration detection.

6. **Reflexes**

i. Tendon reflexes are typically hypoactive, with a pendular quality, in cerebellar disorders; unilateral cerebellar lesions produce ipsilateral hyporeflexia.

ii. Hyporeflexia of the legs is a prominent manifestation of Friedreich ataxia, tabes dorsalis, and polyneuropathies that cause sensory ataxia.

iii. Hyperactive reflexes and extensor plantar responses may accompany ataxia caused by multiple sclerosis, vitamin B12 deficiency, focal brainstem lesions, and certain autosomal dominant spinocerebellar ataxias.

4.1.6. Investigative Studies

- **Blood Tests:** Low levels of vitamin B12 and hematologic abnormalities (such as macrocytic anemia, leukopenia with hypersegmented neutrophils, and thrombocytopenia with giant platelets) in vitamin B12 deficiency, reduced thyroid hormone levels in hypothyroidism, elevated hepatic enzymes and low concentrations of ceruloplasmin and copper in Wilson disease, immunoglobulin deficiency and elevated α-fetoprotein in ataxia-telangiectasia, antibodies to Purkinje cell antigens in paraneoplastic cerebellar degeneration, or mutations linked to certain autosomal dominant spinocerebellar ataxias and Friedreich's ataxia can all be revealed by blood tests.
- Cerebrospinal Fluid: Cerebellopontine angle, brainstem or spinal cord tumors, hypothyroidism, and certain polyneuropathies are associated with elevated protein levels in the cerebrospinal fluid (CSF). Infectious or parainfectious encephalitis, paraneoplastic cerebellar degeneration, and neurosyphilis are all associated with increased protein concentration with pleocytosis. In patients with Creutzfeldt-Jakob disease, CSF levels of 14–3-3 protein are

elevated. Cerebellar hemorrhage is characterized by elevated pressure and bloody CSF, but lumbar puncture is not advised if any of these symptoms are present. Tabes dorsalis is reactive to CSF VDRL, and multiple sclerosis and other inflammatory disorders may exhibit oligoclonal immunoglobulin G (IgG) bands.

- **Brain Imaging:** Cerebellar atrophy linked to degenerative disorders, posterior fossa tumors or malformations, and cerebellar infarction or hemorrhage can all be seen on computed tomography (CT). Magnetic resonance imaging (MRI) is superior to CT in the detection of multiple sclerosis lesions and offers superior visualization of lesions located in the posterior fossa, including tumors of the cerebellopontine angle.
- **Evoked Potentials:** When assessing patients who may have multiple sclerosis, evoked potential testing—particularly of the optic pathways, or visual evoked potentials—may be useful. Brainstem auditory evoked potentials have the potential to detect tumors of the cerebellopontine angle and to pinpoint vestibular disease to the peripheral vestibular pathways.
- **Chest X-ray and Echocardiography:** An echocardiogram or chest X-ray may show signs of cardiomyopathy linked to Friedreich ataxia. A lung tumor in paraneoplastic cerebellar degeneration may also be visible on the chest X-ray.
- **Audiometry:** This can differentiate vestibulocochlear (VIII) nerve, brainstem disease, conductive, and labyrinthine vestibular disorders that are linked to auditory impairment.

  Pure tone hearing tests are abnormal when sounds are transmitted through bone or air with vestibulocochlear (VIII) or labyrinthine nerve disorders, or when sounds are transmitted through air with conductive hearing loss.

  Vestibulocochlear (VIII) nerve lesions significantly impair speech discrimination; labyrinthine disorders lessen this impairment; and brainstem disease or conductive hearing loss do not affect speech discrimination.
- **Electronystagmography:** This can identify and describe nystagmus, including that which is caused by calorie stimulation.

4.2. Peripheral Vestibular Disorders

A list of peripheral vestibular disorders and characteristics that aid in their differential diagnosis is given in Table 4.7.

4.2.1. Benign Positional Vertigo

When one assumes a specific head position, positional vertigo sets in. It is typically linked to peripheral vestibular lesions, but central (cerebellar or brainstem) disease may also be the cause.

- **Pathogenesis:** Approximately 30% of cases of vertigo of peripheral origin are caused by benign positional vertigo. Head trauma is the most commonly found cause, although in most cases, no cause can be found. It is believed that canalolithiasis, or the stimulation of the semicircular canal by debris floating in the endolymph, is the pathophysiologic basis of benign positional vertigo.
- **Clinical Findings:** The syndrome is typified by intense vertigo attacks that

last anywhere from a few seconds to several minutes and may be followed by nausea and vomiting. Any change in head position may cause symptoms, but they are typically worst when the affected ear is down in the lateral decubitus position. Periodic vertigo usually lasts for a few weeks before going away on its own; occasionally, it comes back. Deafness is not a characteristic.

Table 4.7. Differential Diagnosis of Peripheral Vestibular Disorders

	Hearing Loss		Other Cranial Nerve Palsies
	Conductive	Sensorineural	
Benign positional vertigo[1]	−	−	−
Ménière disease[1]	−	+	−
Acute peripheral vestibulopathy[1]	−	−	−
Otosclerosis	+	+	−
Head trauma	±	±	±
Cerebellopontine angle tumor	−	+	±
Toxic vestibulopathy			
Alcohol	−	−	−
Aminoglycosides	−	+	−
Salicylates	−	+	−
Quinine	−	+	−
Vestibulocochlear (VIII) neuropathy			
Basilar meningitis	−	+	±
Hypothyroidism	−	+	−
Diabetes	−	+	±
Paget disease of the skull (osteitis deformans)	−	+	±

[1] Most common causes.

Source: https://dl.mehrsys.ir/pdf-books/Clinical%20Neurology%209%20Edition%20(www.myuptodate.com).pdf.

The Nylen-Bárány or Dix-Hallpike maneuver can help distinguish between peripheral and central causes of positional vertigo during a physical examination. In cases of benign positional vertigo, nystagmus is always present and tends to be unidirectional, rotatory, and delayed by a few seconds after assuming the triggering head position. The nystagmus and vertigo usually resolve within minutes if the position is maintained, and the response diminishes with repeated maneuvers. On the other hand, central positional vertigo is generally milder, and nystagmus may not be present. Additionally, there is no delay, fatigue, or habituation seen in central positional vertigo.

- **Treatment:** Repositioning (Epley) maneuvers are the cornerstone of treatment because they leverage gravity to transfer endolymphatic debris from the semicircular canal into the vestibule, where it can be reabsorbed. In one such maneuver, the patient reclines to a supine position with the head still turned 45 degrees, hanging down over the end of the examination table. The head is turned 45 degrees in the direction of the affected ear (determined clinically, as previously described). The head is then rotated 90 degrees in the other direction, to 45 degrees toward the ear on the other side, while it is still hanging down. The patient then rolls to a lateral decubitus position, hanging down and keeping the head 45 degrees turned toward the unaffected ear while the affected ear is raised. At last, the patient sits up and assumes a prone posture (Figure 4.7).

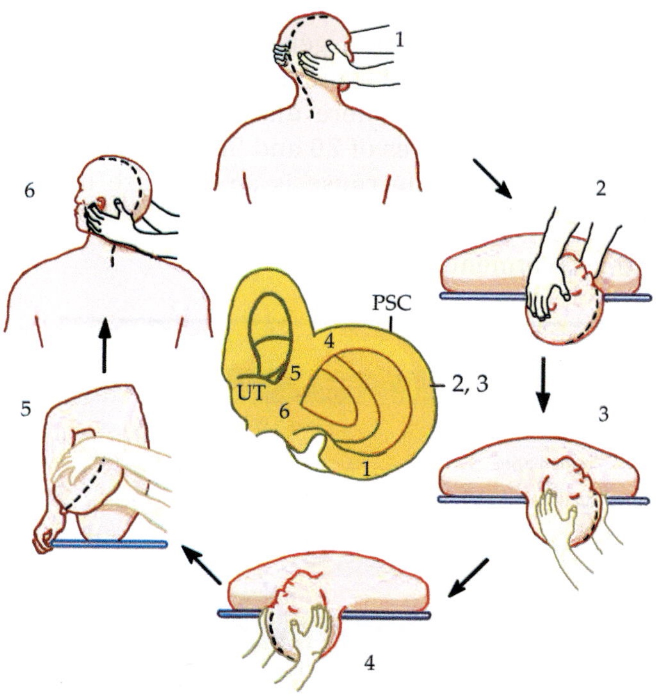

Figure 4.7. Repositioning treatment for benign positional vertigo resulting from canalolithiasis. In the example shown, repositioning maneuvers are used to move endolymphatic debris out of the posterior semicircular canal (PSC) of the right ear and into the utricle (UT), the larger of two membranous sacs in the vestibule of the labyrinth, where this debris can be reabsorbed. The numbers (1–6) refer to both the position of the patient and the corresponding location of debris within the labyrinth. The patient is seated, and the head is turned 45 degrees to the right (1). The head is lowered rapidly to below the horizontal (2); the examiner shifts position (3); and the

head is rotated rapidly 90 degrees in the opposite direction, so it now points 45 degrees to the left, where it remains for 30 seconds (4). The patient then rolls onto the left side without turning the head in relation to the body and maintains this position for another 30 seconds (5) before sitting up (6). This maneuver may need to be repeated until nystagmus is abolished. The patient must then avoid the supine position for at least 2 days.

Source: Used with permission from Baloh RW and from Samuels MA, Feske SK, eds. Office Practice of Neurology. New York, NY: Churchill Livingstone; 1995.

Medications that suppress the vestibule may also be helpful during the acute phase. Vestibular rehabilitation may also be beneficial as it encourages the recruitment of other sensory modalities in order to compensate for vestibular dysfunction.

4.2.2. Ménière Disease

Recurrent episodes of vertigo that last anywhere from minutes to days are the hallmark of Ménière disease. Tinnitus and progressive sensorineural hearing loss also accompany these symptoms.

- **Pathogenesis:** Although familial occurrence has been reported, the majority of cases are sporadic and may exhibit anticipation (earlier onset in successive generations). The COCH (coagulation factor C homology) gene, which codes for cochlin, a component of the extracellular matrix found in the inner ear, appears to be mutated in rare cases. Men are afflicted with sporadic Ménière disease more frequently than women, and it typically manifests between the ages of 20 and 50. Although the pathogenetic mechanism is unknown, it is believed that the cause is an increase in the volume of labyrinthine endolymph (endolymphatic hydrops).

Table 4.8. Drugs Used in the Treatment of Vertigo

Drug	Dosage[1]
Antihistamines	
Meclizine	25 mg PO q4-6h
Promethazine	25-50 mg PO, IM, or PR q4-6h
Dimenhydrinate	50 mg PO or IM q4-6h or 100 mg PR q8h
Anticholinergics	
Scopolamine	0.5 mg transdermally q3d
Benzodiazepines	
Diazepam	5-10 mg IM q4-6h
Sympathomimetics	
Amphetamine	5-10 mg PO q4-6h
Ephedrine	25 mg PO q4-6h

[1] IM, intramuscularly; PO, orally; PR, rectally.

Source: Adapted from Baloh RW, Honrubia V, Kerber KA. Baloh and Honrubia's Clinical Neurophysiology of the Vestibular System. 4th ed. New York, NY: Oxford; 2010.

- **Clinical Findings:** Patients may have already noticed the subtle onset of tinnitus, hearing loss, and a feeling of fullness in the ear at the time of the initial acute attack. Vertigo, nausea, and vomiting are the hallmarks of acute episodes, which can recur every few weeks to years. Ten to 70% of patients experience bilateral involvement as their hearing deteriorates gradually. Vertigo usually gets milder as hearing loss gets worse.

  During an acute episode, a physical examination may reveal spontaneous horizontal or rotational nystagmus, which can change direction. Although spontaneous nystagmus is typically absent between attacks, caloric testing often indicates impaired vestibular function. The hearing loss may not always be noticeable during bedside testing, but audiometry typically shows fluctuating low-frequency pure-tone hearing loss, impaired speech discrimination, and heightened sensitivity to loud sounds.

- **Treatment:** Acute attacks can be treated symptomatically with benzodiazepines, antihistamines, and other medications shown in Table 4.8. Patients may be treated with a low-salt diet and diuretics in between episodes, such as hydrochlorothiazide (50 mg oral daily) plus triamterene (25 mg oral daily), or with betahistine (8–24 mg oral three times daily), an antagonist of the histamine H3 receptor. Vestibular ablation by intratympanic gentamicin, vestibular (VIII) nerve section, or labyrinthectomy may be helpful in persistent, incapacitating cases.

4.2.3. Acute Peripheral Vestibulopathy

This phrase is used to characterize an inapparent cause-related spontaneous attack of vertigo that goes away on its own and isn't accompanied by hearing loss or problems with the central nervous system. It can come on after a feverish sickness and includes conditions such as acute labyrinthitis or vestibular neuronitis.

Vertigo, nausea, and vomiting with an acute onset that usually lasts up to two weeks are the hallmarks of the disorder. Vestibular dysfunction may persist to some degree permanently, and symptoms may recur. The patient looks extremely sick during an attack, usually lies on one side with the affected ear facing up, and is reluctant to move their head. There is constant nystagmus with the fast phase away from the afflicted ear. One or both ears exhibit abnormal vestibular responses to calorie testing, but auditory acuity is normal.

It is important to differentiate acute peripheral vestibulopathy from central causes of acute vertigo, such as posterior cerebral circulation stroke. Vertical nystagmus, altered consciousness, motor or sensory deficit, or dysarthria are indicators of central disease.

A course of 10 to 14 days of prednisone (20 mg orally twice daily), the medications listed in Table 4.8, or both is recommended for the treatment of acute peripheral vestibulopathy.

4.2.4. Otosclerosis

The stapes, an ear ossicle that connects the inner ear to the tympanic membrane and transmits vibrations, becomes immobile, which results in otosclerosis. Its most characteristic feature is conductive hearing loss, although vertigo and sensorineural hearing loss are also possible, and tinnitus is rare. The majority of auditory symptoms start before the age of thirty, and familial occurrence is frequent.

The most common symptoms of vestibular dysfunction are a feeling of positional imbalance and recurrent episodic vertigo, either with or without positional vertigo. Along with more persistent symptoms, attacks may also become more frequent and more severe over time. Attenuated caloric responses, which are typically unilateral, and spontaneous or positional nystagmus of the peripheral type are examples of vestibular abnormalities on examination.

Audiometry can always be used to demonstrate hearing loss. Usually bilateral, it has a mixed conductive-sensorineural nature and affects about two-thirds of patients. It is important to differentiate otosclerosis from Ménière disease in patients exhibiting episodic vertigo, progressive hearing loss, and tinnitus. Positive family history, an early onset tendency, conductive hearing loss, or bilateral symmetric auditory impairment are indicators of otosclerosis. The diagnostic utility of imaging studies is also reported.

Intrathecal dexamethasone, vitamin D, and sodium fluoride therapy may be beneficial. If not, a surgical stapedectomy ought to be taken into account.

4.2.5. Head Trauma

The most frequently found cause of benign positional vertigo is head trauma. Posttraumatic vertigo is usually caused by damage to the labyrinth, but fractures of the petrosal bone can lacerate the vestibulocochlear (VIII) nerve, resulting in vertigo and hearing loss. This kind of fracture is suggested by hemotympanum or CSF otorrhea.

4.2.6. Cerebellopontine Angle Tumor

- **Pathogenesis:** The histologically benign acoustic neuroma is the most common tumor in the cerebellopontine angle, a triangle in the posterior fossa bounded by the lateral pons, petrous ridge, and cerebellum. It usually originates from the neurilemmal sheath of the vestibular portion of the vestibulocochlear (VIII) nerve in the internal auditory canal. It is also known by the names neurilemoma, neurinoma, and schwannoma. Primary cholesteatomas (epidermoid cysts) and meningiomas are less frequent tumors at this location.

  Acoustic neuromas typically appear as solitary lesions in individuals between the ages of 30 and 60, although they can also be a sign of neurofibromatosis. A common autosomal dominant disorder called neurofibromatosis 1 (von Recklinghausen disease) is caused by mutations in the tumor suppressor gene neurofibromin 1 (NF1). Neurofibromatosis 1 is linked to dysplastic bony lesions, axillary or inguinal freckles, cutaneous neurofibromas, optic gliomas, and iris hamartomas in addition to unilateral acoustic neuromas. Mutations in neurofibromin 2 (NF2), an inhibitor of contact-dependent cell proliferation, result in the uncommon autosomal dominant disorder known as neurofibromatosis 2. Bilateral acoustic neuromas are its defining characteristic; these tumors may coexist with other tumors of the central or peripheral nervous systems, such as neurofibromas, meningiomas, gliomas, and schwannomas (Figure 4.8).

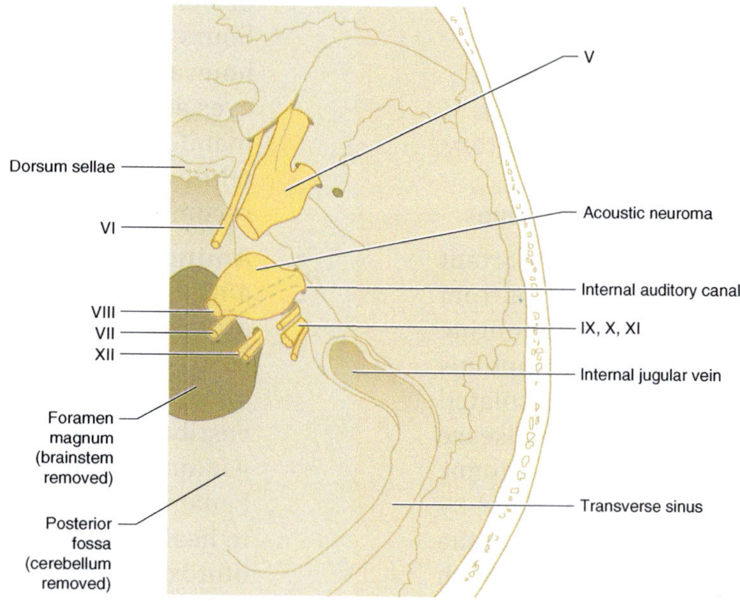

Figure 4.8. Cerebellopontine angle tumor, viewed from above, with the brain removed to permit the cranial nerves and base of the skull to be seen. The tumor, a neuroma arising from the vestibulocochlear (VIII) nerve, may compress adjacent structures, including the trigeminal (V) and facial (VII) nerves, the brainstem, and the cerebellum.

Source: https://dl.mehrsys.ir/pdf-books/Clinical%20Neurology%209%20Edition%20(www.myuptodate.com).pdf.

- **Pathophysiology:** Flow obstruction of the CSF and compression or displacement of the brainstem, cerebellum, and cranial nerves cause symptoms. The vestibulocochlear (VIII) and trigeminal (V) nerves are anatomically related, and as such, they are frequently affected.
- Clinical Findings
  - **Symptoms and Signs:** Usually, the first sign is subtle hearing loss. Patients with headache, vertigo, ataxia of gait, facial pain, tinnitus, fullness in the ear, or facial weakness are less frequently present. Twenty to 30% of patients eventually experience vertigo, although general unsteadiness is more common. The symptoms might not change over months or years, or they might.

  When a patient is examined, the most frequent finding is unilateral sensorineural hearing loss. Ipsilateral facial palsy, a diminished or absent corneal reflex, and sensory loss throughout the face are additional common findings. Less frequently seen symptoms include ataxia, spontaneous nystagmus, various lower cranial nerve palsies, and indications of elevated intracranial pressure. Calorimetric testing is typically used to demonstrate unilateral vestibular dysfunction.

  - **Laboratory Findings:** A sensorineural deficit with high-frequency pure-tone hearing loss, poor speech discrimination, and noticeable tone decay is revealed by audiometry. About 70% of patients have elevated CSF protein, which is typically in the range of 50 to 200 mg/dL. An MRI of the cerebellopontine angle is the most beneficial imaging test. Anomalous brainstem auditory evoked potentials can be caused by acoustic neuromas.

- **Differential Diagnosis:** It's important to differentiate acoustic neuromas from other tumors of the cerebellopontine angle. Patients whose initial symptoms suggest something more than isolated vestibulocochlear (VIII) nerve disease should be evaluated for meningioma. A cholesteatoma may be indicated by early facial weakness, twitching of the face, or conductive hearing loss with normal CSF protein. Another possible symptom of metastatic carcinoma is a lesion in the cerebellopontine angle.
- **Treatment:** Surgery is used to remove all tissue. Bevacizumab is a monoclonal antibody that targets vascular endothelial growth factor (VEGFA) and may be helpful for patients with acoustic neuroma and neurofibromatosis 2. If left untreated, hydrocephalus or brainstem compression can lead to serious consequences.

4.2.7. Toxic Vestibulopathies

- **Alcohol:** Alcohol's differential distribution between the inner ear's cupula and endolymph results in acute positional vertigo. Positional vertigo caused by alcohol usually happens two hours after ethanol consumption is high enough to cause blood levels to exceed 40 mg/dL. Alcohol diffuses into the cupula first, then into the endolymph subsequently, and finally out of the cupula before it exits from the endolymph. This results in two symptomatic phases of vertigo, which can last up to 12 hours total, interspersed with a 1–2 hour asymptomatic period. When the eyes are closed, the clinical syndrome manifests as nystagmus and vertigo while the patient is in a lateral recumbent position.
- **Aminoglycosides:** Antibiotics called aminoglycosides are well-known ototoxins that can cause symptoms related to hearing and vestibular systems. The drugs most likely to cause vestibular toxicity are streptomycin, gentamicin, and tobramycin; amikacin, kanamycin, and tobramycin are linked to hearing loss. Aminoglycosides cause ototoxicity by destroying sensory hair cells, and they are concentrated in the perilymph and endolymph. Preexisting vestibular or cochlear dysfunction, concurrent administration of other ototoxic agents, drug dosage, plasma concentration, length of therapy, and conditions that hinder drug clearance—like renal failure—all increase the risk of toxicity.

Vertigo, nausea, vomiting, and ataxia of the gait may start suddenly; physical manifestations include the Romberg sign and spontaneous nystagmus. Usually lasting one to two weeks, the acute phase is followed by a steady improvement. Prolonged or recurrent aminoglycoside treatment has been linked to progressive vestibular dysfunction that is chronic.

- **Salicylates:** When salicylates are taken long-term and in high doses, they can lead to vertigo, tinnitus, and sensorineural hearing loss, all of which are usually curable by stopping the medication. Damage to the cochlea and vestibular end organs causes symptoms. Headache, tinnitus, vertigo, hearing loss, nausea, vomiting, thirst, hyperventilation, and occasionally a state of confusion are the symptoms of salicylism. Seizures, psychosis, coma, bleeding, fever, skin rash, and dehydration can all be signs of severe intoxication. A high plasma salicylate level (≥0.35 mg/mL) and a combination of respiratory alkalosis and metabolic acidosis were observed in the laboratory. Hemodialysis or peritoneal dialysis, forced diuresis, gastric lavage, activated charcoal, and hemoperfusion are among the treatments.

- **Quinine and Quinidine:** Cinchononism, which is similar to salicylate intoxication in many ways, can be caused by quinine and quinidine. Tinnitus, hearing loss, vertigo, visual impairments (including color vision disorders), nausea, vomiting, abdominal pain, hot flushed skin, and sweating are some of the symptoms. There may be a coma, encephalopathy, fever, and even death. The most common cause of symptoms is overdosage, but they can also be caused by unique reactions to prescribed dosages.
- **Cisplatin:** Antineoplastic medications such as cisplatin are used to treat solid tumors of the testicles, ovary, lung, head and neck, bladder, and other tissues. In many cases, it results in ototoxicity, which is usually bilateral and irreversible. Vestibular dysfunction, hearing loss, and tinnitus could all manifest.

4.2.8. Vestibulocochlear Neuropathy

One rare cause of vertigo is involvement of the vestibulocochlear (VIII) nerve by systemic disease. Vestibulocochlear and other cranial nerve compression can result from bacterial, syphilitic, tuberculous, or sarcoidosis-induced basilar meningitis; however, hearing loss is a more frequent side effect than vertigo. Vestibulochoglear neuropathy is linked to metabolic disorders such as diabetes, hypothyroidism, and Paget disease.

4.3. Cerebellar and Central Vestibular Disorders

Cerebellar dysfunction can be acute or chronic and is a result of many disorders. Central vestibular pathways, in particular Wernicke encephalopathy, vertebrobasilar ischemia or infarction, multiple sclerosis, and posterior fossa tumors, may also be involved in these conditions.

Table 4.9. Differential Diagnosis of Cerebellar Ataxia

Acute
Drug intoxications: ethanol, sedative-hypnotics, anticonvulsants, hallucinogens[1]
Wernicke encephalopathy[1]
Vertebrobasilar ischemia or infarction[1]
Cerebellar hemorrhage[1]
Inflammatory disorders
Chronic
Multiple sclerosis[1,2]
Alcoholic cerebellar degeneration
Phenytoin-induced cerebellar degeneration
Hypothyroidism
Paraneoplastic cerebellar degeneration
Autosomal dominant spinocerebellar ataxias
Ataxia-telangiectasia
Wilson disease
Acquired hepatolenticular degeneration
Creutzfeldt-Jakob disease
Posterior fossa tumor[1]
Posterior fossa malformations[1]

Source: https://dl.mehrsys.ir/pdf-books/Clinical%20Neurology%209%20Edition%20(www.myuptodate.com).pdf.

[1] May also be associated with central vestibular dysfunction.

[2] May also produce sensory ataxia.

This is why disorders of the cerebellum and central vestibular system are taken into consideration together (Table 4.9).

4.3.1. Acute Disorders

- **Drug Intoxication:** Nystagmus, dysarthria, and ataxia of the limbs and gait are examples of pancreas dysfunction, which is a common side effect of ethanol, sedative-hypnotics, anticonvulsants, and hallucinogens. The degree of symptoms is dose-dependent; nystagmus is frequently the result of therapeutic dosages of sedatives or anticonvulsants, but other cerebellar signs suggest toxicity (Figure 4.9).

Confusion is frequently linked to drug-induced cerebellar ataxia; ethanol and sedative medications typically induce somnolence, while hallucinogens can cause agitated delirium. Generally, only general supportive care is required.

- **Wernicke Encephalopathy:**

o **Pathogenesis:** The acute condition known as Wernicke encephalopathy is characterized by the three clinical symptoms of ataxia, ophthalmoplegia, and confusion. It results from malnutrition from any source and is most common in chronic alcoholics. It is caused by thiamine (vitamin B1) deficiency.

o **Clinical Findings:** Ataxia, which primarily or exclusively affects gait, is a result of both cerebellar and vestibular involvement; only about 20% of patients have ataxia in their arms, and 10% in their legs. Rarely is dysarthria reported. Additional observations include bilateral lateral rectus palsy, absence of ankle reflexes, horizontal or combined horizontal and vertical nystagmus, and amnestic syndrome or global confusional state. Bilateral or unilateral vestibular dysfunction is revealed by caloric testing. Hypothermia, pupillary anomalies, and conjugate gaze palsy are further possible outcomes.

o **Diagnosis and Treatment:** In patients who are malnourished and alcoholics, the diagnosis should be suspected; the clinical response to intravenous thiamine (100 mg) confirms the diagnosis. After a few days, ataxia, nystagmus, and confusion usually go away from ocular palsies. The horizontal nystagmus might continue. Only about 40% of patients with ataxia have complete reversibility; for them, a full recovery usually takes weeks to months.

- **Vertebrobasilar Ischemia and Infarction:** Ataxia and vertigo are frequently linked to transient ischemic attacks and strokes in the vertebrobasilar system.

o **Internal Auditory Artery Occlusion:** Unilateral hearing loss and vertigo of central vestibular origin result from occlusion of the internal auditory artery, which supplies the vestibulocochlear (VIII) nerve and can arise from the basilar or anterior inferior cerebellar artery. Nystagmus occurs along with vertigo, with the fast phase directed away from the affected side. The type of hearing loss is sensorineural and unilateral.

o **Lateral Medullary Infarction:** Wallenberg syndrome is caused by lateral medullary infarction, which is typically caused by proximal vertebral artery occlusion. The degree of infarction determines the clinical manifestations (Figure 4.10).

- § Vertigo, nausea, vomiting, and nystagmus result from involvement of the vestibular nuclei.
- § Hoarseness and dysphagia are caused by involvement of the dorsal motor nucleus of the vagus (X) nerve, nucleus solitarius, and nucleus ambiguous.
- § Ipsilateral Horner syndrome, limb ataxia, and loss of all sensation over the face and of light touch and position sense in the limbs are due to involvement of the descending sympathetic tract, inferior cerebellar peduncle, and spinal nucleus and tract of the trigeminal (V) nerve.
- § Contralateral impaired pin and temperature sense in the limbs results from involvement of the spinothalamic tract.

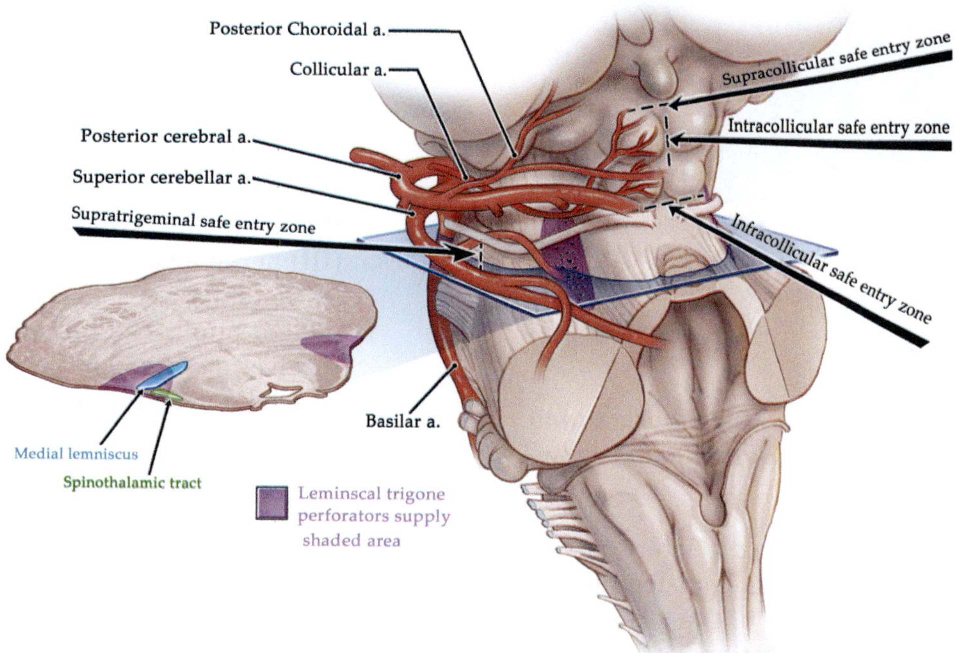

Figure 4.9. Principal arteries of the posterior fossa.

Source: Tomasi SO, Umana GE, Scalia G, Rubio-Rodriguez RL, Raudino G, Rechberger J, Geiger P, Chaurasia B, Yamurlu K, Lawton MT and Winkler PA (2021) Perforating arteries of the lemniscal trigone: A microsurgical neuroanatomic description. Front. Neuroanat. 15:675313. doi: 10.3389/fnana.2021.675313.

- o **Cerebellar Infarction:** Three arteries supply the cerebellum: the posterior inferior cerebellar, anterior inferior cerebellar, and superior cerebellar. Each of these vessels supplies a highly variable territory, both between the two sides in a given patient and from one individual to another. The anterior inferior, posterior inferior, and superior cerebellar arteries normally supply the superior, middle, and inferior cerebellar peduncles, respectively.

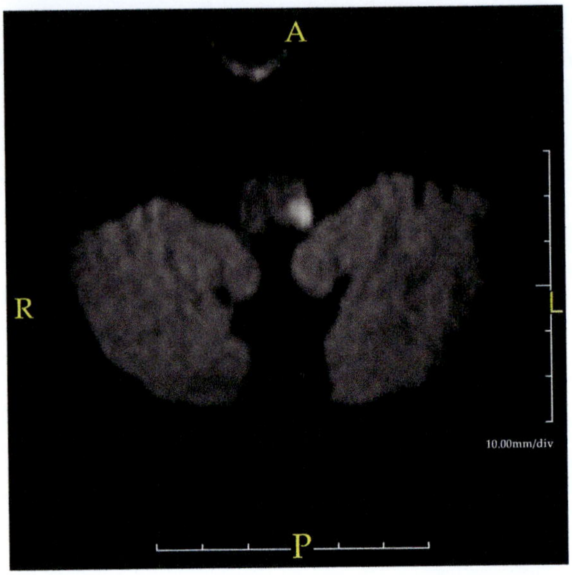

Figure 4.10. *Lateral medullary infarction (Wallenberg syndrome) showing the area of infarction (blue) and anatomic structures affected.*

Source: By John S. To, M.D. – Own work, Public Domain, https://commons.wikimedia.org/w/index.php?curid=1644951.

Ipsilateral limb ataxia, lateropulsion (falling toward or, less frequently, away from the side of the lesion), and hypotonia are indications of cerebellar infarction. Other possible symptoms include facial weakness or sensory loss, vertigo, nystagmus, dysarthria, ocular or gaze palsies, headache, nausea, vomiting, and contralateral hemiparesis or hemisensory deficit. When the superior, anterior, and posterior cerebellar arteries are occluded, it is typically only possible to differentiate them based on related brainstem abnormalities, if at all. Coma and death may ensue from brainstem infarction or compression caused by cerebellar edema.

The diagnosis is made using CT or MRI, which can distinguish between hemorrhage and infarction and should be obtained as soon as possible. A potentially life-saving surgical procedure called decompression and resection of infarcted tissue is indicated by brainstem compression (Figure 4.11).

- **Paramedian Midbrain Infarction:** The oculomotor (III) nerve root fibers and red nucleus are affected by paramedian midbrain infarction, which is caused by blockage of the paramedian penetrating branches of the basilar artery. The outcome, known as Benedikt syndrome, is contralateral limb ataxia (usually affecting only the arm) and ipsilateral oculomotor (III) nerve involvement, which results in medial rectus palsy with a fixed dilated pupil. The red nucleus, which receives a crossed projection from the cerebellum in the ascending limb of the superior cerebellar peduncle, is involved in the cerebellar signs (Figure 4.12).

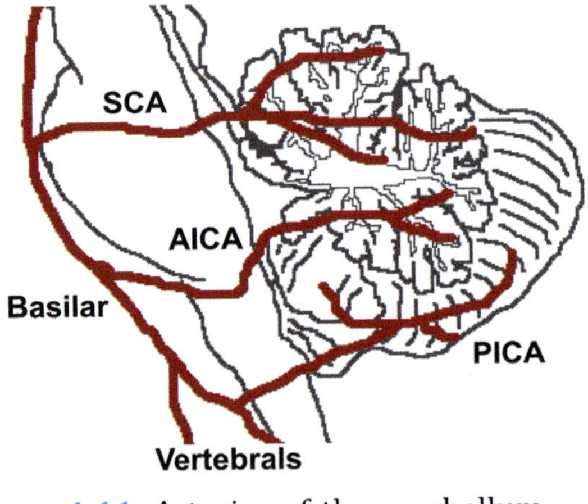

Figure 4.11. Arteries of the cerebellum.

Source: https://en.wikipedia.org/wiki/Anatomy_of_the_cerebellum#/media/File:CerebellumArteries.svg.

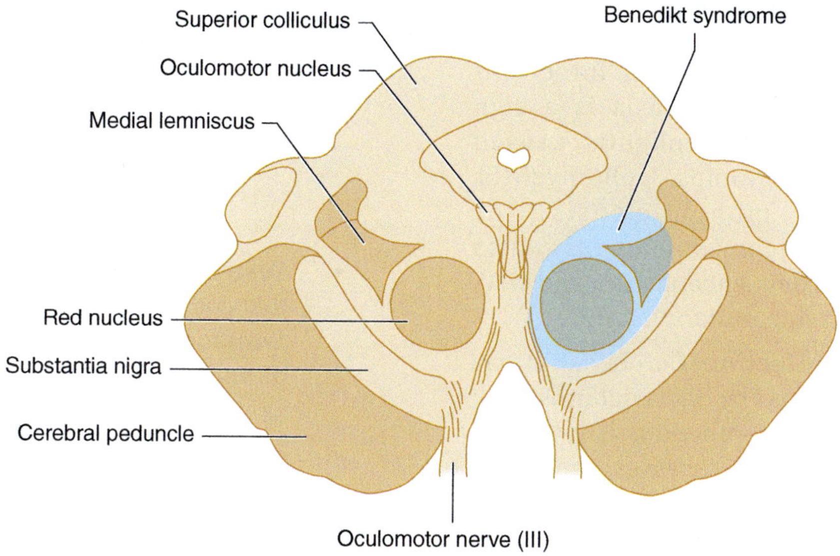

Figure 4.12. Paramedian midbrain infarction (Benedikt syndrome). The area of infarction is indicated in blue.

Source: https://dl.mehrsys.ir/pdf-books/Clinical%20Neurology%209%20Edition%20(www.myuptodate.com).pdf.

- **Cerebellar Hemorrhage**
  - **Pathogenesis:** Hypertensive vascular disease is the most common cause of cerebellar hemorrhage; anticoagulation, arteriovenous malformation, blood dyscrasia, tumors, and trauma are less common causes. Hypertensive cerebellar hemorrhages typically occur in the cerebellum's deep white matter and frequently spread into the fourth ventricle.
  - **Clinical Findings:** An abrupt onset of headache, possibly accompanied by nausea, vomiting, and vertigo, is the result of hypertensive cerebellar hemorrhage. Other symptoms include gait ataxia and impaired consciousness, which typically develop over hours.

    Patients may be comatose, fully awake, or confused at presentation. There may be nuchal rigidity and an increase in blood pressure. The pupils are frequently tiny and react slowly. Both ipsilateral peripheral facial palsy and ipsilateral gaze palsy—with a preference for looking away from the side of the hemorrhage—are frequent. Caloric stimulation with cold water cannot cure gaze palsy. There could be ipsilateral corneal reflex depression and nystagmus. If the patient is conscious, ataxia of posture and gait is evident; ataxia of the limbs is less frequent. Leg spasticity and extensor plantar responses are symptoms of late-stage brainstem compression.
  - **Diagnosis and Treatment:** It is possible for cerebellar hemorrhage to go undiagnosed or be delayed, leading to death, if a patient with hypertension who also has an acute headache or low consciousness does not have their gait evaluated right away. Although lumbar puncture should be avoided if cerebellar hemorrhage is suspected, as it may result in herniation, the CSF is often bloody. CT is used for diagnosis. The hematoma is surgically removed as part of the treatment, which may be lifesaving.

- **Inflammatory Disorders**
  - o **Viral Infection:** Viral infection-induced cerebellar ataxia is a sign of St. Meningoencephalitis caused by varicella, mumps, poliomyelitis, infectious mononucleosis, or lymphocytic choriomeningitis; also known as Louis encephalitis and HIV-associated dementia.
  - o **Bacterial Infection:** Cerebellar ataxia is rarely caused by bacterial infection; however, the cerebellum is home to 10–20% of brain abscesses, and ataxia can also be a sign of meningitis caused by *Haemophilus influenzae* in children or *Listeria monocytogenes* in adults. Cerebellar syndrome can also result from pneumonia caused by *Legionella pneumophila*, even in the absence of meningitis symptoms.
  - o **Acute Cerebellar Ataxia of Childhood:** When a child has acute cerebellar ataxia, it is characterized by severe gait ataxia that usually goes away completely in a few months after an acute viral infection or vaccination.
  - o **Acute Disseminated Encephalomyelitis:** Atherosclerosis resulting from immune-mediated demyelination in the cerebellar white matter can be idiopathic and is frequently accompanied by focal neurologic signs, myelopathy, seizures, and reduced consciousness.
  - o **Fisher Variant of Guillain-Barré Syndrome:** This variant of Guillain-Barré syndrome is characterized by ataxia, ophthalmoplegia, and areflexia. The condition usually manifests as ascending paralysis. The onset of symptoms takes several days. Dysarthria is rare; ataxia mainly affects the trunk and gait, with a lesser degree of involvement in the individual limbs. The CSF protein could be higher. Rare as it is, respiratory insufficiency typically resolves over the course of weeks to months with a gradual and often total recovery.

4.3.2. Chronic Disorders

- **Vestibular Migraine:** Episodic vertigo that coexists with other migraine attack symptoms like headache, photophobia, phonophobia, or visual aura is known as vestibular migraine.
- **Multiple Sclerosis**
  - o **Pathogenesis:** Clinically, multiple sclerosis is defined by neurologic dysfunction that comes and goes at various sites in the central nervous system, including vestibular, cerebellar, and sensory pathways. White matter is primarily affected by demyelination and axonal loss, which are linked to symptoms and indicators.
  - o **Clinical Findings:** One of the most frequent observations is nystagmus. Vertigo happens less frequently and dysarthria more frequently. 10 to 15% of patients present with gait ataxia, which is typically the result of cerebellar involvement. Approximately one-third of patients have cerebellar signs at the time of initial examination, and twice as many patients eventually develop them. Leg ataxia is a common condition that typically affects both legs or all four limbs. It is typically bilateral.
  - o **Diagnosis:** A history of several episodes of neurologic dysfunction that were spaced apart in time is crucial to the diagnosis. Physical findings like optic neuritis, internuclear ophthalmoplegia, or pyramidal signs, as well as laboratory tests, may reveal subclinical lesions. Oligoclonal bands,

elevated IgG, increased protein, or a mild lymphocytic pleocytosis may all be seen in a CSF analysis. Subclinical sites of involvement can also be recorded using evoked responses that are visual, auditory, or somatosensory. MRI or CT scans reveal demyelination.

- **Alcoholic Cerebellar Degeneration**
  - **Pathogenesis:** Chronic alcoholics may develop a cerebellar syndrome due to nutritional deficiencies. Degenerative changes in the cerebellum typically occur in the superior vermis, which is also affected in Wernicke encephalopathy.
  - **Clinical Features:** The majority of cases of alcoholic cerebellar degeneration occur in men, and they typically start in the 40s to 60s. Patients usually have a history of eating inadequately and binge or daily drinking that has lasted for ten years or longer. The majority have also dealt with liver disease, delirium tremens, Wernicke encephalopathy, or polyneuropathy, among other medical consequences of alcoholism. Typically, the disorder begins slowly and worsens over several weeks to months before reaching a dysfunctional plateau. Ataxia can sometimes develop suddenly.

    All patients have some form of gait ataxia, which is nearly always the initial cause for medical attention. About 80% of patients have ataxic legs on the heel-knee-shin test (Figure 4.13).

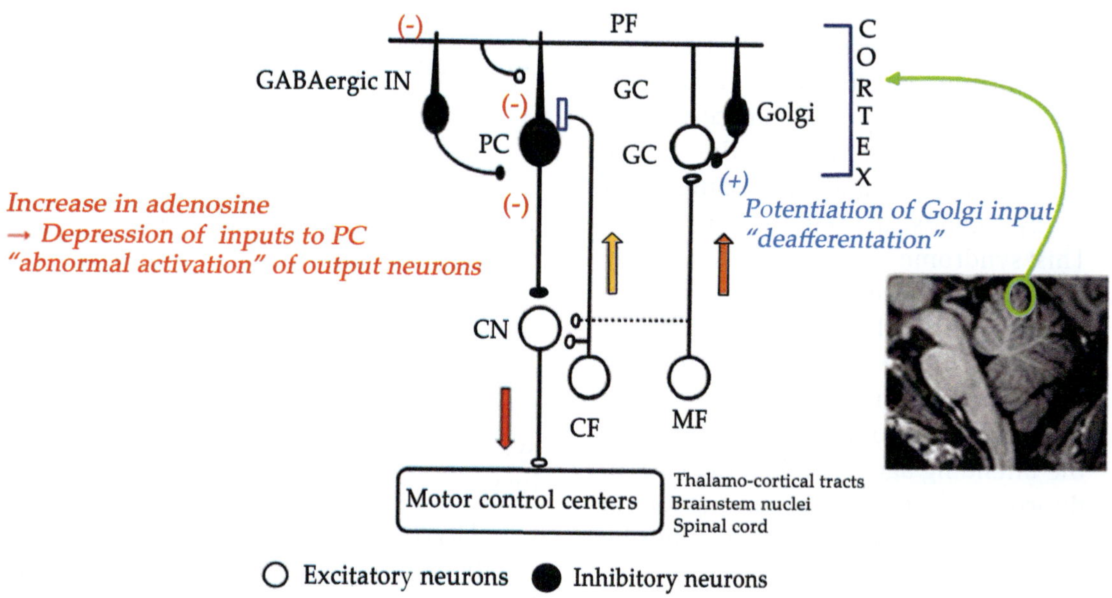

Figure 4.13. Distribution of disease in alcoholic cerebellar degeneration.

Key: MF, mossy fiber; CF, climbing fiber; GC, granule cell; Golgi, Golgi cell; PF, parallel fiber; GABAergic In, GABAergic interneurons; CN, cerebellar nucleus neurons.

Source: Mitoma H, Manto M, Shaikh AG. Mechanisms of Ethanol-Induced Cerebellar Ataxia: Underpinnings of Neuronal Death in the Cerebellum. *International Journal of Environmental Research and Public Health*. 2021; 18(16):8678. https://doi.org/10.3390/ijerph18168678.

Distal sensory deficits in the feet and absent ankle reflexes, resulting from polyneuropathy, are common associated findings. Less commonly occurring symptoms include truncal instability, dysarthria, hypotonia, nystagmus, and ataxia of the arms. Cerebellar atrophy may be seen on CT or MRI, however this is a nonspecific finding.

- o **Treatment:** Although there isn't a specific treatment for this syndrome, patients should take thiamine because it appears to play a role in the pathophysiology of Wernicke encephalopathy, which is closely related. Drinking no alcohol and eating a healthy diet may help stop the disease from progressing.

- **Toxin-Induced Cerebellar Degeneration:** The cerebellum's granule and Purkinje cells are particularly susceptible to different kinds of toxins. These may result in cerebellar degeneration that affects the limbs, trunk, and gait and is accompanied by nystagmus, dysarthria, and ataxia. This syndrome can also be caused by alcohol (discussed above), phenytoin, lithium, amiodarone, fluorouracil, cytarabine, toluene, lead, mercury, and thallium. Treatment for toxin-induced cerebellar syndromes involves stopping the offending agents and, in the case of fluorouracil, giving thiamine (vitamin B1). However, these effects may not be reversible (Figure 4.14).

- **Hypothyroidism:** A subacute or chronically progressive cerebellar syndrome, most common in middle-aged and older women, can be caused by hypothyroidism. The course of symptoms can take months or years. Myxedema and other systemic symptoms typically occur before the cerebellar disorder, though ataxia is sometimes the initial symptom to appear in patients.

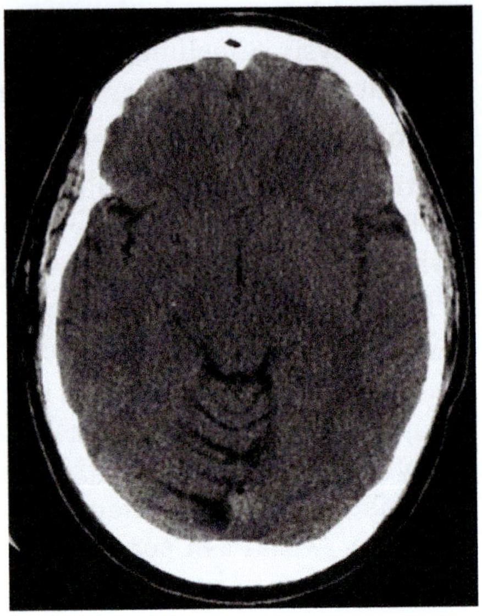

Figure 4.14. CT scan in alcoholic cerebellar degeneration, showing marked atrophy of the cerebellar vermis with relative sparing of the cerebellar hemispheres.

Source: Used with permission from A. Gean.

The most notable discovery is that gait ataxia is present in every population. Asymmetric limb ataxia is another common condition. Nystagmus and dysarthria are less common. Cerebellar involvement may coexist with other neurologic disorders associated with hypothyroidism, such as myopathy, carpal tunnel syndrome, neuropathy, or sensorineural hearing loss.

Thyroid hormone blood levels are lower in laboratory studies, while thyroid-stimulating hormone is elevated and CSF protein is frequently elevated.

When levothyroxine 25–50 μg is taken orally and gradually increased to 100–200 μg/d, replacement therapy typically results in a noticeable but partial improvement.

- **Paraneoplastic Cerebellar Degeneration**

- o **Pathogenesis:** Systemic cancer may

have distant (paraneoplastic) effects that include cerebellar degeneration. The most frequently associated neoplasms are small-cell lung cancer, ovarian cancer, breast cancer, and Hodgkin's disease.

The cerebellar vermis and hemispheres are diffusely affected by paraneoplastic degeneration. Since onconeural antibodies cross-react with antigens from tumor cells and cerebellar Purkinje cells, the pathogenic mechanism appears to be involved in many cases.

- **Clinical Findings:** Cerebellar symptoms usually take months to manifest and can occur either before or after systemic cancer diagnosis. Treatment for the underlying neoplasm has been shown to induce remission, despite the typical steady progression of the condition.

  The most common symptom is dysarthria, and prominent features include ataxia of the gait and limbs. There could be asymmetrical effects on the limbs. Nystagmus is not common. Other neurological system regions affected by paraneoplastic involvement may result in neuropathy, dysphagia, dementia, memory problems, or pyramidal signs.

- **Diagnosis:** Blood tests may occasionally reveal onconeural antibodies, such as those against Yo (ovarian and breast cancer), Hu (small-cell lung cancer), or Ri (breast cancer). Elevated protein or mild lymphocytic pleocytosis may be seen in the CSF.

  It is most challenging to diagnose paraneoplastic cerebellar degeneration when neurologic symptoms appear before underlying cancer is found. The recurrent occurrence of dysphagia and dysarthria serves to differentiate this illness from the cerebellar syndromes caused by hypothyroidism or chronic alcoholism. Arm ataxia further indicates that alcohol is not likely to be the cause. Because cancer patients are more likely to suffer from malnutrition, Wernicke encephalopathy should always be taken into consideration.

- **Treatment:** The treatment targets the underlying tumor and may involve immunotherapy (e.g., plasma exchange, methylprednisolone up to 1 g/dintravenously, prednisone 1 mg/kd/d orally, cyclophosphamide 2 mg/kg/d orally, or rituximab 375 mg/m2 intravenously monthly for 4 months). If necessary, immunotherapy is added to the treatment (Table 4.10).

Table 4.10. Onconeural Antibodies Reported in Research

Patient	Neurological syndrome	Tumor	Antibody	Expected result according to cancer type?
1	Alcoholic neuropathy	NSCLC	CV2 (CRMP5)	Yes
2	Brain metastasis	NSCLC	Yo (PCA1)	No
3	Neurotoxicity ICI	NSCLC	Yo (PCA1)	No
4	Subarachnoid hemorrhage	Ovary	Zic4	No
5	Decreased visual acuity	Ovary	Zic4	No
6	Myasthenia	Thymoma	CV2 (CRMP5)	Yes
7	Morvan syndrome	Thymoma	Yo (PCA1)	No
8	Seizures	Rectum	Yo (PCA1)	No
9	Neuroxicity ICI	Prostate	SOX1	No
10	Neuroxicity ICI	Melanoma	CV2 (CRMP5)	No
11	Decreased visual acuity	CUO	Zic4	No

CUO, carcinoma of unknown origin; ICI, immune checkpoint inhibitors.

Source: Ruiz-García R, Martínez-Hernández E, Saiz A, Dalmau J and Graus F (2020) The Diagnostic Value of Onconeural Antibodies Depends on How They Are Tested. Front. Immunol. 11:1482. doi: 10.3389/fimmu.2020.01482.

- **Autosomal Dominant Spinocerebellar Ataxia:** Spinocerebellar ataxia (SCA) is a collective term for a set of genetically and clinically diverse disorders.
  - **Genetics:** Autosomal dominant SCA can result from at least three different types of mutations: point mutations, expansion of tri- or pentanucleotide repeats in noncoding regions, and expansion of CAG trinucleotide repeats coding for polyglutamine (polyQ) tracts. The most prevalent and well-studied of these are the polyQ disorders, which impact a variety of proteins such as cytoskeletal proteins, enzymes, receptors, and ion channels.

    The underlying trinucleotide expansion in polyQ disorders is unstable and has a tendency to grow larger over time, which is a notable characteristic. This is consistent with the anticipation phenomenon, wherein in subsequent generations there is a decrease in the age at onset, an increase in the severity of the disease, or both.

    Huntington's disease and spinal bulbar muscular atrophy (Kennedy disease) are examples of polyQ disorders in addition to SCAs.
  - **Pathogenesis:** The target protein gains a toxic function as a result of PolyQ expansions. The protein is more susceptible to conformational changes, misfolding, and proteolytic cleavage because of its abnormally long polyQ tract. Consequently, this leads to the generation of protein fragments that have a propensity to aggregate and occasionally move from the cytoplasm into the nucleus. It is believed that a combination of poor proteosomal function, axonal transport, or nuclear function; protein-protein interactions; and direct toxicity of aberrant proteins or their cytoplasmic or nuclear aggregates can cause neuronal dysfunction and death.
  - **Clinical Findings:** Even within a single family, the autosomal dominant SCAs exhibit significant clinical variability. They are typically linked to a cerebellar syndrome that slowly progresses and develops in adults, with gait ataxia being a prominent early feature. Leg ataxia, diplopia, and dysarthria are additional symptoms. Cognitive, pyramidal, extrapyramidal, motor neuron, peripheral nerve, or macular involvement are examples of common extracerebellar findings.

    The SCAs 1, 2, 3, 6, and 7 are the most prevalent. SCA1 causes brainstem involvement, gait ataxia, limb ataxia, and dysarthria, but little cognitive abnormality. SCA2 is distinguished by its correlation with polyneuropathy and slow saccadic eye movements in ataxia and dysarthria. Patients with Portuguese ancestry are more likely to suffer from SCA3 (Machado-Joseph disease), which causes ataxia along with eyelid retraction, decreased blinking, external ophthalmoplegia, dysarthria, dysphagia, and occasionally parkinsonism or peripheral neuropathy. Compared to other SCAs, SCA6 is relatively less severe, advances more slowly, and is primarily limited to cerebellar involvement. SCA7 is characterized by ataxia as well as retinal degeneration that results in blindness.

Cerebellar atrophy and occasionally brainstem atrophy can be seen on CT or MRI scans. Genetic testing, however, provides a conclusive diagnosis. Although there isn't a specific treatment, genetic counseling may be necessary, as well as physical and occupational therapy, as well as ambulation aids.

- **Other Autosomal Dominant Cerebellar Ataxias**
  - **Dentatorubral Pallidoluysian Atrophy:** The dominantly inherited disorder known as dentatorubral pallidoluysian atrophy (DRPLA) is caused by a polyglutamine expansion in the ATN1 gene, which codes for the protein atrophin 1. Ataxia, chorea, dementia, seizures, and myoclonus are all caused by DRPLA. Movement Disorders, Chapter 11, discusses this disorder because of its prominent extrapyramidal features.
  - **Episodic Ataxias:** Autosomal dominant disorders known as episodic ataxias are typified by brief episodes of cerebellar ataxia that can be triggered by stress on the body or mind. Mutations in KCN1A, the gene encoding the Kv1.1 voltage-gated potassium channel, cause episodic ataxia 1 (EA1). Attacks can come in bursts of several minutes or longer, and in between they frequently cause myokymia, an involuntary trembling of the muscles. The α1A subunit of the P/Q-type voltage-gated calcium channel is encoded by the gene CACNA1A, which is also mutated in SCA6 and familial hemiplegic migraine. Mutations in this gene cause EA2. Attacks last for hours on average, longer than in EA2, and in between acute episodes, nystagmus and slowly worsening ataxia continue. Acetazolamide (500 mg taken orally four times per day) frequently prevents or alleviates EA2 acute symptoms. Similar to EA5, this mutation also affects voltage-gated calcium channels; however, in this instance, the β subunit is encoded by CACNB4. Mutations in SLC1A3, which codes for the glial glutamate

transporter EAAT1, cause EA6. Reduced glutamate uptake results in increased excitatory input to the Purkinje cells of the cerebellum. While EA2 involves haploinsufficiency, EA1 and EA6 are thought to impair channel function through dominant negative effects; the mechanism underlying EA5 is unknown (Figures 4.15–4.17).

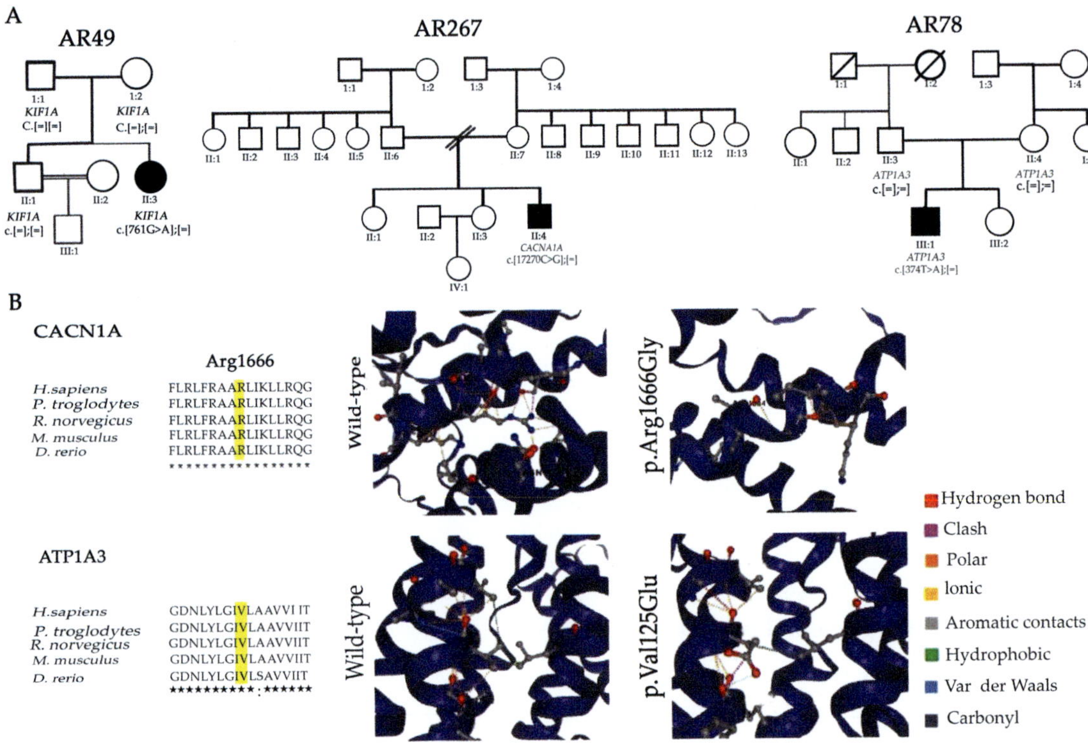

Figure 4.15. Genetic mechanisms in hereditary ataxias. Autosomal dominant ataxias include the spinocerebellar ataxias (SCAs), dentatorubral pallidoluysian atrophy (DRPLA), and the episodic ataxias (EAs). Autosomal recessive ataxias include Friedreich's ataxia (FA), fragile X–associated tremor-ataxia syndrome (FXTAS), and ataxia-telangiectasia (AT). Two distinctive modes of autosomal dominant inheritance are observed in some, but not all, SCAs. An example is pathologic expansion of a CAG trinucleotide repeat in the coding region of an affected gene, which is translated into an abnormally long polyglutamine (PolyQ) tract within the protein (e.g., SCA1, 2, 3, 6, 7, 8, 12, or 17). In another case, there is pathologic expansion of a tri- or pentanucleotide repeat in noncoding regions (NCRs) of the protein, which, although not translated, interferes with protein function (e.g., SCA8, 10, or 31). Two autosomal recessive ataxias, FA and FXTAS, also involve trinucleotide repeats in noncoding regions.

Source: Santos M, Damásio J, Carmona S, Neto JL, Dehghani N, Guedes LC, Barbot C, Barros J, Brás J, Sequeiros J, et al. Molecular Characterization of Portuguese Patients with Hereditary Cerebellar Ataxia. *Cells.* 2022; 11(6):981. https://doi.org/10.3390/cells11060981.

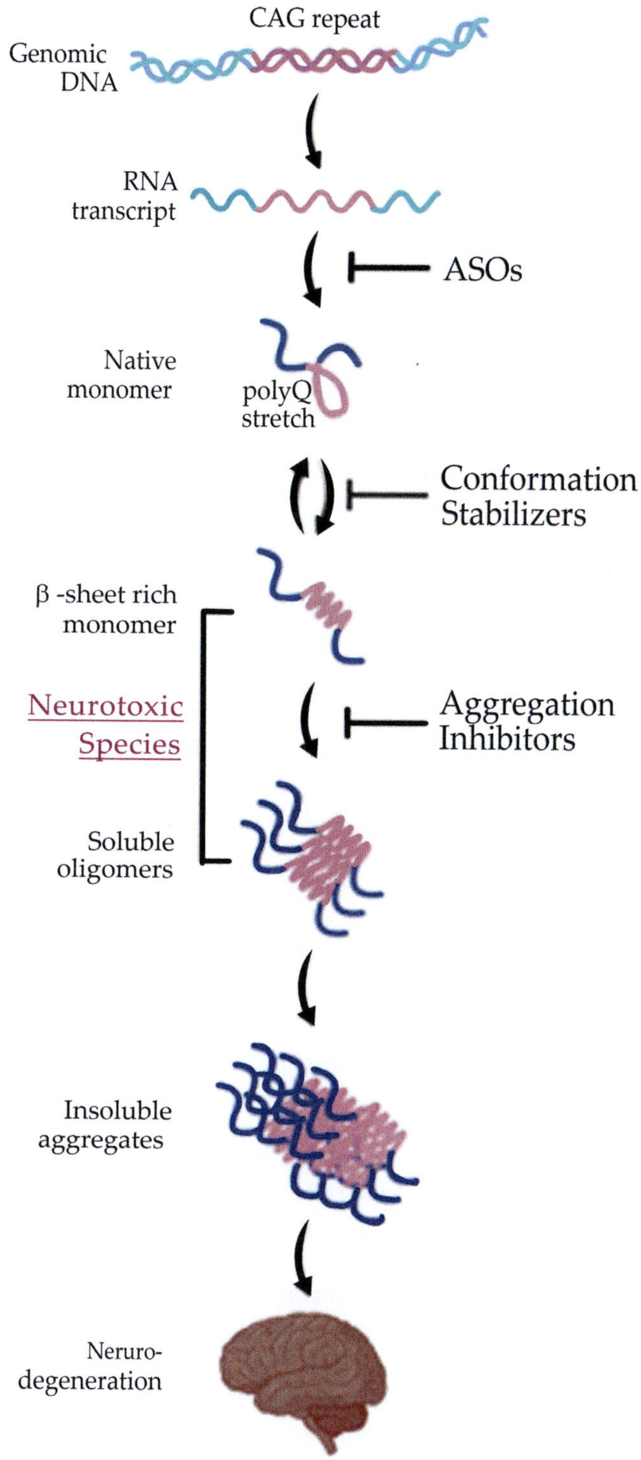
CAG repeat
Genomic DNA
RNA transcript
ASOs
Native monomer
polyQ stretch
Conformation Stabilizers
β -sheet rich monomer
Neurotoxic Species
Aggregation Inhibitors
Soluble oligomers
Insoluble aggregates
Neruro-degeneration

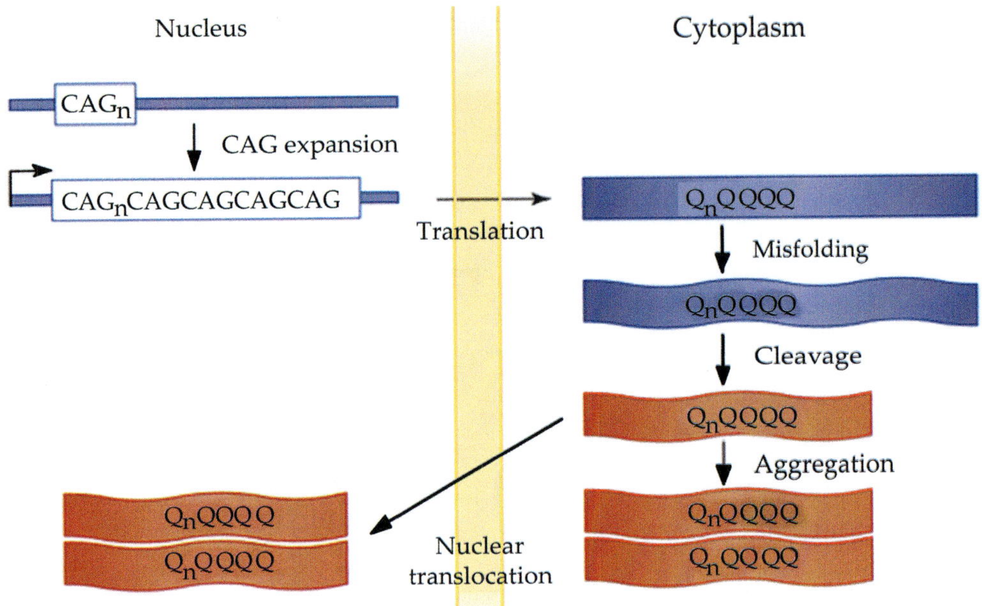

Figure 4.16. Proposed mechanisms of polyQ protein processing and toxicity. In polyQ diseases including several autosomal dominant spinocerebellar ataxias, a gene containing a CAG trinucleotide repeat (CAGn) undergoes mutation by expansion of the repeat. The resulting abnormal protein (QnQQQQ) contains an abnormally long polyQ tract, which induces conformational changes that promote misfolding. The misfolded protein is subject to proteolytic cleavage, which generates abnormal and possibly toxic fragments, which may also have an increased tendency to be translocated from the cytoplasm to the nucleus, to aggregate, or both. As a result of these events, neuronal function is impaired, and neurons may eventually die. How neurotoxicity and neuronal death ultimately occur is unknown, but there may be multiple mechanisms, and these may differ across polyQ diseases. Possible contributing factors include direct toxicity of misfolded and cleaved protein monomers or oligomers, or of cytoplasmic or nuclear aggregates; impaired proteosomal degradation, axonal transport, or nuclear function; and interactions between polyQ proteins and other cellular proteins.

Source: Minakawa EN and Nagai Y (2021) Protein aggregation inhibitors as disease-modifying therapies for polyglutamine diseases. Front. Neurosci. 15:621996. doi: 10.3389/fnins.2021.621996.

- **Ataxia-Telangiectasia**

o **Pathogenesis:** Louis-Bar syndrome, also referred to as ataxia-telangiectasia, is an inherited autosomal recessive illness that manifests in early childhood. The ataxia-telangiectasia mutated (ATM) gene, which codes for a serine/threonine protein kinase connected to phosphatidylinositol 3-kinase, is the source of the mutations that cause it to lose its function. There have been descriptions of substitutions, insertions, and deletions. There is a theory that pathogenesis is related to a malfunction in the repair of DNA double-strand breaks.

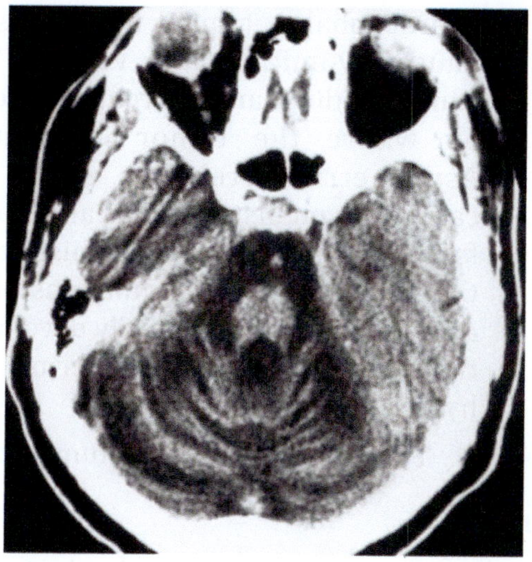

Figure 4.17. CT scan in spinocerebellar atrophy, showing an atrophic cerebellum and brainstem.

Source: Used with permission from A. Gean.

- **Clinical Findings:** Progressive cerebellar ataxia, oculocutaneous telangiectasia, lymphoid tumors, and sinopulmonary infections are the hallmarks of ataxia-telangiectasia. Each patient has a progressive pancerebellar degeneration with gait, limb, and trunk ataxia, dysarthria, and nystagmus. Almost universal findings include choreoathetosis, areflexia, disorders of voluntary eye movement, and loss of vibration and position sense in the legs. It is common to see mental deficiencies in the second decade of life.

  Teenage years are typically when oculocutaneous telangiectasia first manifests. First to be affected are usually the bulbar conjunctivae, then skin areas that have been exposed to the sun, such as the nose, ears, face, antecubital and popliteal fossae. The central nervous system is not affected by the vascular lesions, which hardly ever bleed.

  Immunologic impairment typically manifests later in childhood, with over 80% of patients experiencing recurrent sinus infections. Roughly one-third of patients experience malignancies, which include Hodgkin disease, leukemia, and non-Hodgkin lymphoma.

  Hypogonadism, insulin-resistant diabetes mellitus, and progeric changes in the skin and hair are other common clinical findings. The typical abnormalities observed in the laboratory include elevated levels of carcinoembryonic antigen and α-fetoprotein, as well as decreased levels of circulating IgG2, IgA, and IgE.

  Ataxia-telangiectasia is sometimes confused with Friedreich ataxia, another childhood condition because the vascular and immunologic manifestations appear later than the neurologic symptoms (see later). The early onset (before the age of 4) and absence of kyphoscoliosis, along with the associated choreoathetosis, are characteristics that set ataxia-telangiectasia apart.

  Antibiotics are helpful in the management of infections, but there is no specific treatment for ataxia-telangiectasia. Because this disorder is associated with hypersensitivity to ionizing radiation, X-rays should be avoided.

- **Wilson Disease:** Wilson disease is a disorder of copper metabolism characterized by copper deposition in various tissues, which can cause cerebellar symptoms. Wilson disease arises from mutations in the ATP7B gene, which codes for the β polypeptide of an ATPase that transports copper. It is an autosomal recessive disorder. because the most noticeable neurologic symptoms are typically extrapyramidal.

- **Creutzfeldt-Jakob Disease:** Amnesia is a prion disease that results in dementia. Approximately 60% of patients exhibit cerebellar signs, and 10% of patients exhibit ataxia at presentation. Although there is diffuse cerebellar involvement, the vermis is frequently most severely affected. The loss of Purkinje cells is usually less noticeable than the depletion of granule cells, in contrast to most other cerebellar disorders.

  The primary complaint of patients with cerebellar manifestations of Creutzfeldt-Jakob disease is usually ataxia of the gait. This is typically when dementia becomes apparent, and cognitive dysfunction always appears at some point. About 50% of patients with the ataxic form of Creutzfeldt-Jakob disease initially exhibit nystagmus, dysarthria, truncal ataxia, and limb ataxia. Progressive dementia, myoclonus, and extrapyramidal and pyramidal dysfunction are the hallmarks of the course. Usually, death happens a year after onset.

- **Posterior Fossa Tumors:** When posterior fossa tumors originate in the cerebellum or compress it from the outside, they result in cerebellar symptoms. Astrocytomas and medulloblastomas are the most common types of cerebellar tumors in children, while adult patients are more likely to have metastases from primary sites outside the nervous system (Table 4.11).

  - **Clinical Findings:** Individuals with ataxia or headaches from elevated intracranial pressure are often diagnosed with cerebellar tumors. Common side effects include hydrocephalus, cranial nerve palsies, nausea, vomiting, and vertigo. The clinical findings are different depending on where the tumor is located. Asymmetric cerebellar signs are caused by metastases that are mostly found in the cerebellar hemispheres. On the other hand, medulloblastomas and ependymomas typically develop in the midline, involving the vermis and hydrocephalus early on.

Table 4.11. Tumors of the Cerebellum

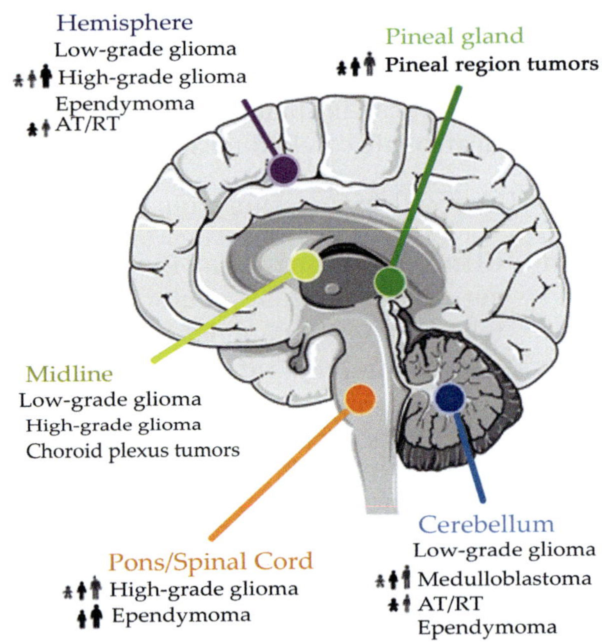

Source: Borgenvik A, Čančer M, Hutter S and Swartling FJ (2021) Targeting MYCN in Molecularly Defined Malignant Brain Tumors. Front. Oncol. 10:626751. doi: 10.3389/fonc.2020.626751.

  - **Diagnosis and Treatment:** The CT scan or MRI is very helpful for diagnosis, as it is with most brain tumors; however, a biopsy may be necessary for histologic characterization. Chemotherapy, radiation, and surgical resection are among the available treatment options. Corticosteroids are helpful in the management of edema caused by tumors.

§ **Metastases:** Cerebellar tumors most commonly occur from the lung and breast and less frequently from other sites, especially in adults. When the patient first exhibits symptoms of involvement of the central nervous system, the location of the primary tumor may or may not be visible. A diagnosis may be reached by a thorough examination of the breasts and skin, a chest X-ray, a urinalysis, and tests to see if there is any occult blood in the stool. Patients with cerebellar metastases typically have a worse prognosis than those with supratentorial lesions. Individuals with primary lung tumors typically have a shorter survival time than those with breast carcinoma.

§ Cerebellar astrocytomas typically affect patients between the ages of 2 and 20, though they can also affect those who are older. These tumors frequently have a cystic appearance and are histologically benign. Increased intracranial pressure symptoms, such as headache and vomiting, usually appear several months before cerebellar dysfunction manifests. Cerebellar astrocytoma may be curable if total surgical resection is achievable.

§ In children, medulloblastoma is common; in adults, it is rare. These tumors seem to arise from dorsal brainstem progenitor cells with activating mutations in the Wnt pathway or cerebellar granule neuron progenitor cells with activating mutations in the Hedgehog signaling pathway. Compared to astrocytomas, medulloblastomas are typically extremely malignant. They may metastasize outside of the nervous system and frequently spread through the ventricles and subarachnoid space. Adult-onset medulloblastomas typically arise laterally, while the majority of childhood medulloblastomas are located in the midline. Symptoms such as headache, vomiting, ataxia, and visual impairment are frequently observed. The majority of tumors are located in one hemisphere, so hemiataxia is a common finding in adults. Other common symptoms include neck stiffness, nystagmus, papilledema, facial palsy, and ataxia of the gait. Within a few months of diagnosis, medulloblastoma results in death if left untreated. Years of survival may be extended with treatment that includes decompression, craniospinal irradiation, and partial surgical resection. Being female and having the tumors develop in adulthood are favorable prognostic factors.

§ Vestibular nerve dysfunction has previously been linked to acoustic neuromas. In addition to the initial symptoms of vertigo and hearing loss, growth of these or other less common tumors of the cerebellopontine angle may cause compression of the ipsilateral cerebellar hemisphere, leading to hemiataxia. Histologically benign, these tumors are frequently completely curable.

§ An uncommon benign tumor that typically affects adults is called hemangioblastoma. It can be a singular anomaly or a characteristic of the dominantly mutated VHL tumor suppressor gene-causing von Hippel-Lindau disease. Von Hippel-Lindau disease is associated with retinal hemangioblastoma, kidney, pancreatic, or other visceral cysts, and polycythemia. Patients usually arrive with headaches, and papilledema, nystagmus, and ataxia are frequently found on examination. Resection surgery is used as treatment.

§ Nine percent of all meningiomas are posterior fossa meningiomas. These benign tumors, which originate from the meninges' arachnoidal cap cells, compress the cerebellum indirectly. In decreasing order of frequency, the posterior surface of the petrous bone, the tentorium cerebelli, the clivus, the cerebellar convexities, and the foramen magnum are the locations of posterior fossa meningiomas. Although tumors of the cerebellopontine angle or clivus may draw attention when they cause symptoms related to the brainstem or cranial nerve, meningiomas typically grow slowly and manifest as headaches. Complete surgical resection is curative when feasible.

§ The walls or choroid plexus of the fourth ventricle are where ependymomas most frequently originate. These are malignant tumors, similar to medulloblastomas, that usually affect children and spread through the ventricular system.

Their position results in early hydrocephalus; cerebellar signs from compression appear later or as mild symptoms. Survival may be extended by surgical resection, craniospinal irradiation, and shunting procedures to relieve hydrocephalus; however, postoperative recurrences and tumor dissemination are frequent.

- **Posterior Fossa Malformations:** Adults who have developmental abnormalities affecting the brainstem and cerebellum may experience vestibular or cerebellar symptoms. The most common cause of this is type I (adult) Arnold-Chiari malformation, which is characterized by the cerebellar tonsils being displaced downward through the foramen magnum. Clinical manifestations of this malformation include brainstem compression, obstructive hydrocephalus, cerebellar involvement, and syringomyelia (a spinal cord cyst, or syrinx). The onset of type II Arnold-Chiari malformation occurs in childhood and is linked to meningomyelocele, which is the protrusion of the spinal cord, nerve roots, and meninges through a fusion defect in the vertebral column.

When cerebellar ataxia occurs in a type I malformation, it typically affects one side of the gait and can occasionally be asymmetric. Hypertension causes vertigo and headaches. Vertigo, nystagmus, and lower cranial nerve palsies may be caused by herniated cerebellar tissue compressing the brainstem. Defective pain and temperature perception are usually distributed in a cape-like manner in cases of syringomyelia. Cerebellar tonsillar herniation seen in CT or MRI scans can be used to diagnose Arnold-Chiari malformation. Surgical decompression of the foramen magnum may be beneficial for patients experiencing headache, neck pain, hydrocephalus, or other symptoms associated with compression of the cerebellum or brainstem. Anticonvulsants and antidepressants may help with neuropathic pain.

4.4. Sensory Ataxias

Usually, lesioning of the dorsal root ganglia (sensory neuronopathy), posterior columns of the spinal cord (myelopathy), or peripheral sensory nerves (sensory neuropathy) results in impaired proprioceptive sensation and sensory ataxia. Clinical manifestations include a slapping or steppage gait, abnormal joint position and vibration sense in the legs and occasionally the arms, and an unstable stance with the Romberg sign.

4.4.1. Sensory Neuropathy or Neuronopathy

Ataxia can be a presenting symptom of sensory neuronopathies (which target dorsal root ganglia) and polyneuropathies that affect large myelinated sensory fibers. Well-known instances include the Fisher variation of Guillain-Barré syndrome, high-dose pyridoxine-induced sensory neuronopathy, and Hu antibody-positive sensory neuronopathy linked to small-cell lung cancer.

4.4.2. Combined Lesions

There are various diseases that can impact both peripheral and central sensory pathways. Examples include neurosyphilis (tabes dorsalis) and combined systems disease from vitamin B12 deficiency, which are explored in other discussions as potential causes of dementia or sensory issues (Table 4.12).

Table 4.12. Causes of Sensory Ataxia

Sensory neuropathy or neuronopathy[1]
Cyanide (cassava plant) poisoning
Dejerine-Sottas disease (HMSN[2] type III)
Diphtheria (delayed radiculoneuropathy)
Immune-mediated neuropathies (GALOP syndrome, anti-MAG antibody syndrome, Miller Fisher syndrome, anti-GD1b antibody syndrome)
Isoniazid
Paraneoplastic sensory neuronopathy (anti-Hu antibodies)
Platinum analogs (cisplatin, carboplatin, oxaliplatin)
Podophyllin poisoning (including etoposide)
Pyridoxine (vitamin B_6) overuse
Refsum disease
Sensory ataxic neuropathy (autosomal dominant)
Sensory ataxic neuropathy with dysarthria and ophthalmoparesis (autosomal recessive)
Taxol
Myelopathy[3]
Acute transverse myelitis
HIV disease (vacuolar myelopathy)
Multiple sclerosis
Tumor or cord compression
Vascular malformations
Combined lesions
Friedreich ataxia
Neurosyphilis (tabes dorsalis)
Nitrous oxide
Vitamin B_{12} deficiency
Vitamin E deficiency (including abetalipoproteinemia)

[1]Involving large, myelinated sensory fibers.
[2]Hereditary motor and sensory neuropathy.
[3]Involving posterior columns.

Source: https://dl.mehrsys.ir/pdf-books/Clinical%20Neurology%209%20Edition%20(www.myuptodate.com).pdf.

4.4.3. Friedreich Ataxia

The most common cause of hereditary ataxia is a childhood-onset autosomal recessive disorder called Friedreich ataxia. It is caused by a large GAA trinucleotide repeat in the noncoding region of the FXN gene, which results in the loss of the functional mitochondrial protein frataxin. Dorsal root ganglia degeneration, large myelinated axons of peripheral sensory nerves, corticospinal tracts, and dentate nuclei of the cerebellum are the main pathologic findings. The spinocerebellar tracts, posterior columns, and dorsal nucleus of Clarke are also secondary findings.

4.4.3.1. Clinical Findings

While around 13 years is the average onset age, and earlier onset is correlated with longer GAA repeats. Progressive gait ataxia is typically the first symptom, followed by limb ataxia, dysarthria, and sensory gait ataxia. A neurologic examination reveals extensor plantar responses, leg (and occasionally arm) weakness, impaired joint position and vibration sense, and knee and ankle areflexia. Pes cavus, or high-arched feet with toe clawing from intrinsic foot muscle weakness and wasting, is a common condition but can also arise in other neurologic disorders (Charcot-Marie-Tooth disease, for example).

Chronic restrictive lung disease may result from severe progressive kyphoscoliosis. Arrhythmia, congestive heart failure, and even death are possible outcomes of cardiomyopathy. Diabetes mellitus and optic atrophy-related visual impairment are additional abnormalities (Figure 4.18).

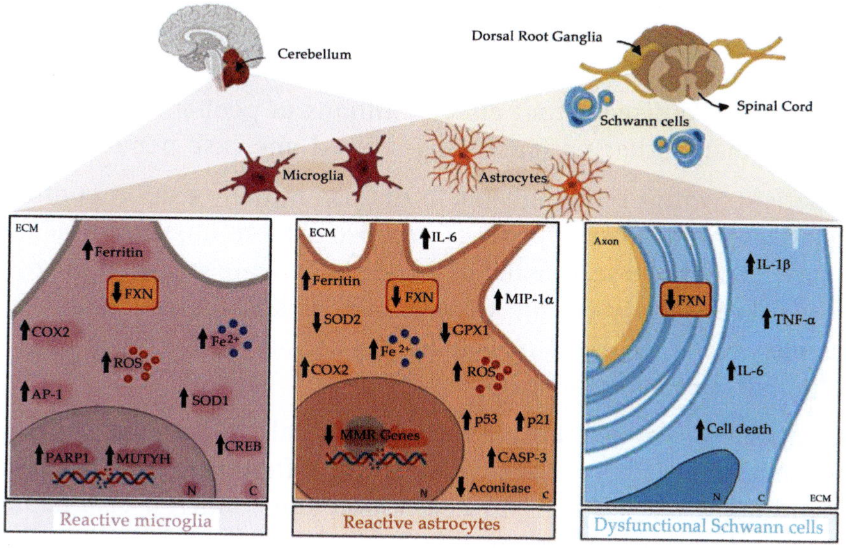

Figure 4.18. Principal sites in disorders producing sensory ataxia.

Source: Apolloni S, Milani M, D'Ambrosi N. Neuroinflammation in Friedreich's Ataxia. *International Journal of Molecular Sciences*. 2022; 23(11):6297. https://doi.org/10.3390/ijms23116297.

As Friedreich's ataxia presents with prominent sensory impairment, areflexia, skeletal abnormalities, and cardiomyopathy, it can typically be distinguished from other cerebellar and spinocerebellar degenerations. Genetic testing provides the final diagnosis.

4.4.3.2. Treatment and Prognosis

As of right now, Friedreich's ataxia's neurological symptoms have no known cure. Idebenone, an antioxidant, might help with the related cardiomyopathy. Orthopedic devices or procedures can help with gait disorders and kyphoscoliosis. The average length of the illness's symptoms is about 25 years, and the average age of death is about 40 years. The most common causes of death are infections and cardiomyopathy.

A Closer Look

Creutzfeldt-Jakob Disease

It is a human prion disease, is called classic CJD. It is a neurodegenerative illness with recognizable symptoms in both diagnosis and treatment. This illness always has a fatal outcome and advances quickly. This disease usually results in death within a year of the onset of illness.

The neurodegenerative illness known as Creutzfeldt-Jakob disease (CJD) progresses quickly and is always fatal. It is thought to be caused by an aberrant form of the prion protein, a cellular glycoprotein. Globally, CJD is a disease that affects millions of people, with estimates of its yearly incidence in the US and many other nations being around one case per million.

About 70% of patients with Creutzfeldt-Jakob disease initially exhibit confusion and memory loss, which all patients eventually experience; 15 to 20% exhibit ataxia and incoordination, which frequently appear early in the disease. Usually in the middle to late stages of the disease, myoclonus triggered by noise or other sensory stimuli (also known as startle myoclonus) manifests. Instead of memory loss, people with vCJD exhibit psychiatric symptoms (such as depression and anxiety). Both forms share similar later symptoms.

While dementia, ataxia, and myoclonus are the most typical symptoms of sCJD, other neurological issues such as hallucinations, seizures, neuropathy, and different movement disorders may also be present. Ocular problems like visual field defects, diplopia, blurred vision, and visual agnosia are frequently seen in individuals with sCJD.

Since there is no known cure for transmissible CJD, prevention is crucial. Wearing gloves and avoiding contact with mucous membranes is required for personnel handling tissues and fluids from patients suspected of having CJD. Skin that has become contaminated can be cleaned by applying four percent sodium hydroxide for five to ten minutes, then thoroughly washing with water.

Materials coming into contact with tissues from patients with suspected or confirmed CJD should be steam autoclaved for one hour at 132°C, or submerged in 1 N (normal) or 10% sodium hypochlorite solution for one hour. Conventional sterilization techniques, such as formalin exposure, don't work.

Summary

- Diseases affecting the cerebellum, peripheral or central vestibular pathways, or proprioceptive sensory pathways can cause disorders of equilibrium.
- The vestibular division of the vestibulocochlear (VIII) nerve or the inner ear labyrinth are both impacted by peripheral vestibular lesions.
- Incoordination or clumsiness in movement that is not caused by weak muscles is known as ataxia.
- Vertigo symptoms could be useful in locating the location of the causing lesion. A problem with the peripheral vestibular apparatus (labyrinth or vestibulocochlear [VIII] nerve) is strongly suggested by hearing loss or tinnitus.
- Orthostatic hypotension is associated with tabes dorsalis, polyneuropathies, and spinocerebellar degenerations.
- An acute confusional state accompanied by ataxia may indicate Wernicke encephalopathy, ethanol or sedative drug intoxication.
- Vestibular disease is usually associated with abnormalities of extraocular (III, IV, and VI) and vestibulocochlear (VIII) nerve function, which frequently coexist with cerebellar lesions.
- Joint position sense is always compromised in the legs and may be compromised in the arms in cases of sensory ataxia.
- The Nylen-Bárány or Dix-Hallpike maneuver can help distinguish between peripheral and central causes of positional vertigo during a physical examination.
- Vertigo, nausea, and vomiting with an acute onset that usually lasts up to two weeks are the hallmarks of the disorder.
- Acoustic neuromas typically appear as solitary lesions in individuals between the ages of 30 and 60, although they can also be a sign of neurofibromatosis.
- Nystagmus, dysarthria, and ataxia of the limbs and gait are examples of pancreas dysfunction, which is a common side effect of ethanol, sedative-hypnotics, anticonvulsants, and hallucinogens.

References

1. Anheim, M., Tranchant, C., & Koenig, M. (2012). The autosomal recessive cerebellar ataxias. *New England Journal of Medicine, 366*, 636–646.
2. Baloh, R. W., Honrubia, V., & Kerber, K. A. (2010). Baloh and Honrubia's Clinical Neurophysiology of the Vestibular System (4th ed.). New York, NY, Oxford: Contemporary Neurology Series.
3. Choi, K. D., Lee, H., & Kim, J. S. (2013). Vertigo in brainstem and cerebellar strokes. *Current Opinion in Neurology, 26*, 90–95.
4. Connor, S. E., & Sriskandan, N. (2014). Imaging of dizziness. *Clinical Radiology, 69*, 111–122.
5. Fife, T. D., & Giza, C. (2013). Posttraumatic vertigo and dizziness. *Seminars in Neurology, 33*, 238–243.

6. Furman, J. M., Marcus, D. A., & Balaban, C. D. (2013). Vestibular migraine: clinical aspects and pathophysiology. *Lancet Neurology, 12*, 706–715.

7. Grazzi, L., & Andrasik, F. (2012). Headaches and Arnold-Chiari syndrome: when to suspect and how to investigate. *Current Pain and Headache Reports, 16*, 350–353.

8. Greenlee, J. E. (2013). Treatment of paraneoplastic cerebellar degeneration. *Current Treatment Options in Neurology, 15*, 185–200.

9. Isenberg-Grzeda, E., Kutner, H. E., & Nicolson, S. E. (2012). Wernicke-Korsakoff-syndrome: under-recognized and under-treated. *Psychosomatics, 53*, 507–516.

10. Jeong, S. H., Kim, H. J., & Kim, J. S. (2013). Vestibular neuritis. Seminars in Neurology, 33, 185–194.

11. Kim, J. S., & Zee, D. S. (2014). Benign paroxysmal positional vertigo. *New England Journal of Medicine, 370*, 1138–1147.

12. Liktor, B., Szekanecz, Z., Batta, T. J., Sziklai, I., & Karosi, T. (2013). Perspectives of pharmacological treatment in otosclerosis. *European Archives of Oto-Rhino-Laryngology, 270*, 793–804.

13. Lin, A. L., & Gutmann, D. H. (2013). Advances in the treatment of neurofibromatosis-associated tumors. *Nature Reviews Clinical Oncology, 10*, 616–624.

14. Magaña, J. J., Velázquez-Pérez, L., & Cisneros, B. (2013). Spinocerebellar ataxia type 2: clinical presentation, molecular mechanisms, and therapeutic perspectives. *Molecular Neurobiology, 47*, 90–104.

15. McKinnon, P. J. (2012). ATM and the molecular pathogenesis of ataxia telangiectasia. *Annual Review of Pathology, 7*, 303–321.

16. Molnar, A., & McGee, S. (2014). Diagnosing and treating dizziness. *Medical Clinics of North America, 98*, 583–596.

17. Orr, H. T. (2012). Cell biology of spinocerebellar ataxia. *Journal of Cell Biology, 197*, 167–177.

18. Parkinson, M. H., Boesch, S., Nachbauer, W., Mariotti, C., & Giunti, P. (2013). Clinical features of Friedreich's ataxia: classical and atypical phenotypes. *Journal of Neurochemistry, 126* (suppl 1), 103–117.

19. Soto-Varela, A., Rossi-Izquierdo, M., Sánchez-Sellero, I., & Santos-Pérez, S. (2013). Revised criteria for suspicion of non-benign positional vertigo. *QJM: An International Journal of Medicine, 106*, 317–321.

20. Strupp, M., & Brandt, T. (2013). Peripheral vestibular disorders. *Current Opinion in Neurology, 26*, 81–89.

21. Syed, I., & Aldren, C. (2012). Meniere's disease: an evidence-based approach to assessment and management. *International Journal of Clinical Practice, 66*, 166–170.

22. van Gaalen, J., & van de Warrenburg, B. P. (2012). A practical approach to late-onset cerebellar ataxia: putting the disorder with lack of order into order. *Practical Neurology, 12*, 14–24.

23. Venti, M. (2012). Cerebellar infarcts and hemorrhages. *Frontiers in Neurology and Neuroscience, 30*, 171–175.

Chapter

DEMENTIA AND AMNESTIC DISORDERS

5

Contents

Introduction

Memory, thinking, behavior, and the capacity to carry out daily tasks are all negatively impacted by dementia and amnestic disorders, which pose serious obstacles to cognitive health. A decline in cognitive function that goes beyond what is typical of normal aging is what defines dementia, a general term covering a range of progressive neurological conditions. Frontotemporal dementia, Lewy body dementia, vascular dementia, and Alzheimer's disease are among the common varieties. Contrarily, amnestic disorders specifically impair memory function, making it difficult to learn, retain, and recall information. Transient global amnesia, one of the most well-known amnestic disorders, is characterized by abrupt, transient memory loss that is frequently caused by stress or other factors. These illnesses have a substantial impact on individuals as well as their families and caregivers. To give affected people the right care and support and enhance their quality of life, it is essential to comprehend the underlying causes, risk factors, diagnostic standards, and available treatments for dementia and amnestic disorders. The management of these disorders and the reduction of their negative effects on cognitive function and general well-being depend heavily on early detection and intervention techniques.

Orientation and Directional Terms

Term	Definition	Illustration
Pseudodementia	Pseudodementia is a term used to describe cognitive impairment that occurs with psychiatric disorders, such as depression and schizophrenia, and mimics neurodegenerative disorders.	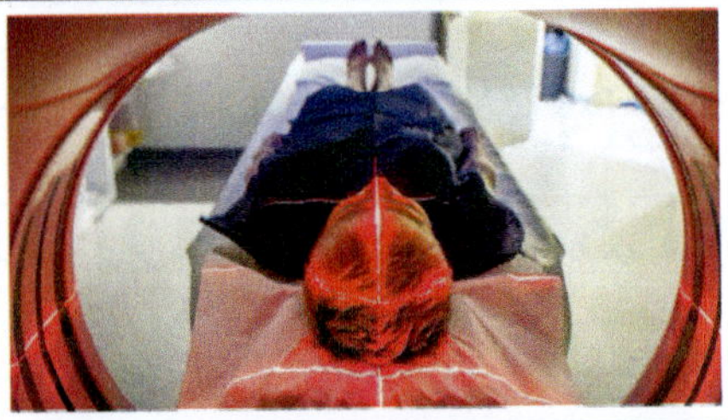
Frontotemporal dementia	Frontotemporal dementia (FTD) is a group of disorders that affect the brain's frontal and temporal lobes, causing them to shrink.	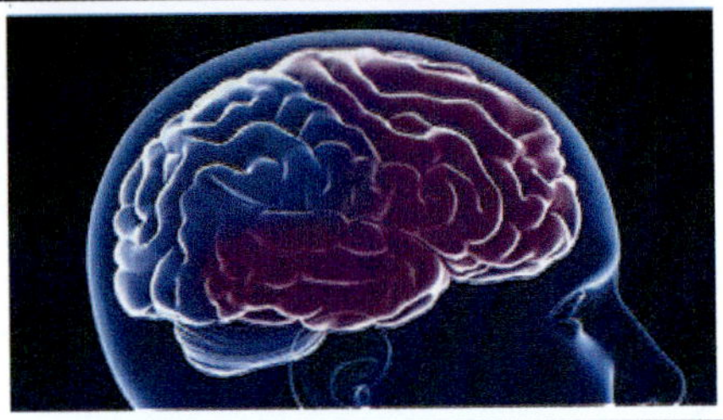
Lewy body dementia	Lewy body dementia (LBD) is a disease associated with abnormal deposits of a protein called alpha-synuclein in the brain.	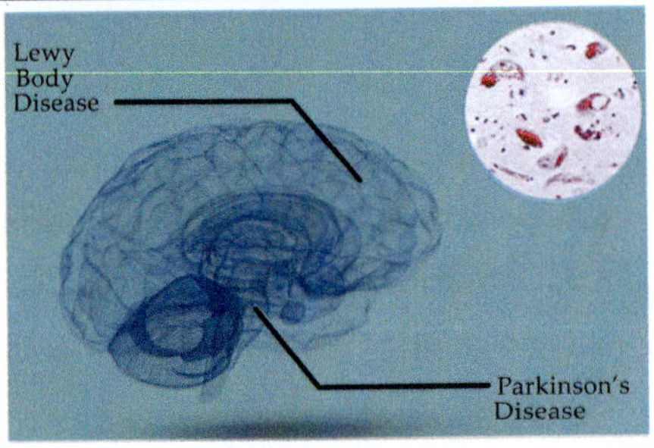
Erythematosus	Erythematosus is a term that refers to the reddish color of facial lesions caused by lupus, also known as systemic lupus erythematosus (SLE).	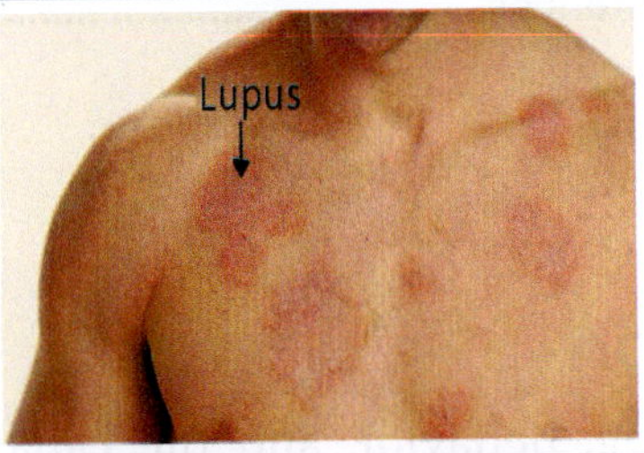
Bradykinesia	Bradykinesia is a symptom of Parkinson's disease that causes slow movement, or progressive hesitations or halts as movements continue.	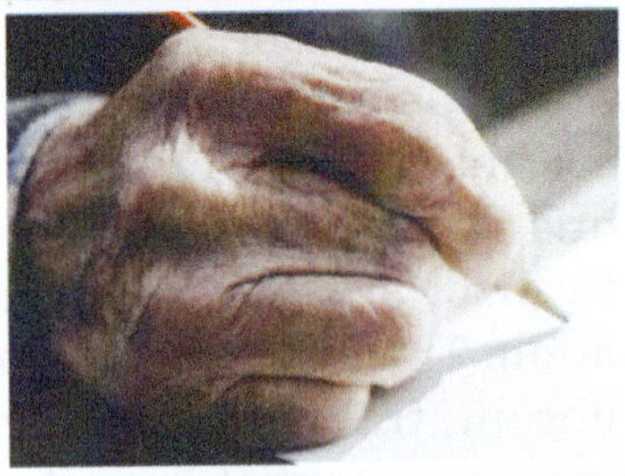

5.1. Dementia Approach to Diagnosis

A generalized, acquired, and typically progressive impairment of cognitive function is called dementia. In contrast to other cognitive dysfunction disorders like coma or confusional states, dementia preserves the patient's level of consciousness, or arousal. While dementia is more common as people age (Figure 5.1), diseases affecting the cerebral cortex, its subcortical connections, or both can cause dementia instead of being an inevitable byproduct of aging. Normal aging can be linked to small changes in neurologic function (Table 5.1) as well as neuroanatomical changes, like enlargement of the cerebral ventricles and cortical sulci observed on magnetic resonance imaging (MRI) or computed tomography (CT) scans (Figure 5.2). These, however, do not point to dementia. When deficits are more severe than typically seen with normal aging but not so severe as to warrant a diagnosis of dementia, the term mild cognitive impairment (MCI) is sometimes used. Nevertheless, the chance of developing dementia is higher in patients with motor cortex injury (MCI)—roughly 10% annually.

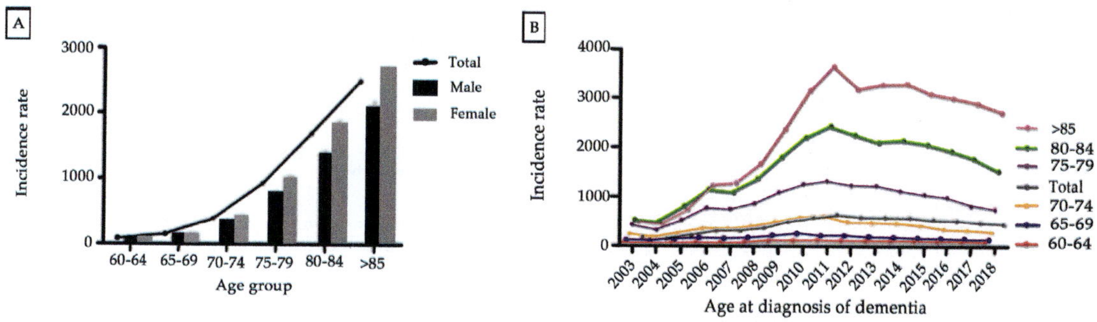

Figure 5.1. Relationship between advancing age and incidence and prevalence of dementia.

Source: Kwon HS, Jeong YW, Kim SH, Park KH, Seo SW, Na HR, Koh S-H, Shim Y, Park MH, Chin J, et al. Annual Incidence of Dementia from 2003 to 2018 in Metropolitan Seoul, Korea: A Population-Based Study. *Journal of Clinical Medicine*. 2022; 11(3):819. https://doi.org/10.3390/jcm11030819.

Smaller-scale cognitive disorders can also happen, as opposed to dementia, which affects various domains of cognitive function. These include deficiencies in motor function (apraxia), sensory integration, or language function (aphasia). This chapter covers memory disturbance, also known as amnestic disorder or amnesia, which is another example of a limited cognitive deficit. Both dementia and normal aging can cause memory impairments; however, in dementia the impairment is more severe and comes with deficits in behavior, reasoning, judgment, and language, among other areas. Certain causes of dementia, most notably Alzheimer's disease, result in a disproportionately early loss of memory and can be hard to differentiate from a simple amnestic condition, at least in the early stages of the condition.

Determining the nature of the issue, which should be categorized as impacting either the content or the level of consciousness (confusional state or coma), is the first step in assessing a patient with cognitive impairment of any kind. Key differences that could help in this distinction-making are listed in Table 5.2. A global cognitive disorder (dementia) should be differentiated from a more focused deficit, like amnesia or aphasia, if the content of consciousness is compromised. This distinction is crucial because the diagnostic strategy is determined by the disorder's classification.

Differentiating dementia from pseudodementia, a psychiatric disorder, can be challenging in certain situations. Finding the precise cause is the last stage in diagnosing dementia or amnestic syndrome. Even intractable causes can have value in being found, even though the main focus should be on treating them. Although only about 10% of dementias are currently curable, the amount of improvement that can be achieved in these cases in terms of both quality and length of life makes the time and money spent finding them worthwhile. A diagnosis may also be necessary in cases of incurable illnesses to inform the patient and family about the prognosis or genetic counseling or to notify medical professionals and family members of the possibility of a transmissible disease.

5.1.1. History

Since dementia is characterized by a decline in cognitive function, it's critical to demonstrate that the patient's level of functioning has decreased. The time course of deterioration; related symptoms like headache, gait disturbance, or incontinence; a family history of a similar condition; coexisting medical conditions; and the use of alcohol and drugs for therapeutic or recreational purposes are some of the data that can be used to determine the cause of dementia (Table 5.3).

Table 5.1. Neurologic Changes in Normal Aging

Gross changes		**Microscopic changes**
Structural Aging • Volume loss • Neurodegeneration in the GM, Demyelination in the WM, Ventricular enlargement • Sulci widening • Cerebrovascular diseases		• Lipofuscin accumulation • Neurofibrillary tangles, amyloid plaque formation • Dendritic tree decrease, axon number decreases, demyelination
Acetylcholine	**Monoamine**	**Neurosteroid**
Biochemical and Metabolic Aging • Dysfunction in the cholinergic system: memory decline • Nicotinic binding ability lost • Nicotinic acetylcholine receptors decrease	• Disturbed dopaminergic pathway • Disturbed serotonergic pathway • Decreased receptors and binding ability	• Decreased testosterone disturbs BBB, and invoke inflammation activity • Decreased androgen and estrogen reduce receptor expression and synapse density.
Changes in the nucleus	**Mitochondrial dysfunction**	**Accumulation of oxidatively damaged molecules**
Cellular and Molecular aging • Alteration in gene expression • Decrease in synaptic function • Increase in stress responses • Telomere shortening	• mtDNA damage • Disturbed ATP production • Apoptosis induced	• ETC damage • Lipid, protein DNA/RNA damage • Disturb cellular metabolic pathway or homeostasis
Impaired lysosome and proteosome function	**Electrophysiological Changes in the Brain by Aging**	**Dysregulation of neuronal calcium homeostasis**
• Autophagy and UPS reduction • Increase cellular wastes	• AP threshold changes: changes in voltage-gated Na^+ channel activation prperties and subtypes expression pattern. • AP amplitude decrease. • AP axonal conduction rate decrease	• Plasma membrane proteins: - Decreased NMDAR function - Post-translational alterations in receptors - Increased VDCC number • Changes in Ca^{2+} influx and disturb cellular Ca^{2+}homeostasis - Cellular organelles - Mitochondria : Depolarization disturbs electrochemical gradients - ER : Ca^{2+}regulating receptors changes. : Changes in calcium-binding protein : Decreased expression and disturbs Ca^{2+}buffering

Source: Lee J and Kim H-J (2022) Normal Aging Induces Changes in the Brain and Neurodegeneration Progress: Review of the Structural, Biochemical, Metabolic, Cellular, and Molecular Changes. Front. Aging Neurosci. 14:931536. doi: 10.3389/fnagi.2022.931536.

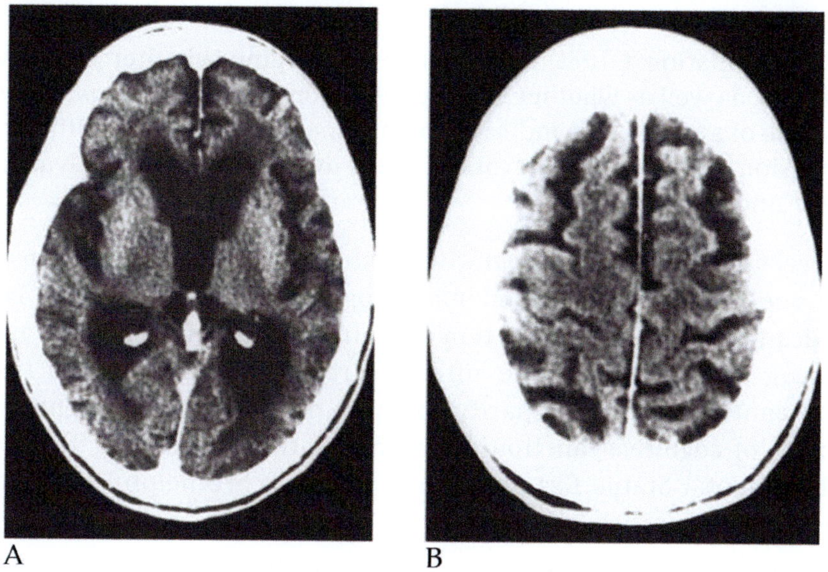

Figure 5.2. CT scan in cerebrocortical atrophy, showing ventricular dilation (A) and prominent cortical sulci (B).

Source.https://doctorlib.info/neurology/clinical-neurology-8/clinical-neurology-8.files/image117.jpg

5.1.2. General Physical Examination

When a general physical examination reveals symptoms of a systemic disease that is the cause of dementia, this information can help determine the etiologic diagnosis. Some signs that are especially useful are included in Table 5.3.

Table 5.2. Differences Between Acute Confusional States and Dementia

Feature	Acute Confusional State	Dementia
Level of consciousness	Impaired	Not impaired, except occasionally late in course
Course	Acute to subacute; fluctuating	Chronic; steadily progressive
Autonomic hyperactivity	Often present	Absent
Prognosis	Usually reversible	Usually irreversible[1]

[1]This is not an inherent feature of dementia but is currently the case.

Source: https://dl.mehrsys.ir/pdf-books/Clinical%20Neurology%209%20Edition%20(www.myuptodate.com).pdf.

5.1.3. Mental Status Examination

The mental status examination (Table 5.4) aids in identifying whether cognitive dysfunction is widespread or localized, as well as whether the degree or content of consciousness is compromised. A disturbance in the state of awareness is indicated by tiredness, lack of focus, difficulty recalling details right away, or confusion about time or location. Until dementia is quite advanced, abnormalities in these regions are uncommon.

In order to ascertain whether the cognitive dysfunction is widespread or limited, tests are conducted one by one across various domains of cognition. These comprise language, memory, parietal lobe abilities (such as picture creation, discrimination between right and left, and object localization in space), and frontal lobe or diffuse cerebral cortical abilities (such as judgment, abstraction, mental content, and the capacity to carry out previously taught actions). Dementia impairs many aspects of cognitive function. When dementia is suspected, the Montreal Cognitive Assessment and Minimental Status Examination (Table 5.5) are helpful bedside screening tests, but they might miss mild cognitive impairment.

Different types of dementia may preferentially impair distinct cognitive domains, and this can offer diagnostic insights. For instance, frontotemporal dementia frequently causes the greatest impairment to language function, but Alzheimer's disease disproportionately affects memory.

Table 5.3. Clinical Features Helpful in the Differential Diagnosis of Dementia

Feature	Most Suggestive of
History	
Unprotected sexual intercourse, intravenous drug abuse, hemophilia, or blood transfusions	HIV-associated dementia
Family history	Huntington disease, Wilson disease
Headache	Brain tumor, chronic subdural hematoma
Vital signs	
Hypothermia	Hypothyroidism
Hypertension	Vascular dementia
Hypotension	Hypothyroidism
Bradycardia	Hypothyroidism
General examination	
Meningismus	Chronic meningitis
Jaundice	Acquired hepatocerebral degeneration
Kayser–Fleischer rings	Wilson disease
Mental status examination	
Prominent memory loss	Alzheimer disease
Aphasia	Frontotemporal dementia (semantic dementia, progressive nonfluent aphasia)
Hallucinations	Lewy body disease
Cranial nerves	
Papilledema	Brain tumor, chronic subdural hematoma
Argyll Robertson pupils	Neurosyphilis
Ophthalmoplegia	Progressive supranuclear palsy
Pseudobulbar palsy	Vascular dementia, progressive supranuclear palsy

Motor	
Limb apraxia	Corticobasal degeneration
Tremor	Lewy body disease, corticobasal degeneration, acquired hepatocerebral degeneration, Wilson disease, HIV-associated dementia
Asterixis	Acquired hepatocerebral degeneration
Myoclonus	Creutzfeldt-Jakob disease, HIV-associated dementia
Rigidity	Lewy body disease, corticobasal degeneration, acquired hepatocerebral degeneration, Creutzfeldt-Jakob disease, progressive supranuclear palsy, Wilson disease
Chorea	Huntington disease, Wilson disease
Other	
Gait apraxia	Normal-pressure hydrocephalus
Hyporeflexia (from associated polyneuropathy)	Neurosyphilis, vitamin B_{12} deficiency, HIV-associated dementia

Source: https://dl.mehrsys.ir/pdf-books/Clinical%20Neurology%209%20Edition%20(www.myuptodate.com).pdf.

Table 5.4. Comprehensive Mental Status Examination

Level of consciousness
Arousability Orientation Attention Concentration
Language and speech
Comprehension Repetition Fluency Naming Reading Writing Calculation Speech
Mood and behavior
Mood Content of thought Hallucinations Delusions Abstraction Judgment
Memory
Immediate recall Recent memory Remote memory
Integrative sensory function
Astereognosis Agraphesthesia Two-point discrimination Allesthesia Extinction Unilateral neglect and anosognosia Disorders of spatial thought
Integrative motor function
Apraxia

Source: https://dl.mehrsys.ir/pdf-books/Clinical%20Neurology%209%20Edition%20(www.myuptodate.com).pdf.

5.1.4. Neurologic Examination

A few conditions that lead to dementia also impair motor or sensory function, coordination, or vision. Establishing an etiologic diagnosis can be aided by identifying such associated neurologic abnormalities. Table 5.3 contains a list of neurologic indicators that could indicate dementia causes.

5.1.5. Laboratory Investigations

Table 5.6 contains a list of laboratory studies that can be used to determine the cause of dementia.

Table 5.5. Minimental Status Examination in the Korean Version of the CERAD (Consortium to Establish a Registry for Alzheimer's Disease) Assessment Packet (MMSE-KC)

Category	Description
Orientation to time	From broadest to most narrow. Orientation to time has been correlated with future decline
Orientation to place	From broadest to most narrow. This is sometimes narrowed down to streets, and sometimes to floor
Registration	Repeating named prompts
Recall	Registration recall
Attention and calculation	Serial sevens, or spelling "world" backwards. It has been suggested that serial sevens may be more appropriate in a population where English is not the first language
Language	Naming a pencil and a watch
Repetition	Speaking back a phrase
Complex commands	Draw pentagonal overlap.
Three-stage commands	Give the patient a piece of plain blank paper and ask him to follow your instructions
Understanding and decision	Understanding and decision

Source: So A, Hooshyar D, Park KW, Lim HS. Early Diagnosis of Dementia from Clinical Data by Machine Learning Techniques. *Applied Sciences.* 2017; 7(7):651. https://doi.org/10.3390/app7070651.

5.2. Dementia

5.2.1. Differential Diagnosis

- **Common Causes of Dementia:** Dementia can be caused by a wide range of illnesses, but only a few do so frequently. The most common causes of dementia in its most common presentation—a gradual decline in cognitive function in an elderly patient (≥65 years of age)—are Parkinson's disease, Lewy body disease, Alzheimer's disease, and vascular dementia (formerly known as "multi-infarct") (Figure 5.3). Numerous patients have both vascular disease and neurodegeneration contributing to their dementia. Furthermore, vascular variables may impact neurodegenerative disease risk or progression. Individuals who first exhibit signs of dementia before the age of 45 are much less likely to have vascular or Alzheimer's disease; instead, a greater variety of neurodegenerative (corticobasal degeneration, multiple sclerosis, systemic lupus erythematosus, vasculitis), inflammatory (multiple sclerosis, prion disease), and infectious (multiple sclerosis) causes must be considered in these patients. The most common cause of dementia that advances quickly over weeks or months is prion (Creutzfeldt-Jakob) disease.

Table 5.6. Laboratory Studies in Dementia

Test	Most Useful in Diagnosis of
Blood	
Hematocrit, mean corpuscular volume (MCV), peripheral blood smear, vitamin B_{12} level	Vitamin B_{12} deficiency
Thyroid function tests	Hypothyroidism
Liver function tests	Acquired hepatocerebral degeneration, Wilson disease
Ceruloplasmin, copper	Wilson disease
FTA or MHA-TP	Neurosyphilis
Cerebrospinal fluid	
VDRL	Neurosyphilis
Cytology	Leptomeningeal metastases
14-3-3 protein	Creutzfeldt-Jakob disease
Aβ42, tau, phospho-tau	Alzheimer disease
HIV mRNA	HIV-associated dementia
CT scan or MRI	Brain tumor, chronic subdural hematoma, vascular dementia, normal-pressure hydrocephalus, Alzheimer disease, frontotemporal dementia
PET Scan	Alzheimer disease
EEG	Creutzfeldt-Jakob disease

Source: https://dl.mehrsys.ir/pdf-books/Clinical%20Neurology%209%20Edition%20(www.myuptodate.com).pdf.

- **Other Causes of Dementia:** Rarely, reversible causes of dementia include intracranial mass lesions, hypothyroidism, vitamin B12 deficiency, normal-pressure hydrocephalus, and neurosyphilis. But because treatment can halt or reverse intellectual decline, it is crucial to diagnose them (Table 5.6).

Genetic counseling can help patients and their families when Huntington disease or other heritable disorders are diagnosed as the cause of their dementia. Antiretroviral medications can be used to treat HIV illness and prevent its spread if Creutzfeldt-Jakob disease or dementia linked to HIV is identified. Progressive multifocal leukoencephalopathy may draw attention to these conditions by signaling underlying immunosuppression caused by leukemia, lymphoma, or HIV infection.

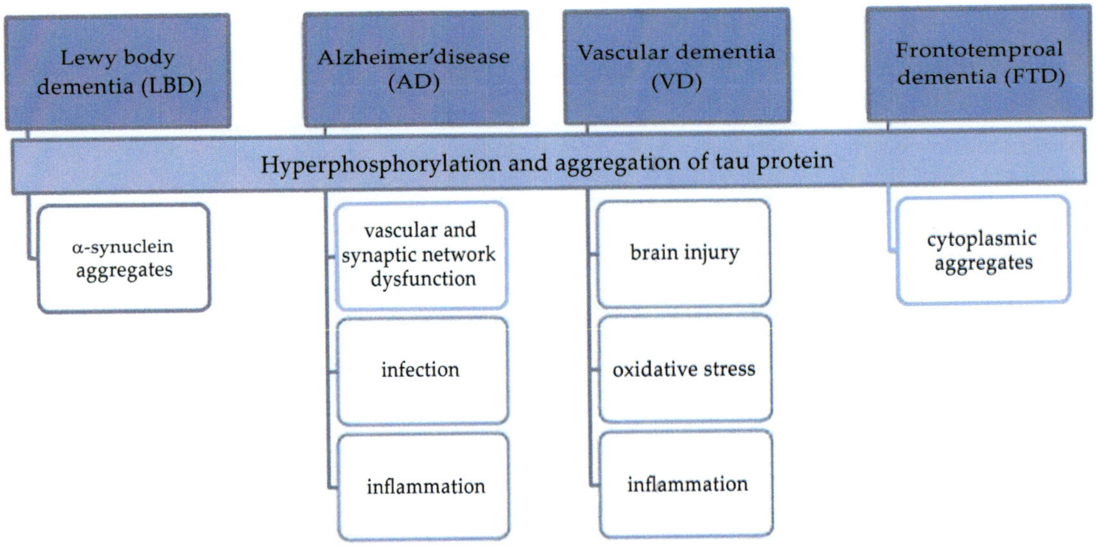

Figure 5.3. Common causes of dementia based on age at presentation and rate of progression.

Source: Zagórska A, Czopek A, Fryc M, Jaromin A, Boyd BJ. Drug discovery and development targeting dementia. *Pharmaceuticals*. 2023; 16(2):151. https://doi.org/10.3390/ph16020151.

About 15% of patients who are referred for a possible dementia evaluation actually have other conditions, or pseudodementias, like depression. Since depression in this context is easily treated, it is crucial to recognize it. Drug abuse, which is frequently blamed for dementia in the elderly, actually causes an acute state of confusion instead of dementia.

5.2.2. Neurodegenerative Proteinopathies

The synthesis of misfolded proteins and their combination to form insoluble aggregates seem to be important pathophysiological factors in many neurodegenerative diseases (Table 5.7). These aberrant proteins may result from acquired or genetic modifications, and their pathologic effects can be caused by a gain of a toxic function, a loss of normal protein function, or a combination of these. Protein aggregates can cause harmful effects on the cell, such as interfering with axonal transport, but they can also serve as a mechanism for sequestering proteins that the proteolytic machinery of the cell is unable to process.

Neurodegenerative proteinopathies have no known underlying cause, except for a small number of hereditary or infectious cases. But these illnesses have a few things in common. Apart from the production of distinctive histopathologic findings (refer to Table 5.7), these disorders can also be linked to cell-to-cell prionic transmission (Figure 5.4), which enables the diseases to proliferate throughout the nervous system and result in distinct anatomic patterns of involvement. The discovery that patients with Parkinson's disease who have fetal tissue grafted into their brains experience the development of the same aberrant protein aggregates in the recipient's brain provides evidence for this mechanism.

5.2.2.1. Alzheimer Disease

- **Epidemiology:** Approximately 60 to 70% of dementia cases are thought to be caused by Alzheimer disease, making it the most prevalent cause of dementia overall.

Table 5.7. Neurodegenerative Proteinopathies

Summary of Most Relevant Modifications of Neurodegeneration Related Proteins with Remarks				
Disease Group	**Protein**	**Disease Type**	**Form**	**Phenotype**
AD	Tau, Aβ	AD	SP/GEN	DEM
Tauopathy (FTLD-Tau *)	Tau	PiD	SP	FTD
		GGT	SP	FTD
		CBD	SP	MD/FTD
		PSP	SP	MD/FTD
		AGD	SP	DEM
		NFT-dementia/PART	SP	DEM
		FTDP-17T	GEN	FTD/MD
TDP-43 proteinopathy	TDP-43	FTLD-TDP (type A–D)	SP/GEN	FTD
		MND-TDP	SP/GEN	MD
		FTLD-MND-TDP	SP/GEN	FTD-MD
FUS (FET)-proteinopathy FTLD/MND-FUS (FET)	FUS/FET	aFTLD-U, NIFID, BIBD	SP	FTD/MD
		MND-FUS	GEN	MD

α-Synucleinopathy	α-Synuclein	PD	SP/ GEN	MD
		DLB	SP/ GEN	DEM/MD
		MSA	SP	MD
Prion disease	PrP	sCJD, VPSPr, sFI	SP	DEM/MD
		iCJD	ACQ	DEM/MD
		vCJD	ACQ	DEM/MD
		Kuru	ACQ	DEM/MD
		gCJD, GSS, FFI, PrP-CAA	GEN	DEM/MD
TRD **	Huntingtin	HD	GEN	MD
	Ataxin 1, 2, 3, 7, CACNA1A, TBP	SCA 1, 2, 3, 6, 7, 17	GEN	MD
	FMRP	FXTAS	GEN	MD
	ARP	SBMA	GEN	MD
	Atrophin-1	DRPLA	GEN	MD
Other forms	Ferritin	Hereditary ferritinopathy	GEN	DEM/MD
	Neuroserpin	Neuroserpinopathy	GEN	DEM
	ABri, ADan, gelsolin, cystatin, transthyretin, Aβ	Hereditary amyloidoses/CAA	GEN	DEM
	Only UPS	FTLD-UPS	GEN	FTD
	Not determined	FTLD-ni	SP	FTD
	Tau, α-Synuclein	NBIA	GEN	DEM/MD
	Tau, a-Synuclein, TDP-43	Various genetic and sporadic diseases ("secondary" proteinopathy forms)	SP/ GEN	DEM/MD

Source: Kovacs GG. Molecular Pathological Classification of Neurodegenerative Diseases: Turning towards Precision Medicine. *International Journal of Molecular Sciences*. 2016; 17(2):189. https://doi.org/10.3390/ijms17020189.

Abbreviations: ACQ: acquired; ARP: androgen receptor protein; AD: Alzheimer disease; AGD: Argyrophilic grain disease; BIBD: Basophilic inclusion body disease; CAA: sporadic cerebral amyloid angiopathy; CACNA1A: α1A subunit of the P/Q-type voltage-gated calcium channel (SCA6; Cytoplasmic aggregates); CBD: Corticobasal degeneration; CJD: Creutzfeldt-Jakob disease (i: iatrogenic, s: sporadic, v: variant, g: genetic); DEM: dementia; DLB: Dementia with Lewy bodies; DRPLA: dentatorubral-pallidoluysian atrophy; sFI: sporadic fatal insomnia; FFI: fatal familial insomnia; FMRP: Fragile X mental retardation protein; FTD: frontotemporal dementia; FTLD: frontotemporal lobar degeneration; aFTLD-U: atypical FTLD with ubiquitinated inclusions; FTLD-UPS: FTLD with inclusions immunoreactive only for the components of the ubiquitine proteasome system; FTLD-ni: FTLD no inclusion specified; FTDP-17T: Frontotemporal dementia and parkinsonism linked to chromosome 17 caused by mutations in the *MAPT* (tau) gene; FXTAS: Fragile X associated tremor and ataxia syndrome (here also astroglial inclusions); GEN: genetic; GGT: globular glial tauopathy; GSS: Gerstmann-Sträussler-Scheinker disease; HD: Huntington disease; INIBD: intranuclear inclusion body diseases; MD: movement disorder; MND: Motor neuron disease; MSA: multiple system atrophy; NBIA: neurodegeneration with brain iron accumulation; NIFID: Neurofilament intermediate filament inclusion disease; PD: Parkinson's disease; PiD: Pick disease; PrP: prion protein; PSP: Progressive supranuclear palsy; SCA: spinocerebellar ataxia; SBMA: spinal and bulbar muscular atrophy; SP: sporadic; TBP: TATA-Box binding protein (SCA17); TRD: trinucleotide repeat expansion disorder: refers to genetic disorder and associated with different proteins; VPSPr: variably protease-sensitive prionopathy. * FTLD is not typical in AGD or PART; ** only SCAs with protein inclusions.

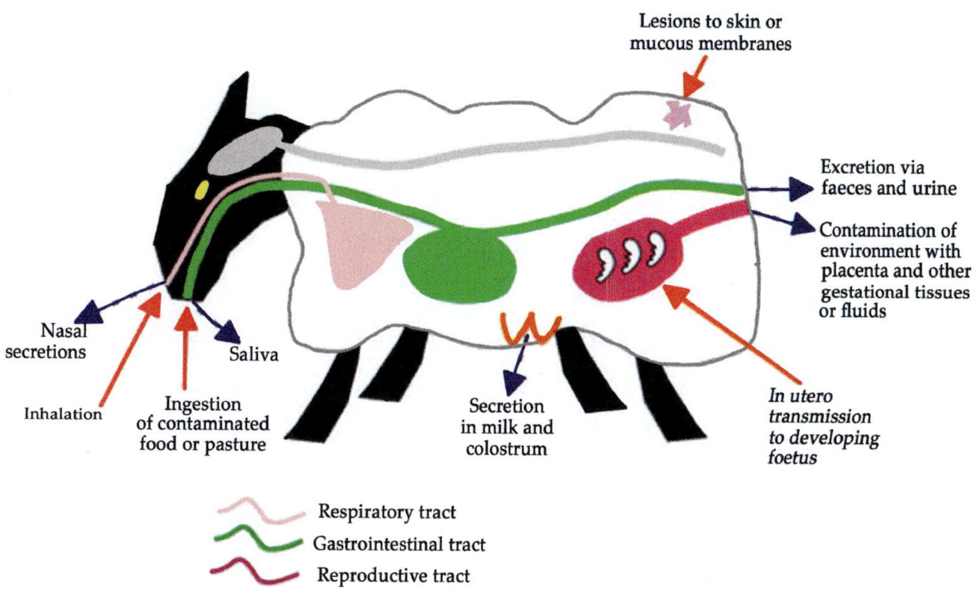

Figure 5.4. Cell-to-cell (prionic) transmission of neurodegenerative proteinopathies. Abnormal proteins associated with neurodegenerative disease may misfold, leading to the formation of protein aggregates; misfolded proteins, protein aggregates, or both may be toxic and contribute to neuronal dysfunction. In addition, toxic protein aggregates may be transferred between cells to propagate the disease.

Source: Mabbott NA. How do PrPSc Prions Spread between Host Species, and within Hosts? *Pathogens*. 2017; 6(4):60. https://doi.org/10.3390/pathogens6040060.

About 15% of people 65 years of age or older and approximately 45% of people 85 years of age or older suffer from Alzheimer's disease. Over 5 million cases occur in the US, and there are about 30 million cases globally. After adjusting for age, the frequency of occurrence is the same for men and women. Nonetheless, women make up about two thirds of Alzheimer patients due to their longer lifespans.

- **Pathology:** Characteristic histopathologic features, particularly neuritic (senile) plaques and neurofibrillary tangles, are what characterize Alzheimer's disease. β-amyloid (Aβ) and other proteins, such as presenilin 1, presenilin 2, α1-antichymotrypsin, apolipoprotein E, α2-macroglobulin, and ubiquitin, are found in extracellular deposits known as neuritic plaques. Cerebral amyloid angiopathy can also be caused by plaques in the walls of the meningeal and cerebral blood vessels. Intracellular deposits of hyperphosphorylated tau, a protein associated with microtubules, and ubiquitin are known as neurofibrillary tangles.
- **Etiology:** Alzheimer's disease is a progressive, degenerative illness that is typically sporadic and has no known cause. In rare instances, it is caused by a genetic defect (see below). Two proteins, tau and Aβ, have abnormal metabolism, deposition, or clearance, and these processes seem to be closely related to pathogenesis.
- **Pathogenesis:**
  - **Genetics:** Presenilin 1 (PS1), presenilin 2 (PS2), or β-amyloid precursor protein (APP) are three functionally related membrane proteins that can be mutated to cause Alzheimer disease, which affects about 1% of patients (Table 5.8). For these patients, the disease usually manifests itself between the ages of thirty and sixty. It is believed that an extra copy of the APP gene, which is found on chromosome 21, causes early Alzheimer's disease (mean onset at age 50) in patients with Down syndrome (trisomy 21). Sporadic Alzheimer's disease lacks a known cause, but familial Alzheimer's disease gene defects implicate both the neurotrophic protein APP and the presenilins, which are involved in APP metabolism.

    The inheritance pattern of isoforms ε2, ε3, and ε 4 of the apolipoprotein E (APOE) gene also affects the risk of Alzheimer's disease. The risk increases approximately threefold with a single apolipoprotein Eε4 (APOE4) allele and approximately twelvefold with two copies of APOE4. Additionally, the age at onset is lowered by approximately five years per copy of APOE4. APOE2 seems to offer somewhat better protection against Alzheimer's disease than APOE4. Although the exact mechanism by which the APOE genotype alters an individual's susceptibility to Alzheimer's disease is unknown, the APOE protein may bind to Aβ.
  - **Aβ and Neuritic Plaques:** The main component of neuritic plaques and the substance deposited in the cerebral and meningeal blood vessels during Alzheimer's disease is amyloid (Aβ). The transmembrane protein APP is cleaved by proteases to yield the 38–43 amino acid peptide known as Aβ (Figure 5.5). Aβ-secretase, which does not produce Aβ,

β-secretase (BACE; β-site APP cleaving enzyme), and γ-secretase cleave APP normally, producing primarily a 40-amino acid fragment (Aβ40), which is secreted and removed from the brain. An excessive amount of Aβ42, a longer version of the molecule with a higher propensity to aggregate, is produced in Alzheimer's disease. Presenilins 1 and 2 have an effect on the activity of γ-secretase.

The involvement of APP mutations in certain familial cases and the neurotoxicity of Aβ in certain situations provide evidence for a causal role of Aβ in Alzheimer's disease. Nevertheless, there is little relationship between the degree of dementia in Alzheimer's disease and the amount of amyloid plaque deposition in the brain. This discrepancy could be explained by the possibility that the toxic agent is soluble Aβ oligomers rather than insoluble plaques. Another theory is that Aβ aggregation indirectly causes Alzheimer's disease by, for example, encouraging the development of neurofibrillary tangles that contain tau.

Table 5.8. Principal Genes Implicated in Alzheimer's Disease

Gene	SNP	**Chromosome position**	**Protein**	**EOAD/ LOAD**	**Proposed function**	**Implicated pathways**
ABCA7	rs3764650 rs4147929	19p13.3	ATP-binding cassette transporter A7	LOAD	Lipid homeostasis	Cholesterol metabolism; immune response
ADAM10	rs61751103 rs145518263	15q21.3	A disintegrin and metalloprotease family, AMAD10	LOAD	Proteolytic cleavage of integral membrane proteins	Aβ metabolism
APOE	rs429358 rs7412	19q13.2	Apolipoprotein E	LOAD	Mediates binding, internalization, and catabolism of lipoproteins	Cholesterol metabolism
APP	–	21q21.3	Amyloid precursor protein	EOAD	Neurite outgrowth, adhesion, and axonogenesis	Aβ metabolism
BIN1	rs744373 rs7561528	2q14	Bridging Integrator 1	LOAD	Regulation of endocytosis of synaptic vesicles	Cell adhesion and endocytosis; tau metabolism
CASS4	rs7274581	20q13.31	Cas scaffolding protein family member 4	LOAD	Docking protein in tyrosine-kinase signaling involved in cell adhesion and spreading	Cytoskeleton and axonal transport

CD2AP	rs9296559 rs9349407	6p12	CD2-associated protein	LOAD	Scaffold molecule regulating actin cytoskeleton	Cell adhesion and endocytosis; tau metabolism
CD33	rs3865444	19q13.3	Cluster of differentiation 33	LOAD	Mediates sialic acid-dependent binding to cells	Immune response
CELF1	rs10838725	11p11	CUGBP and Elav-like family member 1	LOAD	Regulates pre-mRNA splicing	Tau metabolism
CLU	rs11136000, rs2279590, rs7012010, rs7982, rs9331888	8p21-p12	Clusterin	LOAD	Chaperone; regulation of cell proliferation	Cholesterol metabolism Immune response
CR1	rs6656401 rs3818361	1q32	Complement receptor 1	LOAD	Mediates cellular binding of immune complexes that activate complement	Immune response
DSG2	rs8093731	18q12.1	Desmoglein 2	LOAD	Mediates cell–cell junctions between epithelial and other cell type	Cytoskeleton and axonal transport
EPHA1	rs11771145	7q34	EPH Receptor A1	LOAD	Brain and neural development; angiogenesis, cell proliferation, and apoptosis	Cell adhesion and endocytosis; immune response
FERMT2	rs17125944	14q22.1	Fermitin Family Member 2	LOAD	Actin assembly and cell shape and mediator of angiogenesis	Tau metabolism
HLA-DRB5/ DRB1	rs9271192	6p21.3	Major histocompatibility complex, class II, DR beta 5- DR beta 1	LOAD	Immunocompetence and histocompatibility	Immune response
INPP5D	rs35349669	2q37.1	Inositol polyphosphate-5-phosphatase	LOAD	Negative regulator of myeloid cell proliferation and survival	Immune response
MEF2C	rs190982	5q14.3	Myocyte enhancer factor 2C	LOAD	Controls synapse formation	Immune response

MS4A4/MS4A6E	rs983392 rs670139	11q12.1	Membrane-spanning 4-domains, subfamily A, member 4A/6E	LOAD	Signal transduction	Immune response
NME8	rs2718058	7p14.1	NME/NM23 family member 8	LOAD	Ciliary functions	Cytoskeleton and axonal transport
PICALM	rs3851179 rs541458	11q14	Phosphatidylinositol binding clathrin assembly protein	LOAD	AP2-dependent clathrin-mediated endocytosis	Cell adhesion and endocytosis; tau metabolism
PSEN1	–	14q24.3	Presenilin 1	EOAD	Component of catalytic subunit of gamma-secretase complex	Aβ metabolism
PSEN2	–	1q31-q42	Presenilin 2	EOAD	Component of catalytic subunit of gamma-secretase complex	Aβ metabolism
PTK2B	rs28834970	8p21.1	Protein tyrosine kinase 2 beta	LOAD	Induction of long term potentiation in hippocampus	Endocytosis
SLC24A4/RIN3	rs10498633	14q32.12	Solute carrier family 24, member 4/ Ras and Rab interactor 3	LOAD	Brain and neural development	Neural development, synapse function, endocytosis
SORL1	rs11218343	11q23.2-q24.2	Sortilin-related receptor containing LDL receptor class A repeats	LOAD	APOE receptor; binds LDL and RAP and mediates endocytosis of the lipids to which it binds	Cholesterol Metabolism; Cell adhesion and endocytosis
TREM2	rs75932628	6p21.1	Triggering Receptor Expressed on Myeloid Cells 2	LOAD	Induces phagocytosis of apoptotic neurons, and regulates Toll-like receptor mediated inflammatory responses, and microglial activation	Immune response
ZCWPW1	rs1476679	7q22.1	Zinc finger, CW type with PWWP domain 1	LOAD	Epigenetic regulation	Epigenetic regulation

Source: Sun Q, Xie N, Tang B, Li R and Shen Y (2017) Alzheimer's disease: From genetic variants to the distinct pathological mechanisms. Front. Mol. Neurosci. 10:319. doi: 10.3389/fnmol.2017.00319.

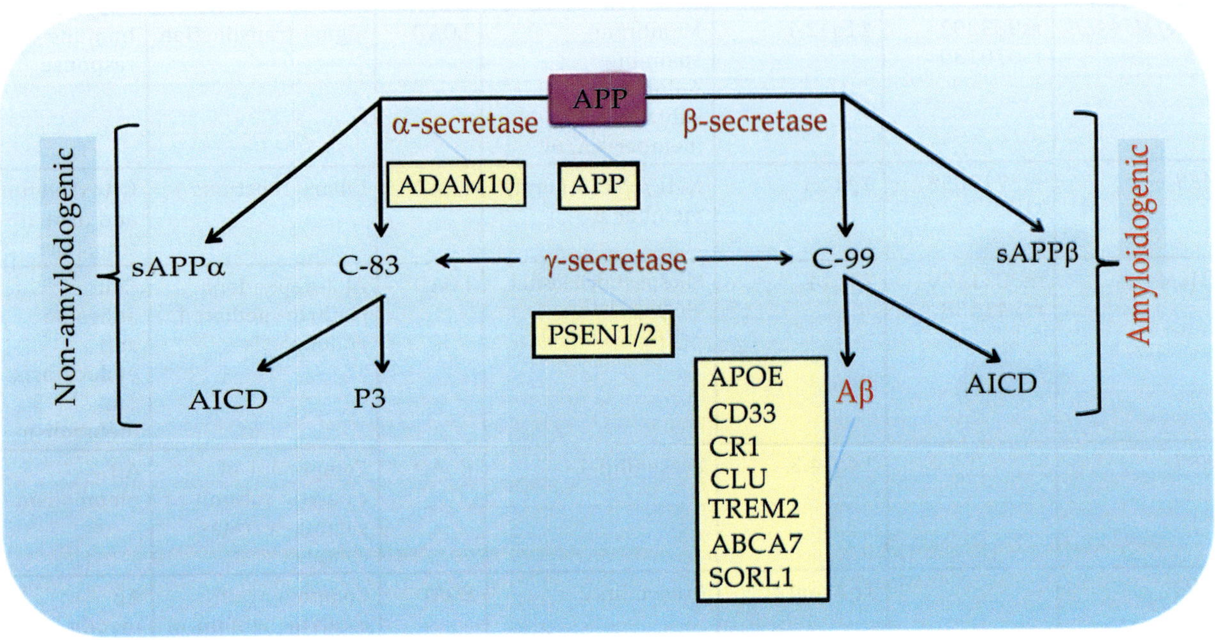

Figure 5.5. Normal and pathologic (amyloidogenic) processing of APP and Aβ. APP, a membrane-spanning protein, is normally cleaved by α-secretase (α), or by β-secretase (β) and then γ-secretase (γ, a protein complex that includes presenilin 1 or 2, nicastrin, anterior pharynx defective 1 homolog [APH1], and presenilin enhancer 2 [PEN2]) to generate β-amyloid (Aβ), a secreted protein. APP mutations associated with familial Alzheimer's disease shift Aβ production from a nontoxic 40-amino acid to a toxic (amyloidogenic) 42-amino acid form, which has a greater tendency to form amyloid deposits. Aβ normally undergoes enzymatic breakdown (by neprilysin [NEP], insulin-degrading enzyme [IDE], or endothelin-converging enzyme [ECE-1]) and clearance from the brain. However, it can also aggregate to form oligomers of increasing size, which are thought to be neurotoxic. sAPP, soluble APP; C83 and C99, C-terminal fragments of APP; AICD, APP intracellular domain.

Source: Sun Q, Xie N, Tang B, Li R and Shen Y (2017) Alzheimer's disease: From genetic variants to the distinct pathological mechanisms. Front. Mol. Neurosci. 10:319. doi: 10.3389/fnmol.2017.00319.

- **Tau and Neurofibrillary Tangles:** Tau is a cytoplasmic protein that attaches itself to tubulin to stabilize microtubules, cytoskeletal structures that support intracellular transport and aid in maintaining cell structure. When tau is hyperphosphorylated and separates from microtubules in Alzheimer's disease and other tauopathies, the microtubules break down and the hyperphosphorylated tau clumps together to form neurofibrillary tangles (Figure 5.6). It's unclear how this affects neuronal function, but it might be related to a problem with axonal transport. The findings that the quantity of neurofibrillary tangles closely corresponds with the severity of the disease and that dementia can also be produced by other tauopathies (such as frontotemporal dementia), in which Aβ processing is normal, provide evidence for a causal role for tau pathology in Alzheimer's disease.

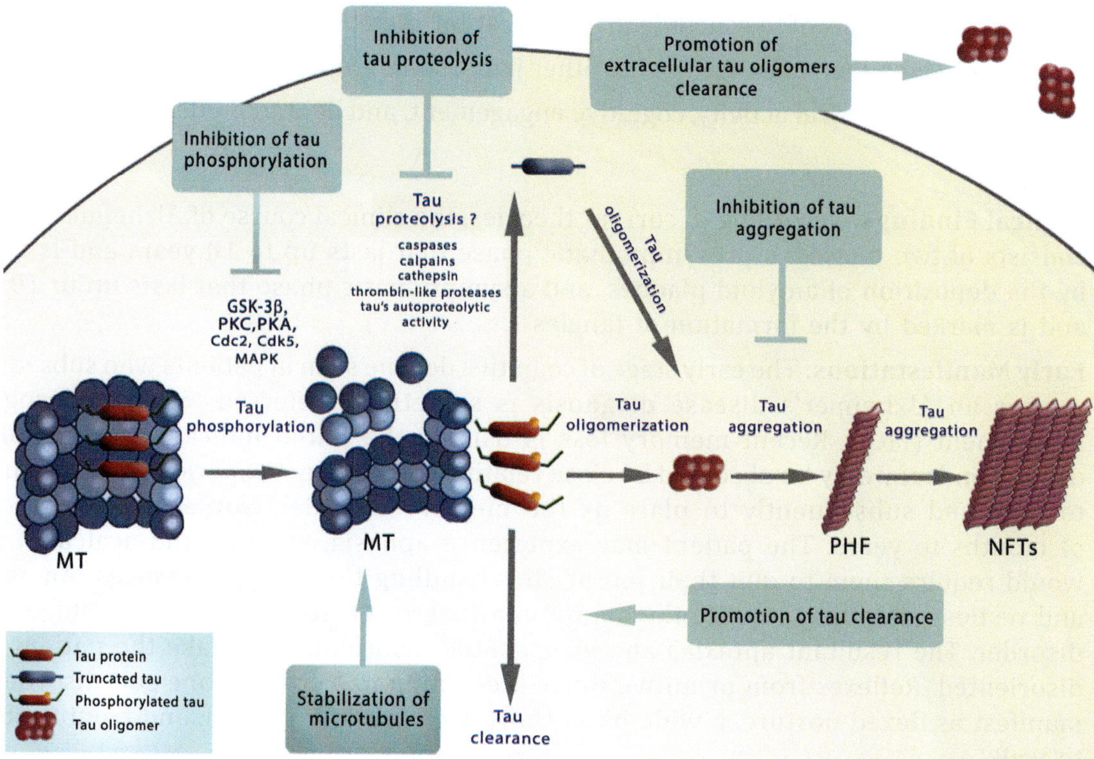

Figure 5.6. Tau hyperphosphorylation and neurofibrillary tangle formation.

Source: Šimić G, Babić Leko M, Wray S, Harrington C, Delalle I, Jovanov-Milošević N, Bažadona D, Buée L, De Silva R, Di Giovanni G, et al. Tau Protein Hyperphosphorylation and Aggregation in Alzheimer's Disease and Other Tauopathies, and Possible Neuroprotective Strategies. *Biomolecules.* 2016; 6(1):6. https://doi.org/10.3390/biom6010006.

- o **Synaptic Dysfunction:** Alzheimer's disease is associated with early dysfunction and eventual loss of synapses, which primarily affects excitatory transmission in the cerebral cortex and the hippocampus. These alterations could be a factor in memory loss.
- o **Neuronal Loss and Brain Atrophy:** Alzheimer's disease causes a preferential loss of certain neuronal populations, such as cholinergic neurons in the basal forebrain and glutamatergic neurons in the entorhinal cortex and the CA1 sector of the hippocampal. There is focal brain atrophy in the impacted regions.
- o **Vascular Involvement:** There is debate over the potential role of vascular pathology in Alzheimer's disease. The overlap of APOE genotype and other risk factors for vascular disease and Alzheimer's disease, as well as the role of blood vessels in amyloid pathology, provide evidence for this relationship.

- **Risk Factors:** The APOE4 gene, female sex, and advancing age are the variables most strongly linked to an increased risk of Alzheimer's disease. Some studies have also linked a family history of Alzheimer's to depression, smoking, diabetes, hypertension, low educational attainment, and a fatty diet. In addition to APOE4, a number of other genes have been found to alter risk, however, their impacts are not very significant.

There is insufficient proof to conclude that medication, diet, or lifestyle modifications can lower the risk of Alzheimer's disease. On the other hand, some evidence supports low-fat and vegetable-rich diets, physical activity, cognitive engagement, and light to moderate alcohol consumption.

- **Clinical Findings:** According to current theories, the clinical course of Alzheimer's disease consists of two phases: a presymptomatic phase that lasts up to 10 years and is marked by the deposition of amyloid plaques, and a symptomatic phase that lasts up to 10 years and is marked by the formation of tangles (Figure 5.7).

o **Early Manifestations:** The early stage of cognitive decline seen in patients who subsequently receive an Alzheimer's disease diagnosis is sometimes referred to as mild cognitive impairment (MCI). Recent memory loss is usually the initial indication of Alzheimer's disease and may only be observed by close relatives. The patient experiences disorientation to time and subsequently to place as the memory disorder worsens over the course of months to years. The patient may experience aphasia, anomia, and acalculia, which would require them to quit their job or stop handling the family's finances. An agitated and restless state may replace the depression that was evident in the early stages of the disorder. The resultant apraxias and visuospatial disorientation make the patient easily disoriented. Reflexes from primitive times are common. A frontal lobe gait disorder may manifest as flexed posture, a wide base, short, slow, shuffling steps, and trouble starting to walk.

o **Late Manifestations:** In the latter stages, mental symptoms, such as psychosis with paranoia, hallucinations, or delusions, may be prominent, and previously maintained social graces are lost. Sometimes people have seizures. At this point, an examination may reveal bradykinesia and rigidity. Hemiparesis, myoclonus, incontinence, spasticity, and extensor plantar responses are rare and typically late symptoms of the disease. A bedridden state, incontinence, and mutism are the terminal symptoms.

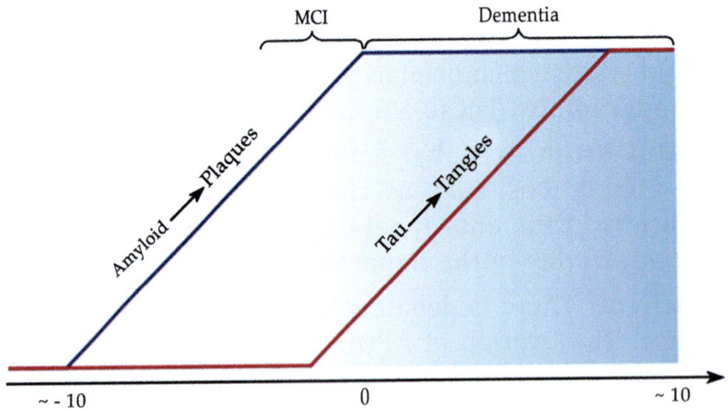

Figure 5.7. Relationship between plaques, tangles, and clinical progression of Alzheimer's disease (AD). MCI, mild cognitive impairment.

Source: https://dl.mehrsys.ir/pdf-books/Clinical%20Neurology%209%20Edition%20(www.myuptodate.com).pdf

In the final months of life, eating disorders, fever episodes, dyspnea, pneumonia, and pain are common complications. Death usually happens five to ten years after the onset of symptoms.

- **Investigative Studies:** Other disorders, such as those that are treatable or reversible, can be ruled out by laboratory tests. Cognitive testing could help differentiate between dementia caused by Alzheimer's disease and other conditions. Cortical atrophy, particularly in the medial temporal lobe, and enlarged ventricles are frequently observed on CT or MRI scans of Alzheimer's disease patients; however, these abnormalities are nonspecific. The temporal and parietal lobes may show signs of hypometabolism and hypoperfusion when subjected to PET scanning. Two more specialized PET tracers are [11C] Pittsburgh compound B (PIB), which binds to amyloid plaques, and [18F]FDDNP, which labels neurofibrillary tangles and amyloid plaques. Alzheimer's disease biomarkers that have been found to be useful are the levels of Aβ42, tau, and phospho-tau in the cerebrospinal fluid (CSF).
- **Differential Diagnosis:** Early-stage Alzheimer's disease can mimic other conditions like depression or isolated memory problems like Korsakoff amnestic syndrome. It is necessary to differentiate between Lewy body dementia, vascular dementia, Creutzfeldt-Jakob disease, and other dementing conditions to identify more advanced Alzheimer's disease.
- **Treatment:** There is currently no proven treatment that can stop the progression of the disease or reverse existing deficits. Memantine, an NMDA-type glutamate receptor antagonist medication (Table 5.9), may, however, provide a slight improvement for individuals withAlzheimer's to severe Alzheimer's disease.

Cholinergic replacement therapy has also been used to treat the symptoms of cognitive dysfunction because cholinergic neuronal pathways degenerate and choline acetyltransferase is depleted in the brains of Alzheimer's disease patients (Table 5.9). It has been demonstrated that acetylcholinesterase inhibitors, such as galantamine, donepezil, rivastigmine, and tacrine, slightly improve cognitive function tests. Tacrine causes side effects such as diarrhea, vertigo, and nausea and vomiting. It also raises serum transaminase levels. One benefit of donepezil is its once-daily dosage schedule and improved side-effect profile.

Table 5.9. Disease Modifying Agents for the Treatment of Alzheimer's Disease in Clinical Trials

Disease Modifying Agents	Mechanism of Action
Phase 3 Clinical Trials	
Aducanumab	Monoclonal antibody—targets β-amyloid and removes it.
Gantenerumab	Monoclonal antibody—binds and removes β-amyloid.
CAD106b	Amyloid vaccine—stimulates production of antibodies against β-amyloid.
BAN2401	Monoclonal antibody—reduces protofibrillar β-amyloid.
TRx0237 (LMTX)	Tau protein aggregation inhibitor.
AGB101	Low-dose levetiracetam—improves synaptic function and reduces amyloid-induced neuronal hyperactivity

ALZT-OP1 (cromolyn + ibuprofen)	Mast cell stabilizer and anti-inflammatory—promotes microglial clearance of amyloid
Azeliragon	RAGE (Receptor for Advanced Glycation End-products) antagonist—reduces inflammation and amyloid transport into the brain
BHV4157 (troriluzole)	Glutamate modulator—reduces synaptic levels of glutamate and improves synaptic functioning
Masitinib	Tyrosine kinase inhibitor—modulates inflammatory mast cell and reduces amyloid protein and tau phosphorylation
Phase 2 Clinical Trials	
Crenezumab	Monoclonal antibody—targets soluble oligomers and removes β-amyloid
ABBV-8E12	Monoclonal antibody—prevents tau propagation
ABvac40	Active immunotherapy—targets β-amyloid and removes it
BAN2401	Monoclonal antibody—removes amyloid protofibrils and reduces amyloid plaques
BIIB092	Monoclonal antibody—removes tau and reduces tau propagation
LY3002813 (donanemab)	Monoclonal antibody—removes amyloid by recognizing aggregated pyroglutamate form of Aβ
LY3303560 (zagotenemab)	Monoclonal antibody—neutralizes soluble tau aggregates
Semorinemab (RO7105705)	Monoclonal antibody—removes extracellular tau
APH-1105	Alpha-secretase modulator—reduces amyloid
Daratumumab	Monoclonal antibody—immunomodulatory that targets CD38 and regulates microglial activity
Dasatinib + Quercetin	Tyrosine kinase inhibitor (dasatinib) + flavonoid (quercetin)—reduces senescent cells and tau aggregation
IONIS MAPTRx (BIIB080)	Epigenetic, Tau Antisense oligonucleotide—reduces tau production
Lithium	Neurotransmitter receptors ion channel modulator—improves neuropsychiatric symptoms
Nilotinib	Tyrosine kinase inhibitor—promotes clearance of amyloid and tau proteins
Posiphen	Selective inhibitor of APP—reduces amyloid, tau, and α-synuclein production
PTI-125	Filamin A protein inhibitor—reduces tau hyperphosphorylation, synaptic dysfunction, and stabilizes soluble amyloid and the α7 nicotinic acetylcholine receptor interaction
PQ912	Glutaminyl cyclase (QC) enzyme inhibitor—reduces amyloid plaques and pyroglutamates Aβ production
Riluzole	Glutamate receptor antagonist—reduces glutamate-mediated excitotoxicity
Thiethylperazine (TEP)	Activates ABCC1 (ATP binding cassette subfamily C member 1 transport protein)—removes amyloid

Phase 1 Clinical Trials	
BIIB076	Monoclonal antibody—removes tau and reduces tau propagation
Lu AF87908	Monoclonal antibody—removes tau
anle138b	Aggregation inhibitor—reduces tau aggregation
RO7126209	Monoclonal antibody—removes amyloid
TPI-287	Stabilizes tubulin-binding, microtubule, and reduces cellular damage mediated by tau

Source: Breijyeh Z, Karaman R. Comprehensive Review on Alzheimer's Disease: Causes and Treatment. *Molecules.* 2020; 25(24):5789. https://doi.org/10.3390/molecules25245789.

Currently being studied are metal chelators, secretase inhibitors, and vaccines against β-amyloid as experimental treatments. Medications classified as antipsychotics, antidepressants, and anxiolytics may help manage behavioral issues linked to Alzheimer's disease. There is, however, little proof of their efficacy, and in certain situations (olanzapine, risperidone) the use of these medications is linked to an increased risk of stroke in older patients.

- **Prognosis:** Patients are typically able to continue social, recreational, and limited professional activities while still living at home during the early stages of the illness. Early diagnosis can give patients the time they need to manage their finances, plan an orderly retirement from the workforce, and talk with doctors and family members about how to handle any future medical issues. Patients with advanced stages of the illness might need to be treated with psychoactive medications and receive care in a nursing home. It is imperative to safeguard these patients and prevent them from causing harm to themselves or their loved ones through careless actions or choices. Infection or death usually takes place five to ten years after the onset of symptoms.

5.2.2.2. Frontotemporal Dementia

A group of dementing disorders known as frontotemporal dementia (FTD) are genetically and clinically heterogeneous; they cause degeneration of the frontal and temporal lobes and have a preferential effect on behavior and language. These are the ways that FTD is different from Alzheimer's disease, which mainly affects the temporal and parietal lobes and results in significant memory impairment. Tau-containing inclusions are seen in both Alzheimer's disease and frontotemporal dementia (FTD); however, only Alzheimer's disease exhibits abnormal amyloid processing and plaques.

- **Epidemiology:** After Alzheimer's disease and vascular dementia, FTD is believed to be the third most common cause of dementia. Between 50 and 60 years old is the typical onset age.
- **Pathology:** The frontal and temporal lobes atrophy is a hallmark of FTD. Histopathologic observations include gliosis, characteristic intracellular protein inclusions, and loss of neurons. Unlike paired helical filaments, tau inclusions in front-end dementia (FTD) are twisted, ribbon-like structures that include neurofibrillary tangles, amorphous deposits (pretangles), and, in certain situations, Pick bodies. The hippocampal, subcortical nuclei, brainstem, cerebellum, and spinal cord can also occasionally contain inclusions.

- **Etiology:** FTD is primarily an unpredictable neurodegenerative illness that strikes occasionally. However, between 20 and 40% of patients report a history of neurodegenerative disease in their family, and about 10% seem to inherit frontotemporal dementia in an autosomal dominant manner.
- **Pathogenesis**
  - o **Genetics:** Most inherited cases seem to be caused by mutations in three genes: progranulin (GRN), chromosome 9 open reading frame 72 (C9ORF72), and the microtubule-associated protein tau (MAPT). While GRN mutations result in function loss through haploinsufficiency, MAPT mutations are thought to primarily cause disease through toxic gain of function. The most frequent cause of FTD, C9ORF72 mutations, result in expanded noncoding GGGCCC hexanucleotide repeats. Impaired RNA processing causes an accumulation of abortive transcripts and sequestration of RNA-binding proteins like nucleolin. Genes encoding valosin-containing protein (VCP), charged multivesicular body protein 2B (CHMP2B), TAR-DNA binding protein (TARDP), or fused in sarcoma (FUS) are less frequently mutated, resulting in FTD.
  - o **Intracellular Inclusions:** These include progranulin-, TDP-43-, and ubiquitin-positive inclusions in patients with GRN mutations; p62-, ubiquitin-, and unconventionally translated dipeptide repeat-positive inclusions in patients with C9ORF72 mutations; and ubiquitin- and FUS-positive inclusions in patients with FUS mutations. Patients with MAPT mutations are also at risk for tau-containing inclusions, which manifest as neurofibrobrillary tangles or amorphous deposits. The part played by the inclusions in the pathogenesis of each disease is unknown.
  - o **Neuronal Dysfunction, Neuronal Loss, and Brain Atrophy:** Uncertainty surrounds the proportion of the FTD clinical picture attributable to aberrant neuronal function versus neuronal loss. Eventually, there is significant brain atrophy that primarily affects the frontal and anterior temporal lobes, along with gliosis and neuronal loss.
- **Clinical Findings**
  - o Behavioral variant frontotemporal dementia is characterized by prominent behavioral changes, including altered interpersonal interactions and personal conduct (e.g., apathy and disinhibition), blunted emotions, and lack of insight. These behavioral abnormalities overshadow more modest cognitive defects, such as impaired judgment, inattention, or disorganization. This syndrome can be seen in patients with tau, TDP-43, C9ORF72, or FUS pathology.
  - o Semantic dementia produces fluent (receptive) aphasia with impaired comprehension and anomia and occurs with disease affecting the dominant temporal lobe. It is most common in patients with TDP-43 pathology.
  - o Progressive nonfluent aphasia produces expressive aphasia with preserved comprehension and results from the predominant involvement of the dominant frontal lobe. It is most common in patients with tau pathology
  - o Overlap syndromes occur in cases in which FTD is combined with features of parkinsonism (corticobasal degeneration or progressive supranuclear palsy or motor neuron disease (amyotrophic lateral sclerosis). Parkinsonian syndromes are seen most often in patients with tau pathology, whereas motor neuron involvement is associated with TDP-43 or C9ORF72 pathology.

- **Investigative Studies:** Frontal and temporal lobe atrophy is seen on MRI (Figure 5.8), and hypometabolism may be seen in these areas on PET. Right-sided atrophy predominates in behavioral disorders, whereas left-sided atrophy predominates in language variants. In both cases, the abnormalities are frequently asymmetric. Certain patients with a positive family history may have mutations, as revealed by genetic testing.

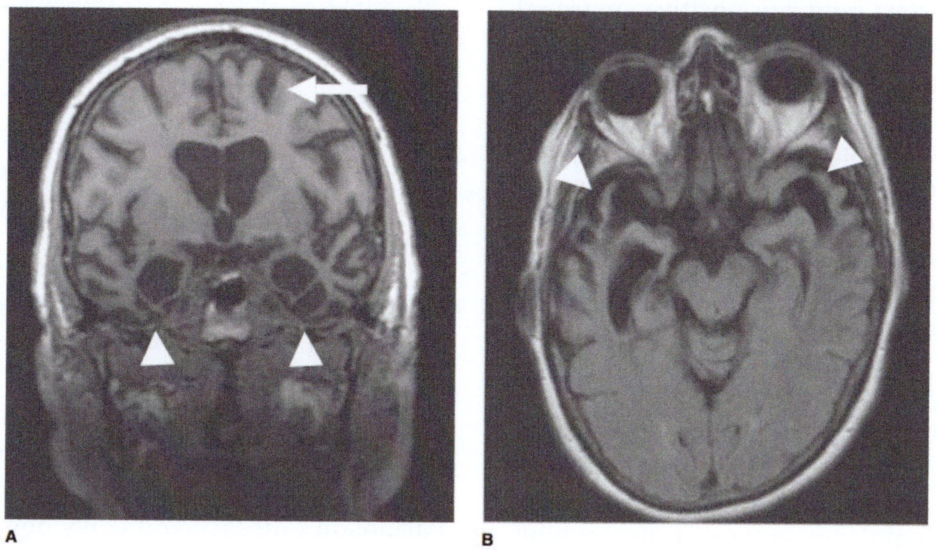

Figure 5.8. Axial (A) and coronal (B) FLAIR MRI in frontotemporal dementia showing regional atrophy of the frontal (arrow) and temporal (arrowheads) lobes.

Source: Used with permission from J. Handwerke.

- o **Differential Diagnosis:** Unlike Alzheimer's disease, the clinical picture of frontotemporal dementia (FTD) does not revolve around memory impairment, and it usually manifests at an earlier age. When dementia strikes before the age of sixty, it is suggested that the diagnosis is dementia with aphasia or behavioral disturbance as the main abnormality. A primary psychiatric disorder may be mistaken for FTD with changed behavior, and language variations may raise concerns about stroke. It's important to differentiate FTD linked to motor neuron disease or parkinsonism from conditions like Parkinson's disease or amyotrophic lateral sclerosis.
- o **Treatment:** It hasn't been demonstrated that memantine and anticholinesterase medications, which are used to treat Alzheimer's disease, work well for FTD. Trazadone and selective serotonin reuptake inhibitors are two antidepressants that may be helpful in treating behavioral symptoms. Carbidopa/levodopa or dopamine receptor agonists may be helpful for patients with parkinsonian features (corticobasal degeneration or progressive supranuclear palsy).
- o **Prognosis:** With FTD, the length of illness varies greatly (2–20 years), which is consistent with the disorder's clinical heterogeneity.

5.2.2.3. Corticobasal Degeneration

A tauopathy associated with tau pathology and FTD is corticobasal degeneration. It results in depigmentation of the substantia nigra, asymmetric frontoparietal cortical atrophy, ballooned neurons, and tau-positive neuronal and glial inclusions. The classic corticobasal syndrome includes extrapyramidal rigidity, bradykinesia, postural tremor, unilateral limb (usually arm) clumsiness, and functional impairment resulting from a combination of apraxia, sensory loss, and myoclonus. This syndrome also reflects the involvement of both the cerebral cortex and basal ganglia. The alien-hand sign is characterized by limb apraxia and sensory loss, with the limb appearing to move on its own. Common psychiatric symptoms include agitation, depression, irritability, and apathy. Apart from corticobasal degeneration, progressive supranuclear palsy and frontotemporal dementia can also exhibit corticobasal syndrome. Antiparkinsonian drugs usually have no effect on rigidity or bradykinesia.

5.2.2.4. Progressive Supranuclear Palsy

Steele-Richardson-Olszewski syndrome, also known as progressive supranuclear palsy (PSP), is an idiopathic degenerative disease that mainly affects the cerebral cortex, subcortical gray matter, and brainstem. It shares pathological characteristics with tau-positive FTD and corticobasal degeneration, including tau-positive intracellular inclusions. Supranuclear ophthalmoplegia (particularly affecting downgaze), pseudobulbar palsy, axial dystonia with or without extrapyramidal rigidity of the limbs, and dementia are the classic clinical features. because PSP typically manifests as a Parkinsonian-like movement disorder.

5.2.2.5. Lewy Body Disease

In about one-third of cases, dementia coexists with Parkinson's disease, a neurodegenerative disorder marked by tremor, rigidity, bradykinesia, and postural instability that can be inherited or occur randomly. Individuals diagnosed with Parkinson's disease with dementia are those whose dementia appears at least a year after the onset of motor symptoms; dementia with Lewy bodies is the diagnosis made for patients whose dementia appears before or within a year of the onset of motor symptoms. Nevertheless, pathologically, it is impossible to distinguish between these two diagnoses, and sometimes both are referred to as Lewy body disease.

Round, eosinophilic, intracytoplasmic neuronal inclusions (Lewy bodies) in the brainstem and cerebral cortex are the histopathological hallmarks of Lewy body disease. Since α-synuclein, which is also present in Lewy bodies in Parkinson's disease without dementia, is present in these inclusions, both Parkinson's disease and Lewy body disease are categorized as synucleinopathies.

Cognitive decline without noticeable early memory impairment is a symptom of Lewy body disease. Characteristics include erratic mental capacity, distinct visual hallucinations, and Parkinsonian symptoms, particularly bradykinesia and rigidity.

Antiparkinsonian drugs are used to treat Lewy body disease's motor manifestations; however, some research indicates that memantine or anticholinesterase medications, which are used to treat Alzheimer's disease (Table 5.9), may also help treat dementia linked to Lewy body disease.

5.2.3. Huntington Disease

An autosomal dominant neurodegenerative disease called Huntington's disease is typified by dementia, chorea, and mental symptoms. The expanded CAG trinucleotide repeat of the huntingtin (Htt) gene, which codes for a polyglutamine tract, is the root cause. There is atrophy in the brain with HTT aggregation in cytoplasmic and nuclear inclusions, affecting the putamen, cerebral cortex, and caudate nucleus. In about 25% of cases, dementia occurs before chorea, but it usually manifests after mental symptoms have been present for a few years. Deficits in memory and executive function (such as judgment) are common, while language is usually saved for later in the course.

5.2.3.1. Creutzfeldt-Jakob (Prion) Disease

Rapidly progressive dementia accompanied by variable focal degeneration of the cerebral cortex, basal ganglia, cerebellum, brainstem, and spinal cord is the hallmark of Creutzfeldt-Jakob disease (CJD). It can be genetic, infectious, or sporadic (affecting about 85% of cases). It is caused by a proteinaceous infectious particle called a prion. In the latter scenario, CJD can spread through the ingestion of contaminated beef (variant CJD) or through contact with prion-contaminated tissue or surgical instruments (iatrogenic CJD). Rarely are cases of documented human-to-human transmission (via cortical electrode implantation, corneal transplantation, or human growth hormone administration) reported. The brain, spinal cord, eyes, lungs, lymph nodes, kidneys, spleen, liver, and CSF all contain the infectious agent, but not other bodily fluids.

There is roughly one case for every million people in the population each year. In contrast to the genetically acquired disease, which typically manifests before the age of 55, the sporadic disease typically affects patients who are older than 40 and has a mean age at onset of about 60 years. Only 5 to 10% of cases involve more than one family member, and conjugal cases are uncommon.

- **Pathogenesis:** A mutation in the PRNP gene, which codes for the prion protein cellular isoform (PrPC), a protein with unclear function, causes familial CJD, an autosomal dominant disorder. A conformational shift in PrPC results in the aberrant prion protein known as the scrapie isoform, or PrPSc, in sporadic CJD. After that, PrPC is transformed into more PrPSc using PrPSc as a template. PrPSc enters the brain from an external source in infectious CJD. The accumulation of aberrant PrPSc prions in brain tissue is the outcome in each instance. Without the use of nucleic acids, PrPSc can replicate because it can induce the PrPSc conformation in PrPC prions.

Additionally, prions have been linked to animal illnesses as well as three other uncommon human conditions (Table 5.10): kuru, a degenerative illness that affects Fore-speaking tribes in New Guinea and is thought to be transmitted by cannibalism; Gerstmann-Straussler syndrome, a familial disorder characterized by ataxia and dementia; and fatal familial insomnia, a disorder that causes disruptions in sleep as well as autonomic, motor, and endocrine functions.

- **Clinical Findings:** A diffuse central nervous system (CNS) disorder or a more localized dysfunction could be the clinical picture (Table 5.11). Almost all cases have dementia, which can start as a focal cortical disorder like aphasia, apraxia, or agnosia, or as mild global cognitive impairment. It usually takes several months for the condition to progress to akinetic mutism or a coma. Anxiety, euphoria, depression, labile affect, delusions, hallucinations, and behavioral or personality changes are examples of common psychiatric symptoms. There is no fever.

Table 5.10. Prion Diseases

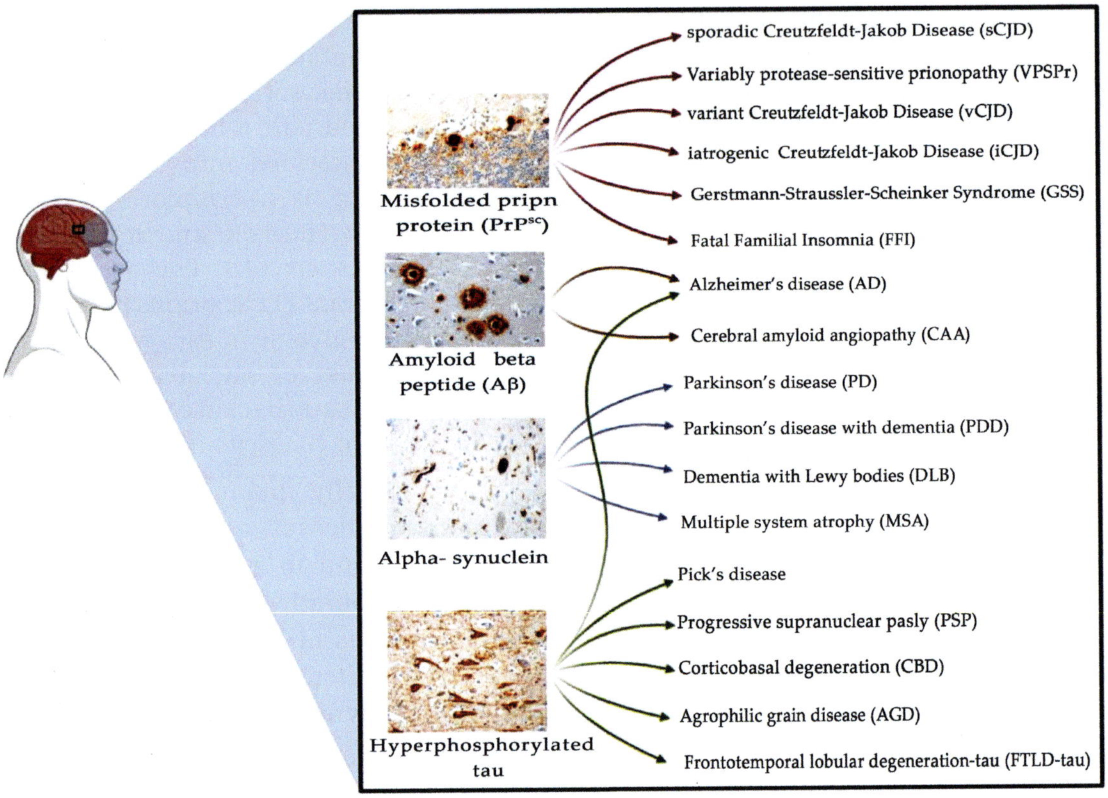

Source: Ritchie DL, Barria MA. Prion diseases: A unique transmissible agent or a model for neurodegenerative diseases? *Biomolecules.* 2021; 11(2):207. https://doi.org/10.3390/biom11020207.

The most common clinical manifestations, aside from cognitive abnormalities, are cerebellar signs, pyramidal signs, rigidity, bradykinesia, tremor, dystonia, chorea, or athetosis, as well as myoclonus, which is frequently caused by a startle. Less frequently, there are seizures, cranial nerve palsies, and visual field defects.

The disease known as "mad cow disease," or bovine spongiform encephalopathy, can infect humans and cause a unique form of CJD. This variation is distinguished by diffuse amyloid plaques, early onset (usually in adolescence or early adulthood), consistent cerebellar involvement, and prominent early psychiatric abnormalities.

Table 5.11. Diagnostic Criteria for Probable and Definite Categories of Prion Diseases

		Probable Disease			**Definitive Disease**		
CJD	**sCJD**	Rapidly progressive cognitive impairment AND typical **EEG** (generalized periodic complexes) OR typical **MRI** (high signal in caudate/ putamen or at least two cortical regions either on DWI or FLAIR) OR positive **14–3-3** AND two of the following: -Myoclonus -Visual or cerebellar problems -Pyramidal or extrapyramidal features -Akinetic mutism	OR	Progressive neurological syndrome AND positive **RT-QuIC** in CSF or other tissues.	Progressive neurological syndrome AND neuropathologically OR immunocytochemically OR biochemically confirmed.		
	gCJD	Progressive neuropsychiatric disorder AND definite or probable CJD in 1st degree relative	OR	Progressive neuropsychiatric disorder AND pathogenic *PRNP* mutation	Definitive CJD AND definitive or probable CJD in 1st degree relative	OR	Definitive CJD AND pathogenic *PRNP* mutation

<table>
<tr><td></td><td>vCJD</td><td colspan="3">Progressive neuropsychiatric disorder with duration of illness >6 months, no history of potential iatrogenic exposure, no evidence of gCJD and no alternative diagnosis suggested by routine investigations AND positive tonsil biopsy OR bilateral pulvinar high signal on MRI AND atypical appearance of sCJD on EEG in the early stages AND four of the following:
-Early psychiatric symptoms (depression, anxiety, apathy, withdrawal, delusions)
-Persistent painful sensory symptoms (frank pain or dysaesthesia)
-Ataxia
-Myoclonus, chorea or dystonia
-Dementia</td><td>Progressive neuropsychiatric disorder AND neuropathological confirmation (spongiform change and extensive PrP deposition with florid plaques throughout the cerebrum and cerebellum)</td></tr>
<tr><td></td><td>iCJD</td><td colspan="3">Progressive cerebellar syndrome in a recipient of human cadaveric-derived pituitary hormone OR sporadic CJD with a recognized exposure risk</td><td>Progressive cerebellar syndrome or sporadic CJD with a recognized exposure risk AND neuropathological confirmation</td></tr>
<tr><td>VSPr</td><td></td><td>Cognitive impairment and/or two of the following:
-Psychiatric symptoms
-Parkinsonism
-Aphasia
-Ataxia
-Myoclonus</td><td>AND</td><td>Less than 8 years duration AND absence of alternative etiology or phenotype divergence from atypical neurodegenerative dementias</td><td>Progressive neurological syndrome AND neuropathological confirmation</td></tr>
</table>

sFI and FFI		Organic sleep disturbances. If not yet clinically apparent, a polysomnography has to be performed. At least two of the following: -Psychiatric symptoms (visual hallucinations, personality changes, depression, anxiety, aggressiveness, disinhibition, listlessness) -Ataxia -Visual symptoms -Myoclonus -Cognitive/mnesic deficits	AND	One of the following: -Loss of >10 kg during the last 6 months -Vegetative signs (hyperhidrosis, newly diagnosed arterial hypertonia, tachycardia, constipation, hyperthermia) -Husky voice	Progressive neurological syndrome AND neuropathological confirmation
GSS		Progressive cerebellar syndrome, cognitive impairment and/or sensory symptoms AND pathogenic *PRNP* mutation			Progressive neurological syndrome AND neuropathological confirmation (amyloid deposits immunoreactive for PrP are the morphological hallmark of GSS)
HDL-1		Abnormal involuntary movements, coordination difficulty, dementia, personality changes and psychiatric symptoms AND pathogenic *PRNP* mutation			Kuru and multicentric plaques that stain with anti-prion antibodies

CJD: Creutzfeldt-Jakob disease; sCJD: sporadic Creutzfeldt-Jakob disease; EEG: electroencephalogram; MRI: magnetic resonance imaging; RT-QuIC: Real-Time Quacking-Induced conversion (RT-QuIC); CSF: cerebrospinal fluid; gCJD: genetic Creutzfeldt-Jakob disease; vCJD: variant Creutzfeldt-Jakob disease; iCJD: iatrogenic Creutzfeldt-Jakob disease; VSPr: Variably protease-sensitive prionopathy; sFI: sporadic fatal insomnia; FFI: fatal familial insomnia; GSS: Gerstmann-Sträusller-Scheinker; PrP: prion protein; HDL-1: Huntington disease-like syndrome. Bold words are for emphasis.

Source: Altuna M, Ruiz I, Zelaya MV, Mendioroz M. Role of Biomarkers for the Diagnosis of Prion Diseases: A Narrative Review. *Medicina*. 2022; 58(4):473. https://doi.org/10.3390/medicina58040473.

- **Investigative Studies:** Periodic sharp waves or spikes on the electroencephalogram (EEG) are possible (Figure 5.9); these are not present in the previously described variant form. Both CSF protein and 14–3-3 protein levels may be elevated (≤100 mg/dL). Hyperintense signals in the basal ganglia on T2-weighted MRI scans are possible (Figure 5.9). The final diagnosis can be made by immunodetection of PrPSc in brain tissue taken during a biopsy, cerebrospinal fluid, or, in cases where the condition runs in the family, by looking for mutant forms of PrPC in lymphocyte DNA.
- **Differential Diagnosis:** It's important to distinguish CJD from many other conditions. Alzheimer's disease is frequently taken into account, particularly in individuals who have a less fulminant course and few cerebellar and extrapyramidal symptoms. Progressive supranuclear palsy, Parkinson's disease, or cerebellar degeneration may be suspected when there is significant subcortical involvement. An intracerebral mass lesion is a possibility if there are striking focal signs. Acute metabolic disorders, such as sedative drug withdrawal, can mimic chronic limb ischemia by causing altered mentation and myoclonus.
- **Prognosis:** There isn't a treatment available right now. The illness usually progresses relentlessly and is always fatal. Most infrequent cases end in death within a year of the onset of symptoms. Families with the disease may experience a longer course of the condition (1–5 years), depending on the specific mutation present.

5.2.4. Cerebrovascular Disease

5.2.4.1. Vascular Dementia

After Alzheimer's disease, vascular disease is usually regarded as the second most common cause of dementia, and many patients have characteristics of both conditions. Individuals diagnosed with this condition may present with multiple large (diameter >1 cm) cortical infarcts; multiple small (e.g., lacunar) infarcts affecting subcortical white matter, basal ganglia, or thalamus; multiple intracerebral hemorrhages (e.g., cerebral amyloid angiopathy); or combinations of these.

Vascular dementia is typically sporadic, but there are also known hereditary causes. These include cerebral arteriopathy with subcortical infarcts and leukoencephalopathy (CADASIL, caused by mutations in NOTCH3) and autosomal dominant cerebral amyloid angiopathy, which is typically caused by mutations in the amyloid precursor protein gene.

- **Clinical Findings:** Patients with vascular dementia typically present with a history of hypertension, a progressive decline in cognitive abilities, a relatively sudden onset of dementia, and focal neurologic symptoms or indicators. The neurologic examination may reveal focal motor and sensory deficits, ataxia, gait apraxia, hyperreflexia, extensor plantar responses, and pseudobulbar palsy with dysarthria, dysphagia, and pathologic emotionality (pseudobulbar affect). Generally speaking, memory impairment is less severe than in Alzheimer's disease. But depending on the underlying pathologic process, this picture changes. As a result, patients with hemorrhage may have a noticeable headache, and those with strategic infarcts may present more acutely.

- **Investigative Studies:** The MRI (Figure 5.10) is more sensitive than the CT scan at identifying abnormalities such as multiple large infarcts, multiple small (lacunar) infarcts, areas of low density in subcortical white matter, or combinations of these findings.

Particularly in younger patients or those without a history of hypertension, more laboratory testing should be done to rule out cardiac emboli, polycythemia, thrombocytosis, cerebral vasculitis, and meningovascular syphilis as causes of multiple infarctions.

- **Treatment:** If hypertension is detected, it should be addressed to lower the risk of future heart attacks and prevent damage to other organs. There is no evidence that antiplatelet medications or statins can decrease the occurrence or advancement of vascular dementia.

5.2.4.2. Chronic Subdural Hematoma

Patients with chronic subdural hematoma are typically between the ages of 50 and 70, and they frequently have mild head trauma. Long-term hemodialysis, anticoagulation, alcoholism, cerebral atrophy, epilepsy, and ventricular shunts are additional risk factors. After trauma, symptoms might not appear for several months. About one sixth of cases have bilateral hematomas.

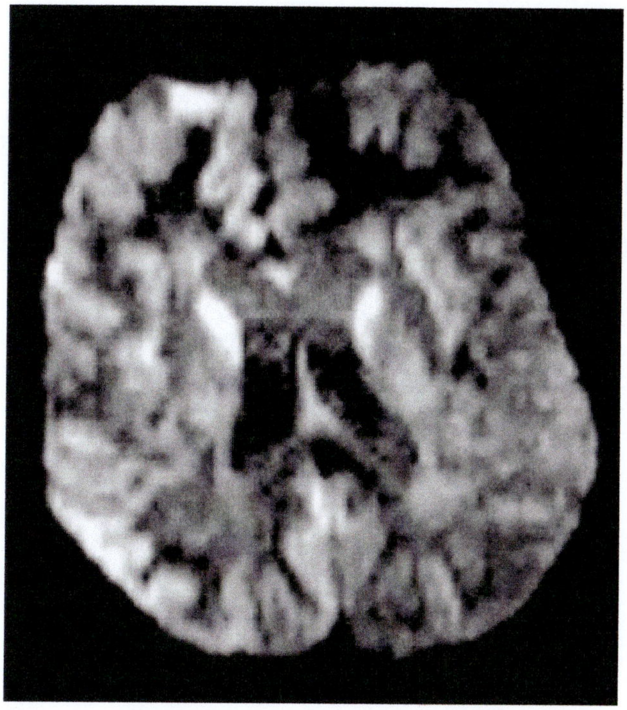

A

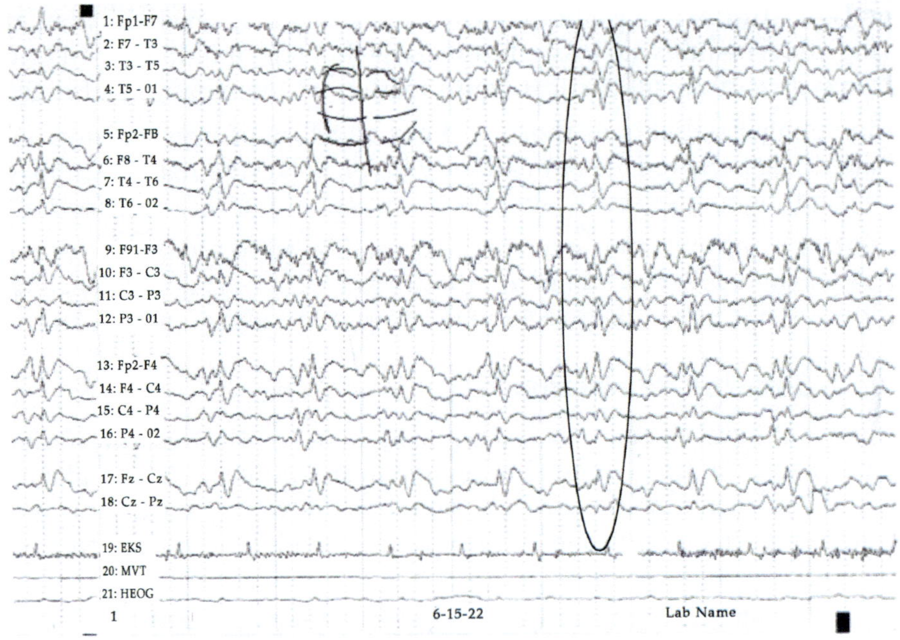

B

Figure 5.9. Diffusion-weighted image of the brain in Creutzfeldt-Jakob disease, showing characteristic hyperintensities (white) in the basal ganglia and cortical ribbon (A), and EEG with typical triphasic waves in all leads (B), which occur repetitively about once every second.

Source: https://dl.mehrsys.ir/pdf-books/Clinical%20Neurology%209%20Edition%20(www.myuptodate.com).pdf.

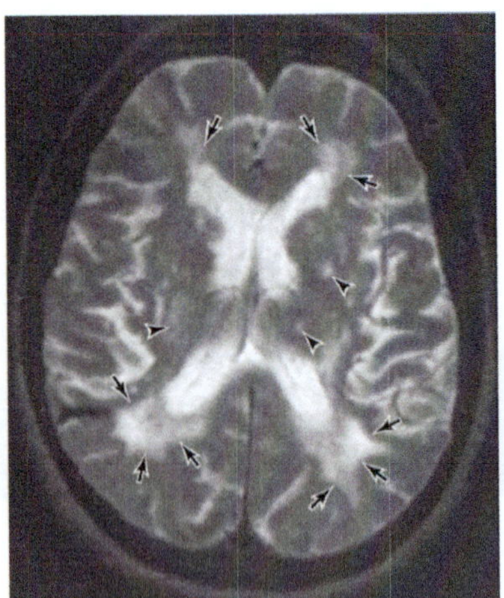

Figure 5.10. T2-weighted MRI in vascular dementia, showing foci of abnormal high signal intensity adjacent to the lateral ventricles (arrows) and within the basal ganglia (arrowheads).

Source: https://dl.mehrsys.ir/pdf-books/Clinical%20Neurology%209%20Edition%20(www.myuptodate.com).pdf.

- **Clinical Findings:** Most patients typically experience a headache as the first symptom. This may be followed by confusion, dementia, hemiparesis, and vomiting. The most commonly observed signs include cognitive disturbance, hemiparesis, papilledema, and extensor plantar responses. Aphasia, visual field defects, and seizures are rare but possible occurrences.

On a CT scan, the hematoma is typically visible as an extra-axial, crescent-shaped, low-density region with ipsilateral cortical sulci obliteration and frequently ventricular compression (Figure 5.11). It is important to carefully examine the scan to look for indications of bilateral subdural collections. A contrast infusion may make isodense collections more visible.

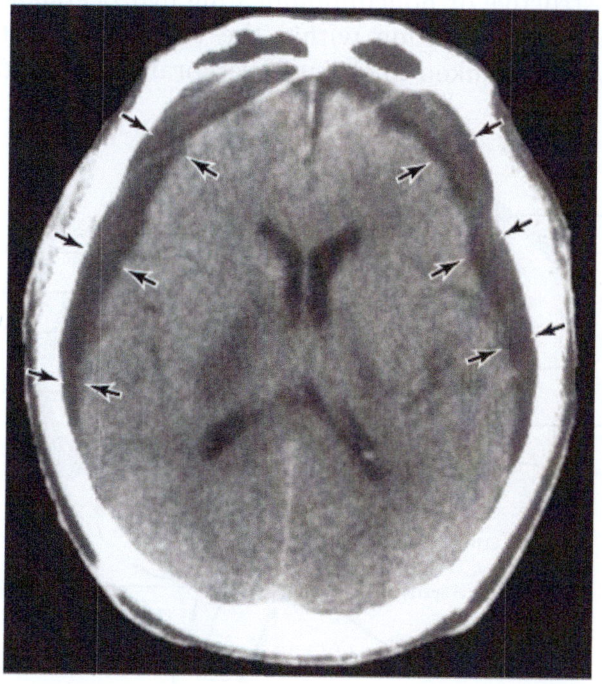

Figure 5.11. CT scan in chronic subdural hematoma, showing bilateral low-density collections between the inner table of the skull and the cerebral hemispheres (arrows).

Source: https://dl.mehrsys.ir/pdf-books/Clinical%20Neurology%209%20Edition%20(www.myuptodate.com).pdf.

- **Treatment:** Symptomatic hematomas should be surgically removed unless otherwise indicated by health issues or spontaneous improvement. Methods include burr-hole or twist-drill craniostomy and craniotomy. It has not been demonstrated that corticosteroid or preventative anticonvulsant therapy is helpful.

5.2.5. Other Cerebral Disorders

5.2.5.1. Normal-Pressure Hydrocephalus

A possibly curable cause of dementia, normal-pressure hydrocephalus is typified by the clinical trifecta of dementia, gait apraxia, and incontinence. It could be idiopathic or the result of diseases like meningitis or subarachnoid hemorrhage that obstruct the absorption of CSF. Usually preceded by incontinence and gait disorder, the dementia has a gradual and mild onset. Global cognitive dysfunction develops later, after mental slowness and apathy initially appear. While memory loss is common, aphasia and agnosia are uncommon.

- **Pathophysiology:** Normal-pressure hydrocephalus is sometimes referred to as nonobstructive hydrocephalus (since the CSF flow between the ventricles is unaffected) or communicating hydrocephalus (because the lateral, third, and fourth ventricles continue to communicate). The arachnoid granulations in the subarachnoid space above the cerebral hemispheres are thought to be the source of the impaired CSF absorption (Figure 5.12). On the other hand, obstructive or noncommunicating hydrocephalus results from a blockage of cerebral spinal fluid circulation within the ventricular system, such as a tumor or intraventricular cyst. It is linked to elevated cerebral spinal fluid pressure, headache, and papilledema.

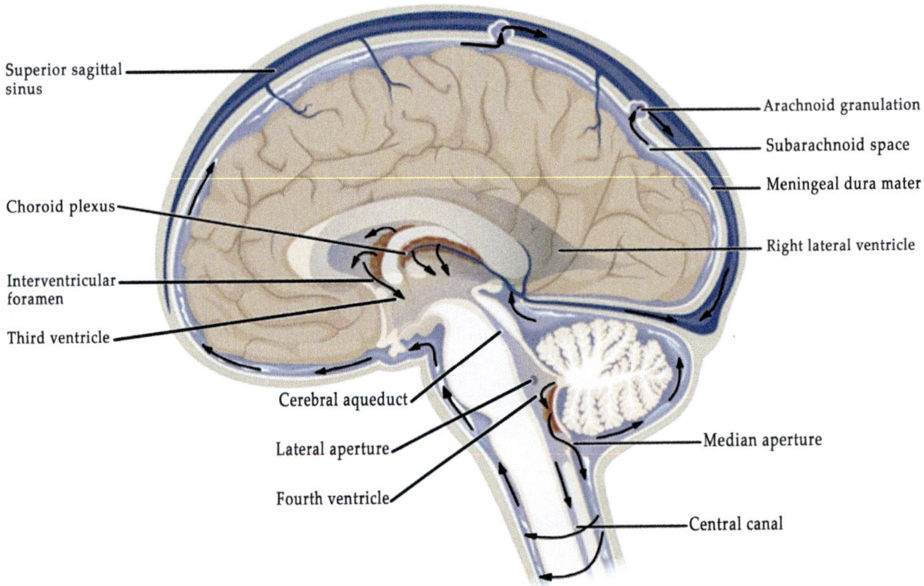

Figure 5.12. Circulation of cerebrospinal fluid (CSF). CSF is produced by the choroid plexus, which consists of specialized secretory tissue located within the cerebral ventricles. It flows from the lateral and third ventricles through the cerebral aqueduct and fourth ventricle and exits the ventricular system through two laterally situated foramina of Luschka and a single, medially located foramen of Magendie. CSF then enters and circulates through the subarachnoid space surrounding the brain and spinal cord. It is ultimately absorbed through arachnoid granulations into the venous circulation.

Source: https://courses.lumenlearning.com/suny-dutchess-anatomy-physiology/chapter/circulation-and-the-central-nervous-system/.

- **Clinical Findings:** The first signs of normal-pressure hydrocephalus are frequent gait disorders, which typically take months to develop. This usually manifests as gait apraxia, which is characterized by a lack of weakness or ataxia but causes unsteadiness when standing and difficulty starting a walk (magnetic gait). The patient can kick a ball, walk, cycle, and trace figures with their feet when they are sitting or lying down, but they are unable to do so when their legs are bearing weight. When walking, the patient usually looks like they are glued to the ground and moves slowly in shuffling motions. There may occasionally be pyramidal symptoms, such as hyperreflexia, spasticity, and extensor plantar responses. Grip reflexes in the hands and feet as well as motor perseveration—the improper repetition of motor activity—may manifest. Psychomotor slowing, inattention, and problems with decision-making and spatial recognition are all signs of dementia. Fecal incontinence is rare; urinary incontinence develops later and patients may not be aware of it.

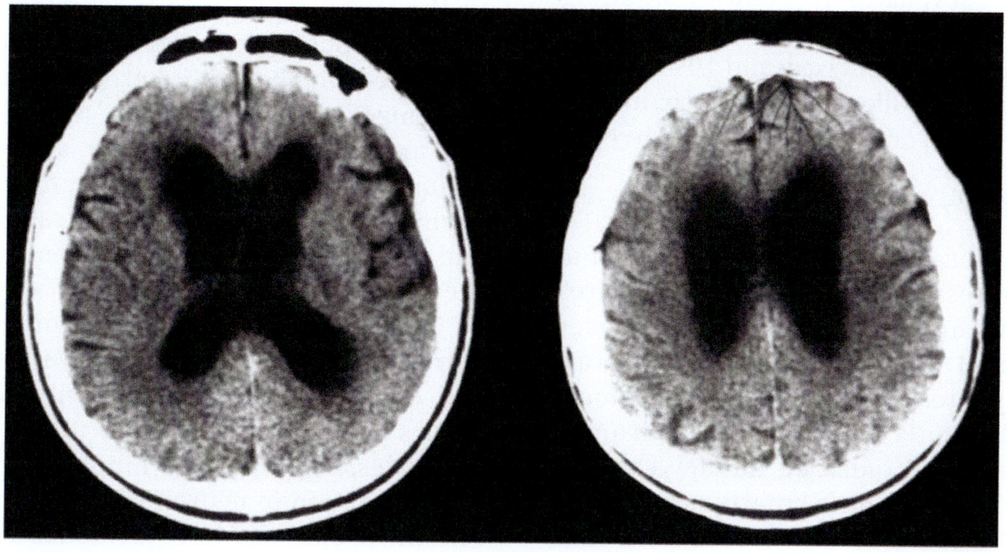

Figure 5.13. CT scan at two transverse levels in normal-pressure hydrocephalus, showing enlarged lateral ventricles without enlargement of the cortical sulci.

Source: https://dl.mehrsys.ir/pdf-books/Clinical%20Neurology%209%20Edition%20(www.myuptodate.com).pdf.

- **Investigative Studies:** Normal or low opening pressure is revealed by lumbar puncture. Usually, the lateral ventricles are enlarged on the CT scan or MRI, but the cortical sulci are not as prominent (Figure 5.13). Isotope accumulation in the ventricles, delayed clearance, and failure of ascent over the cerebral convexities are classical signs of radionuclide cisternography. However, patients who respond to shunting may not always exhibit this pattern. The best indicator of a positive clinical response to shunting is likely to be a brief improvement in gait, cognitive testing, or sphincteric function following the removal of 30 to 50 mL of CSF by lumbar puncture (tap test) or external lumbar drainage of 750 to 1,000 mL of CSF over 72 hours (see Treatment).
- **Differential Diagnosis:** Alzheimer's disease frequently has a longer course, and an MRI or CT scan may reveal enlarged cortical sulci and prominent focal cortical dysfunction. The gait disorder can mimic Parkinsonism, but it can be differentiated from it by extrapyramidal rigidity, tremor, and reaction to antiparkinsonian drugs. If pseudobulbar palsy, focal sensorimotor signs, a history of stroke, or a stepwise course of the disorder are observed, vascular dementia should be suspected. Vascular lesions should be visible on an MRI or CT scan in these situations.

- **Treatment:** Some patients respond well to ventriculoatrial, ventriculoperitoneal, or lumboperitoneal shunting, particularly those who have hydrocephalus due to meningitis or subarachnoid hemorrhage. About 70% of patients with idiopathic normal-pressure hydrocephalus respond to shunting. About 15% of patients need to have their shunts revised, and 10% develop problems like infection, seizures, or subdural or intracerebral hemorrhage.

5.2.5.2. Brain Tumor

A variety of local and diffuse effects, such as edema, compression of nearby brain structures, elevated intracranial pressure, decreased cerebral blood flow, and disruption of brain connectivity, are combined by brain tumors to cause dementia and related syndromes. Chemotherapy and radiation therapy can also impair cognitive function in brain tumor patients. Gliomas originating in the corpus callosum, frontal or temporal lobes, are the tumors most likely to cause generalized cerebral syndromes. Even though these lesions frequently invade subcortical white matter, they rarely cause many focal neurologic symptoms at first.

Apathy, poor concentration, prominent mental slowness, and mild personality changes are hallmarks of brain tumor-related dementia. Early signs of memory impairment, aphasia, or agnosia may be evident depending on the areas involved. In the end, headaches, seizures, or focal sensorimotor disturbances are caused by brain tumors.

Meningeal neoplasia can also result in symptoms and signs of dysfunction at several sites in the nervous system, as well as dementia, which is frequently accompanied by headaches. Cytologic analysis of the CSF is used to establish the diagnosis.

5.2.5.3. Chronic Traumatic Encephalopathy

Repeated or severe head trauma can lead to progressive cognitive impairment and, in rare cases, dementia. Neurofibrillary tangles containing hyperphosphorylated tau, β-amyloid deposits in diffuse or neuritic plaques or in blood vessels, and α-synuclein-positive Lewy bodies are examples of histopathologic features. Dementia pugilistica, a condition traditionally associated with boxers, is becoming more widely recognized in other athletes and veterans of the armed forces who have suffered head trauma. Headache, difficulty focusing and paying attention, depression, erratic behavior, and short-term memory problems are some of the initial symptoms. Dementia accompanied by aggressive behavior and trouble finding words is the result of executive dysfunction and other cognitive impairments. Suicidality occurs often. Diffuse axonal injury, enlarged ventricles, and cortical or hippocampal atrophy can all be seen in neuroimaging studies. About one-third of cases have evidence at autopsy of another neurodegenerative disease, such as motor neuron disease, Alzheimer's disease, Lewy body disease, or frontotemporal dementia.

5.2.6. Systemic Disorders

5.2.6.1. Infection

- **HIV-Associated Neurocognitive Disorders:** Numerous HIV-associated neurocognitive disorders can result from brain infection with the human immunodeficiency virus (HIV-1). These consist of HIV-associated dementia (moderate to severe cognitive and functional impairment), mild to moderate neurocognitive disorder, and asymptomatic neurocognitive impairment (demonstrated only by cognitive testing). Since combination antiretroviral therapy was introduced, the incidence of HIV-associated dementia has decreased, but as patients live longer, its prevalence has increased. Intravenous drug use, female gender, and advanced age are risk factors.

- o **Pathogenesis:** Blood-borne macrophage-tropic retrovirus, which infects macrophages, microglia, and astrocytes but not neurons, invades the brain and causes HIV-associated dementia. Although the virus may stay dormant and asymptomatic for years, it appears to enter the central nervous system (CNS) early in systemic HIV-1 infection. As an alternative, it may result in HIV-1 meningitis with transient symptoms (see Chapter 4, Confusional States). The neurotoxic effects of viral proteins as well as soluble factors released by inflammatory cells such as chemokines and cytokines are some of the pathogenesis's hypothesized mechanisms.
- o **Pathology:** The brainstem, thalamus, subcortical white matter, and basal ganglia are all affected by perivascular infiltration by macrophages, multinucleated giant cells, and astrogliosis in HIV-associated dementia. The frontal and temporal cortex, as well as the basal ganglia, may show signs of neuronal loss. Vacuolar myelopathy may also impact the spinal cord.
- o **Clinical Findings:** HIV-associated dementia typically develops slowly and is accompanied by abnormalities in cognition, behavior, and motor function. These include tremors, gait abnormalities, reading and writing difficulties, memory loss, and apathy. Antiretroviral medication has also been linked to cortical deficits, including decreased learning and executive function as well as Parkinsonian traits. Examining the patient may reveal cerebellar ataxia, extensor plantar responses, hyperreflexia, and primitive reflexes.
- o **Investigative Studies:** HIV-associated dementia cannot be definitively diagnosed through a laboratory test. Oligoclonal bands, modest, usually mononuclear pleocytosis (≤50 cells/μL), and mild to moderate elevation of protein (≤200 mg/dL) can all be seen in CSF. By displaying diffuse signal abnormalities in subcortical white matter along with cortical and subcortical atrophy, MRI can help rule out other HIV-related neuropathologic processes, such as opportunistic infection (Figure 5.14).
- o **Treatment:** Combination antiretroviral therapy, as described for HIV-1 meningitis, should be given to patients with HIV-associated cognitive disorders.

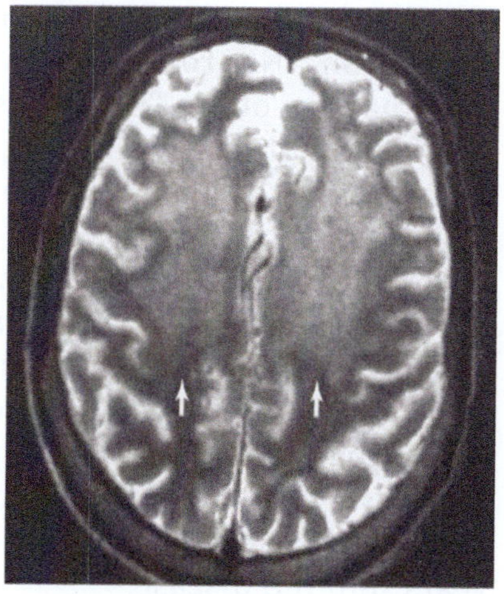

Figure 5.14. T2-weighted MRI in HIV-associated dementia, showing increased signal intensity (arrows) in subcortical white matter.

Source: https://dl.mehrsys.ir/pdf-books/Clinical%20Neurology%209%20Edition%20(www.myuptodate.com).pdf.

- o **Prognosis:** The course could be comparatively stable, progressively worsening, or suddenly made worse by another illness. Median survival has increased from a few months to several years with combination antiretroviral therapy.

- **Neurosyphilis:** Treponema pallidum, the causative agent of syphilis, is spread through intercourse in about one-third of cases involving infected people. While common during the prepenicillin era, dementia resulting from neurosyphilis (general paresis) is now uncommon.

- o **Clinical Findings:**

- § Localized skin lesions (chancres) are the hallmark of primary syphilis, and they typically manifest one month after exposure. T. hematogenously spreads. Within one to six months, pallidum causes the symptoms and indicators of secondary syphilis, such as fever, rash, alopecia, anogenital skin lesions, and mucous membrane ulceration. Neurologic symptoms don't happen often. The earliest type of neurosyphilis with symptoms, meningeal syphilis, develops two to twelve months after the initial infection and is characterized by headache, stiff neck, nausea, vomiting, and involvement of the cranial nerves, particularly those of the II, VII, or VIII. Meningovascular syphilis typically manifests as a transient ischemic attack or stroke and is diagnosed 4–7 years into the disease.

- § General paresis and tabes dorsalis are the syndromes caused by late (parenchymatous) neurosyphilis. These can manifest alone or in combination (taboparesis); both can coexist with optic atrophy. A persistent meningoencephalitis caused by an active spirochetal infection is known as general paresis. Gradual memory loss or changes in personality, or behavior are the first signs. Global intellectual decline with grandiosity, depression, psychosis, and focal weakness come next. Strokes, seizures, or incontinence are examples of terminal features. A neurologic examination may reveal pyramidal signs, dysarthria, facial expression deficiency, and tremor of the face and tongue. When tabes dorsalis and general paresis coexist, it is known as taboparesis. Argyll Robertson pupils, lancinating (stabbing) pains, areflexia, posterior column sensory deficits with sensory ataxia and Romberg sign, incontinence, impotence, hypertrophic joints (Charcot), and hyperextended knees (genu recurvatum) are among the indications and symptoms of tabes dorsalis. There may also be optic atrophy.

- o **Investigative Studies:** A treponemal blood test should be obtained in all suspected cases because non-treponemal blood tests (Venereal Disease Research Laboratory [VDRL] or rapid plasma reagin [RPR]) can be negative. Treponemal serologic blood tests (fluorescent treponemal antibody absorbed [FTA-ABS] or microhemagglutination Treponema pallidum [MHATP]) are reactive in almost all patients with active neurosyphilis. If this is nonreactive, neurosyphilis can be ruled out; if reactive, lumbar puncture should be done to confirm the diagnosis and obtain a baseline CSF profile for evaluating the effectiveness of treatment. A lymphocytic pleocytosis and reactive nontreponemal CSF serology (e.g., VDRL) are observed in the CSF in cases of active neurosyphilis, except end-stage tabes dorsalis and early meningeal and meningovascular syphilis. Increased γ-globulin, protein elevation, and the presence of oligoclonal bands are among the other abnormalities found in CSF. Unilateral or bilateral medial temporal lobe T2 high-intensity abnormalities, with or without associated atrophy, may be seen on the MRI in cases of general paresis.

  - **Treatment:** The same treatment used previously for syphilitic meningitis is applied to general paresis. Shortly after therapy commences, a transient fever and leukocytosis may happen (Herxheimer reaction). Retreatment is necessary if the CSF does not return to normal within six months.
  - **Prognosis:** After treatment, general paresis may get better or stabilize, but in certain cases, it gets worse. Although it is unlikely that patients with persistently reactive CSF serologic tests and no pleocytosis will benefit from penicillin therapy, they are typically treated anyhow.

- **Progressive Multifocal Leukoencephalopathy:** Immunosuppressed patients who experience reactivation of the JC virus infection—which is typically asymptomatic—develop progressive multifocal leukoencephalopathy (PML). These include those receiving treatment for multiple sclerosis, Crohn's disease, or psoriasis with efalizumab, as well as those with lymphoma, leukemia, or HIV infection. The condition affects oligodendrocytes, which results in diffuse and patchy demyelination of the cerebellum, brainstem, and cerebral hemispheres.

The majority of patients experience a subacute and progressive course that culminates in death within 3 to 6 months, with a mortality rate of approximately 20% among those receiving natalizumab. Years after treatment, PML linked to natalizumab or efalizumab manifests. There is no fever or systemic symptoms. Focal cortical dysfunction and dementia are common. Hemiparesis, visual impairments, aphasia, dysarthria, and sensory impairment are among the symptoms. There are rarely headaches and ataxia, and there are no seizures.

The CSF is normally normal, although there may be a slight increase in protein, white blood cell count, or pressure. Multifocal white matter abnormalities are visible on the MRI or CT scan (Figure 5.15). Brain biopsies can be used to confirm a diagnosis when there is uncertainty.

For patients with HIV infection, treatment for PML consists of combination antiretroviral therapy, while patients on natalizumab undergo plasma exchange in addition to medication discontinuation.

5.2.6.2. Metabolic Disorders

- **Alcoholism:** Dementia may result from some alcoholism-related complications. These include states of nutritional deficiency, chronic subdural hematoma from head trauma, and acquired hepatocerebral degeneration from alcoholic liver disease.

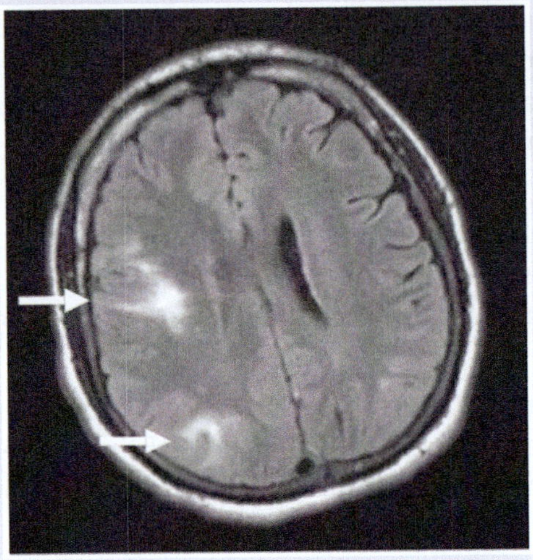

Figure 5.15. Axial FLAIR MRI in progressive multifocal leukoencephalopathy, showing abnormally high signal intensity (arrows) in white matter of the right parietal and occipital lobes.

Source: https://dl.mehrsys.ir/pdf-books/Clinical%20Neurology%209%20Edition%20(www.myuptodate.com).pdf.

- o Nicotinic acid (niacin) deficiency, which causes pellagra, damages neurons in the brainstem, cerebellum, anterior horns of the spinal cord, basal ganglia, and cerebral cortex. Diarrhea, glossitis, anemia, and erythematous skin lesions are signs of systemic involvement. Dementia, psychosis, confused states, pyramidal, extrapyramidal, and cerebellar signs, polyneuropathy, and optic neuropathy can all result from neurologic involvement. Nicotinamide is the treatment, however even with this, the neurologic deficits may not improve.
- o Marchiafava-Bignami syndrome is primarily seen in malnourished alcoholics and is typified by necrosis of the corpus callosum and subcortical white matter. It may follow an acute, subacute, or chronic course. Dementia, spasticity, dysarthria, gait abnormality, and coma are examples of clinical features. MRIs and CT scans can occasionally be used to make the diagnosis. While there isn't a specific treatment available, it is advised to stop drinking and improve one's diet. A patient's prognosis is unpredictable; one could pass away, endure dementia, or recover.
- o Although it has been suggested that ethanol's direct toxicity on the brain causes alcoholic dementia, the brains of demented alcoholics do not exhibit any particular abnormalities. It is more likely that one of the metabolic and traumatic disorders previously mentioned, or a misdiagnosis of Korsakoff syndrome, will cause dementia in alcoholics.

- **Hypothyroidism:** Chronic organic psychosis or reversible dementia are other conditions that can result from hypothyroidism (myxedema). Dementia is a widespread illness marked by irritability, memory loss, and mental slowness. There are no focal cortical deficits. Psychiatric symptoms are often noticeable and include suicidal thoughts and actions, mania, depression, paranoia, and auditory and visual hallucinations.

  Myxedema patients may experience paresthesia, weakness, vertigo, tinnitus, headaches, or hearing loss. Examination may reveal cerebellar ataxia, dysarthria, or deafness. The delayed relaxation of the tendon reflexes is the most intriguing discovery.

- **Vitamin B12 Deficiency:** One uncommon cause of organic psychosis and reversible dementia is a vitamin B12 deficiency. Dementia can manifest with or without hematologic and other neurologic symptoms, similar to the acute confusional state linked to vitamin B12 deficiency (though decreased vibratory sensation and proprioception in the lower extremities are common). In addition to mental slowness, poor concentration, and memory disturbance, the dementia is characterized by global cognitive dysfunction; aphasia and other focal cortical disorders are not present. Psychotic symptoms are common and include auditory and visual hallucinations, paranoid psychosis, and depression.

5.2.6.3. Organ Failure

- **Dialysis Dementia:** This is an uncommon condition that affects people who get long-term hemodialysis. Myoclonus, dysarthria, and seizures are examples of clinical features. These are sporadic at first, but eventually, they become permanent, and dementia takes over. Diazepam can reverse the paroxysmal high-voltage slowing seen in the EEG, which is characterized by mixed spikes and slow waves. The incidence of the syndrome has decreased with the removal of trace metals from the dialysate. Renal hypoperfusion episodes during hemodialysis may also be linked to cognitive dysfunction and related subcortical white matter lesions on MRI.
- **Non-Wilsonian Hepatocerebral Degeneration:** One rare consequence of chronic hepatic cirrhosis with either spontaneous or surgical portosystemic shunting is acquired (non-Wilsonian) hepatocerebral degeneration. The inability of the liver to detoxify ammonia may be the cause of the symptoms. In about one-sixth of patients, neurological symptoms appear before hepatic symptoms.
    - o **Clinical Findings:** The majority of the time, chronic liver disease has systemic symptoms. Over the course of one to nine years, the neurologic syndrome is variable but progressive, and episodes of acute hepatic encephalopathy may occur periodically. The most typical symptoms include dementia, dysarthria, and signs of the cerebellum, extrapyramidal, and pyramidal regions. Mental slowness, apathy, trouble focusing and paying attention, and memory problems are symptoms of dementia. Cerebellar signs include dysarthria, ataxia of the limbs, and abnormal gait; nystagmus is uncommon. Athetosis, dystonia, chorea, rigidity, and resting tremor can all result from extrapyramidal involvement. Paraparesis is uncommon; asterixis, myoclonus, hyperreflexia, and extensor plantar responses are typical.

      Laboratory investigations reveal elevated blood ammonia and aberrant hepatic blood chemistries, but there is no correlation between the degree of abnormality and the severity of neurologic symptoms. Lesions in the subcortical white matter and basal ganglia may be seen on an MRI. With the exception of occasionally mildly elevated protein and increased glutamine, the CSF is normal.
    - o **Differential Diagnosis:** Wilson disease can be identified by its abnormal copper metabolism, Kayser-Fleischer rings, and earlier onset. Alcoholic cerebellar degeneration does not present with extrapyramidal or pyramidal signs; instead, it primarily affects gait.
    - o **Treatment and Prognosis:** Low-protein diets, lactulose, neomycin, liver transplants, portosystemic shunts, and

improvement following levodopa or bromocriptine therapy have all been reported to help patients. Either variceal hemorrhage or progressive liver failure leads to death.

- **Wilson Disease:** Wilson disease, also known as hepatolenticular degeneration, is an uncommon but curable autosomal recessive genetic copper metabolism disorder that manifests as extrapyramidal symptoms and dementia. Mutations in the ATP7B gene, which codes for the β polypeptide of an ATPase that transports copper, cause the illness.

5.2.7. Pseudodementia

The most common disorder to be confused with dementia is depression. Making this distinction is crucial because depression is a common and treatable condition. Mental slowness, apathy, self-neglect, withdrawal, irritability, problems with memory and concentration, and behavioral and personality changes are characteristics of both dementia and depression. Furthermore, depression may coexist with dementia as separate disorders, depression in later life may be a sign of dementia in the future, and depression itself may be a feature of dementing illnesses. Table 5.12 contains a list of clinical characteristics that aid in differentiation. It is important to seek psychiatric consultation when depression is being considered. Depression should be treated directly if it cannot be resolved by treating an underlying illness or by switching medications. Electroconvulsive therapy, antidepressant medications, and psychotherapy are among the treatments.

5.3. Amnestic Syndromes

Amnestic syndrome is a memory disorder that can arise alone or as a symptom of acute confusion, dementia, or both.

Table 5.12. Dementia Versus Pseudodementia of Depression: Distinguishing Features

Dementia	Depression
Insidious onset	Abrupt onset
Progressive deterioration	Plateau of dysfunction
No history of depression	History of depression may exist
Patient typically unaware of extent of deficits and does not complain of memory loss	Patient aware of and may exaggerate deficits and frequently complains of memory loss
Somatic complaints uncommon	Somatic complaints or hypochondriasis common
Variable affect	Depressed affect
Few vegetative symptoms	Prominent vegetative symptoms
Impairment often worse at night	Impairment usually not worse at night
Neurologic examination and laboratory studies may be abnormal	Neurologic examination and laboratory studies normal

Source: https://dl.mehrsys.ir/pdf-books/Clinical%20Neurology%209%20Edition%20(www.myuptodate.com).pdf.

It is possible to think of memory as a complex function with various components. Declarative (conscious) memory comprises episodic (personal) and semantic (factual) memory over a longer period of time, as well as working memory, which allows for the rapid manipulation of newly presented information. Nondeclarative, or unconscious, memory consists of emotional memory that gives objects or events affective significance, as well as procedural memory needed to perform learned and seemingly automatic tasks.

The stages of information registration, storage, and retrieval can also be thought of as comprising memory. The parahippocampal region of the medial temporal lobe, the hippocampus, and the neocortical association areas are thought to play key roles in memory processing, according to autopsy and imaging studies. The inability to create new memories is a clinical manifestation of short-term memory impairment caused by bilateral damage to these regions. Retrieving previously learned information is part of long-term memory, which is comparatively preserved. This may be because ingrained memories are stored more widely. Confabulation is the attempt by some patients with amnestic syndromes to make up memories to fill in blanks. These false recollections can be complex fabrications or real memories that have been misplaced in time. However, in most cases, the most enduring and deeply ingrained memories—like one's own name—are unaffected by organic memory disorders. On the other hand, dissociative (psychogenic) amnesia may significantly or solely impair these private recollections.

5.3.1. Acute Amnesia

5.3.1.1. Head Trauma

Amnestic syndrome is almost always linked to head injuries that cause unconsciousness. Patients seen soon after such an injury may behave in an apparently normal automatic manner, but they also show signs of confusion, including anterograde amnesia (Figure 5.16), in which they are unable to integrate new memories. Furthermore, there is retrograde amnesia that spans a variable amount of time before the trauma.

Regaining full consciousness also brings back the capacity to create new memories. On the other hand, things that happen during the confusional interval usually fade from memory forever. Islands of memory during a coherent interval between trauma and unconsciousness or times of reduced impairment during a fluctuating posttraumatic confusional state are exceptions. The most distant memories come back first as the period of retrograde amnesia gets shorter. The length of disorientation and the degree of both permanent retrograde and posttraumatic amnesia are generally correlated with the severity of the injury.

5.3.2. Hypoxia or Ischemia

Amnestic syndromes can arise from conditions that cause cerebral hypoxia or ischemia, such as carbon monoxide poisoning or cardiac arrest because these insults selectively affect the hippocampal neurons involved in memory formation. Patients who have been in a coma for more than 12 hours are more likely to experience amnesia. An isolated short-term memory disorder is caused by a significant impairment in the ability to integrate new memories while maintaining a comparatively high level of registration and remote memory. There could be a period of retrograde amnesia that existed before the insult. Patients confabulate occasionally and show a lack of concern about their impairment. Amnesia following cardiac arrest may coexist with cerebral watershed syndromes, such as bibrachial paresis, cortical blindness, or visual agnosia, or it may be the only sign of neurologic dysfunction. Recoveries usually take a few days, though deficiencies might linger.

Depressive symptoms are often linked to amnestic syndromes caused by carbon monoxide poisoning. Extrapyramidal and focal cortical dysfunction are among the other abnormalities. Elevated levels of hemoglobin, cardiac arrhythmia, and cherry-red skin and mucous membranes are indicators of acute carbon monoxide poisoning. The dentate nuclei and basal ganglia may exhibit lucencies on a CT scan of the brain. Oxygen therapy involves either normo- or hyperbaric delivery.

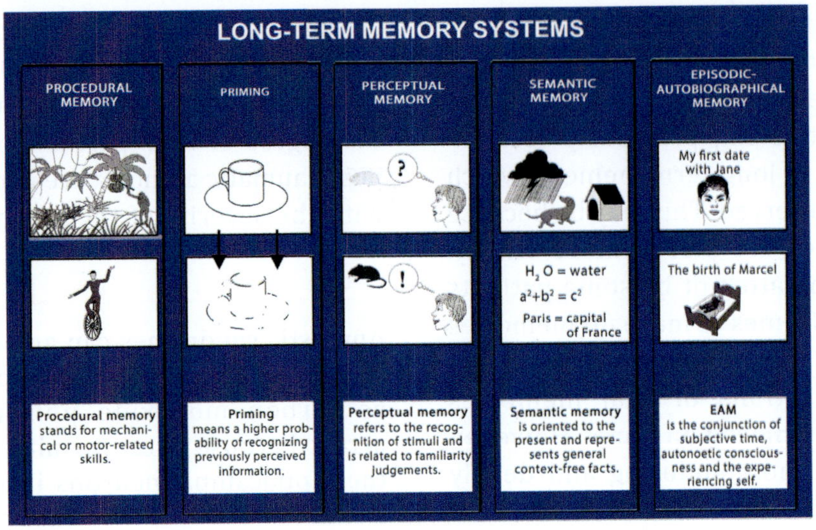

Figure 5.16. Retrograde and anterograde amnesia in posttraumatic memory disorders. Head trauma may produce transient coma, followed by a confusional state during which the patient is unable to form new memories. With recovery, this ability is restored, but there is persistent amnesia for the period of coma and confusion (anterograde amnesia) and for a variable period preceding the trauma (retrograde amnesia); the latter deficit may improve with time.

Source: Staniloiu A, Markowitsch HJ. The Remains of the Day in Dissociative Amnesia. *Brain Sciences*. 2012; 2(2):101–129. https://doi.org/10.3390/brainsci2020101.

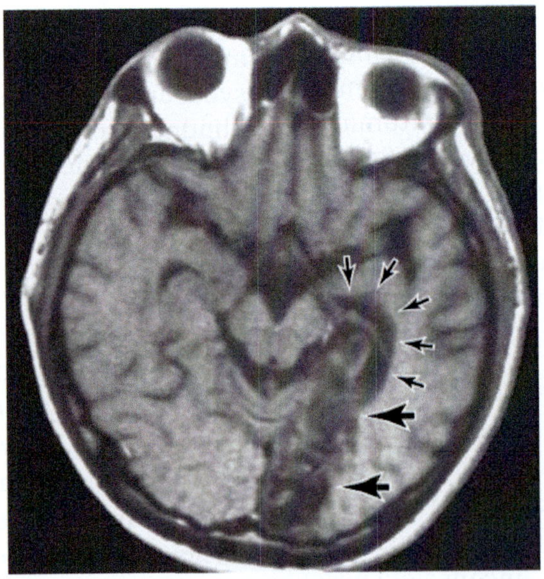

Figure 5.17. T1-weighted MRI in a patient with an old left posterior cerebral artery occlusion, showing tissue loss in the medial temporal (small arrows) and occipital (large arrows) lobes and associated dilation of the temporal and occipital horns of the lateral ventricle.

Source: Used with permission from A. Gean.

5.3.2.1. Bilateral Posterior Cerebral Artery Occlusion

The occipital cortex, thalamus, posterior internal capsule, and medial temporal lobe are all supplied by the posterior cerebral artery (Figure 5.17). An amnestic syndrome that is either temporary or permanent can result from ischemia or infarction in this region, usually when it is bilateral. These conditions are frequently caused by emboli in the vertebrobasilar system.

Usually, unilateral or bilateral hemianopia is linked to the amnestic syndrome. Other symptoms that may be present include visual agnosia, alexia without agraphia, anomia, sensory abnormalities, or indications of upper midbrain dysfunction, particularly impaired pupillary light reflex. Selective impairment of recent memory is common, while remote memory and registration are largely preserved.

The CT scan displays lucencies in any combination of the aforementioned regions, which may or may not be enhanced by the use of contrast material.

5.3.2.2. Transient Global Amnesia

Patients in their middle or later years are more likely to experience the acute memory loss syndrome known as transient global amnesia. There have been several theories regarding the cause, including transient cerebral ischemia, spreading depression (waves of decreased electrical activity in the cerebral cortex), and physical or psychological stress. Less than 10% of patients experience recurrence of the disorder.

Short-term memory is impacted by transient global amnesia, which can linger up to 24 hours. Patients may frequently ask questions regarding their whereabouts, the time, and the nature of what they are experiencing, displaying signs of agitation and confusion. Personal identity knowledge is retained, along with distant memories and registration. However, the inability to form new memories explains the patient's repeated questions. Retrograde amnesia may exist for a variable amount of time prior to the episode, but it diminishes as the episode ends. Symptoms that are often experienced include headache, nausea, and vertigo.

Transient global amnesia differs from the majority of other amnestic syndromes in that the patient expresses clear concern about the condition. Signal abnormalities affecting the CA1 field of the hippocampal may be visible on high-resolution MRI.

5.3.2.3. Alcoholic Blackouts

Large-scale, brief ethanol intake by both alcoholics and non-alcoholics can result in "blackouts," which are brief amnestic episodes unrelated to seizures, head trauma, Wernicke-Korsakoff syndrome, or generalized confusion. The hallmark of these spells is the incapacity to create new memories, without compromising short-term or long-term memory. Although there is no specific treatment needed for the disorder because it is self-limiting, it is advisable to reduce ethanol intake and treat Wernicke encephalopathy with thiamine.

5.3.2.4. Wernicke Encephalopathy

A thiamine deficiency causes Wernicke encephalopathy, which typically manifests as acute confusion, ataxia, and ophthalmoplegia. However, amnesia may be the primary or only cognitive disturbance, particularly if other cognitive abnormalities improve and thiamine treatment is started. because rather than just isolated amnesia, patients with Wernicke encephalopathy typically present with global confusion.

5.3.2.5. Dissociative (Psychogenic) Amnesia

Amnesia could be a sign of malingering or a dissociative disorder. Such patients frequently have a history of mental illness, additional mental symptoms, or an emotional stressor that preceded the illness. An isolated or disproportionate loss of traumatic or stressful personal memories is the hallmark of dissociative amnesia.

Typically, dissociative amnesia is restricted to the moments immediately following a traumatic event or selectively affects certain events during that time but not others. Generalized amnesia, continuous amnesia for events from some time in the past up to and including the present, and amnesia limited to specific categories of information are less common patterns. It is extremely uncommon for patients with organic amnesia to be unable to recall even their own name. It is possible to maintain orientation to time and place even in the face of such disorientation to people. Furthermore, recent memories might be less affected than distant memories; organic diseases cause the opposite pattern of amnesia that is typically observed. A hypnotic examination or one conducted following amobarbital sodium administration could prove beneficial in proving that the amnesia is psychogenic.

5.3.3. Chronic Amnesia

5.3.3.1. Alcoholic Korsakoff Amnestic Syndrome

Thiamine deficiency is thought to be the cause of the Korsakoff amnestic syndrome, which manifests in chronic alcoholism and other malnutrition states. Typically, it is preceded by one or more Wernicke encephalopathy episodes, though this history may not always be present. Bilateral dorsomedial thalamic nuclei degeneration may be connected to the memory impairment. About three-fourths of patients recover from Wernicke encephalopathy, and after that, they experience an amnestic syndrome of varying severity that is frequently accompanied by polyneuropathy and other residual symptoms like nystagmus or gait ataxia. The fundamental flaw is the incapacity to create new memories, which severely impairs short-term memory. Although less so, long-term memory is frequently impacted as well. Registration is still valid. Most patients are indifferent and have little understanding of their illness. They might try to convince the doctor that they are not impaired and try to justify their blatant forgetfulness. Confabulation is frequently present but not always so.

Thiamine can be given to Wernicke encephalopathy patients right away to prevent Korsakoff syndrome. Although existing deficits are unlikely to be reversed, patients with established Korsakoff syndrome should also receive thiamine to prevent the progression of deficits.

5.3.3.2. Postencephalitic Amnesia

After recovering from acute viral encephalitis, especially from the herpes simplex virus, patients may develop a persistent amnestic syndrome. The main characteristic of the syndrome is an inability to create new memories, which is similar to that caused by chronic alcoholism. Less so than more recent memories, distant memories are unaffected, and registration is unharmed. Confabulation is possible. Complete amnesia for the duration of the acute encephalitis is common.

Other limbic system disease symptoms may also be present in patients. They include the following: impotence, hyperphagia, repetitive stereotyped motor activity, flatness of mood, indifference, docility, inappropriate jocularity, sexual allusions, and the lack of goal-oriented activity. It is possible to experience complex partial seizures with or without secondary generalization.

5.3.3.3. Brain Tumor

An uncommon cause of amnestic syndrome is brain tumors. This kind of presentation is possible for tumors that compress or reside within the third ventricle. The symptoms of amnestic syndrome are similar to those of Korsakoff syndrome and can include papilledema, headaches, endocrine disruptions, lethargy, and visual field abnormalities. Memory loss may also result from brain tumor chemotherapy, radiation therapy to the head, or surgery. An MRI or CT scan is used to diagnose brain tumors. Treatment options include radiation, surgery, or a combination of the two, based on the kind and location of the tumor.

5.3.3.4. Paraneoplastic and Cell-Surface Directed Antibody-Mediated Limbic Encephalitis

Inflammation and degeneration of the CNS's gray matter regions can happen whether or not systemic cancer is present. An amnestic syndrome is a common symptom when limbic structures are mostly affected (limbic encephalitis). Autoimmune responses to intracellular or cell-surface neuronal antigens are linked to limbic encephalitis in a large number of patients. Antibodies directed against intracellular antigens of intact cells are not likely to cause disease because circulating antibodies cannot access them, but they are still useful as diagnostic markers. On the other hand, cell surface antigens may act as the main targets of autoimmunity because they are accessible to circulating antibodies.

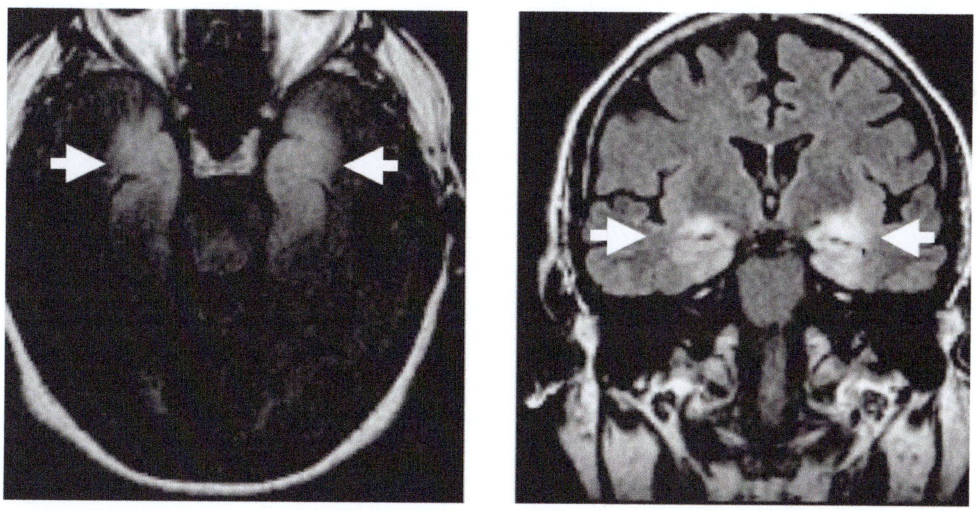

Figure 5.18. FLAIR MRI with axial (A) and coronal (B) views in limbic encephalitis, showing increased signal (arrows) in the medial temporal lobes.

Source: https://dl.mehrsys.ir/pdf-books/Clinical%20Neurology%209%20Edition%20(www.myuptodate.com).pdf.

The most common association between paraneoplastic limbic encephalitis and small-cell lung cancer is that the condition usually manifests before the underlying cancer is diagnosed. The gray matter of the hippocampus, cingulum, piriform cortex, inferior frontal lobes, insula, and amygdala are affected by perivascular lymphocytic cuffing, reactive gliosis, neuronal loss, and microglial proliferation, according to histopathologic findings. The onset of symptoms takes several weeks. Significant impairment of recent memory is present, along with sparing of registration and less involvement of remote memory; confabulation can occasionally happen. There is a chance for mood disorders, dementia, delusions, hallucinations, sleep disturbances, and complex partial or generalized seizures. Cerebellar, pyramidal, bulbar, and peripheral nerve abnormalities may also arise, depending on the degree of involvement of gray matter regions beyond the limbic system.

A slight mononuclear pleocytosis and slightly elevated protein may also be seen in the CSF. On an EEG, diffuse slowing or bitemporal slow waves and spikes can occasionally be observed. The medial temporal lobes of an MRI may show abnormal signal intensity (Figure 5.18). Most patients have elevated serum or CSF levels of antineuronal antibodies, which are helpful as diagnostic markers, as well as mononuclear cell pleocytosis and CSF protein. The most prevalent of these, anti-Hu, is typically linked to small-cell lung cancer and is directed against an intracellular antigen. In paraneoplastic limbic encephalitis, which is typically linked to lung cancer, as well as in limbic encephalitis that is unrelated to cancer, antibodies against cell-surface AMPA and GABAB receptors have also been seen. Some patients with non-cancerous limbic encephalitis also have antibodies against another cell-surface antigen, LGI1, which is a component of a voltage-gated potassium channel complex. These patients frequently also have hyponatremia and seizures.

There are three types of paraneoplastic amnestic syndrome: remitting, progressive, and static. It is crucial to rule out other conditions that can be treated, such as herpes simplex virus encephalitis. Given that cancer patients are prone to nutritional deficiencies and that thiamine administration may prevent worsening, it is important to consider Korsakoff syndrome.

Treatment options include plasma exchange, intravenous immunoglobulin, corticosteroids, and underlying cancer treatment.

A Closer Look

Amyloids

Amyloids are an aggregate of misfolded proteins that form fibrillary structures due to a variety of factors, such as errors in normal folding processes and hereditary or de novo mutations of the proteins. This protein's aberrant misfolding may cause it to form insoluble polymers or become resistant to proteolysis. Consequently, the tissue sustains damage due to the extracellular or intracellular deposition of amyloid. We refer to this illness as amyloidosis.

Protein fibrils make up over 90% of the amyloid deposition, with the remaining 10% being made up of proteoglycans, glycoproteins, or serum amyloid P components. Since the fibril structure of over thirty species of amyloid protein that have been previously identified is similar, the proteins may have a similar appearance when deposited inside an organ. Electron microscopy is used to observe the structure of amyloid, revealing fibrils with a diameter of roughly 7–10 nm. Additionally, β-pleated sheet structures were revealed by infrared spectroscopy and X-ray crystallography within the fibrils.

Every kind of amyloid has a propensity to accumulate in a particular tissue or organ depending on its chemical makeup and place of origin. However, when different types of amyloid are deposited within the same organ, the clinical signs and symptoms of those types can be strikingly similar. Furthermore, upon microscopical examination of the affected organ, the deposited amyloid will exhibit identical homogeneous amorphous materials with a bright pink color. Apple-green birefringence on Congo red stain with polarization and fluorescence microscopy can be used to confirm this. Despite sharing a similar morphologic appearance and clinical picture, the type of amyloid greatly influences the prognosis and course of treatment. Determining the amyloid type is therefore crucial.

With a few exceptions, amyloid deposition occurs in the same way within the same tissue regardless of the protein composition. In a gross sense, amyloidosis deposition can manifest as organomegaly and nodules. Occasionally, it can also exhibit a firm consistency color shift from pale gray to waxy. Under a standard hematoxylin–eosin stain, bright pink amorphous material deposition in extracellular space is most frequently seen under a microscope. Although they are uncommon, peculiar intracellular and spheroid-type amyloid depositions can be observed.

The gold standard for verifying the presence of amyloid protein has been Congo red stain since its accidental discovery by Hans Hermann Bennhold in 1922. The amyloid gives off a reddish-pink, orange, or salmon-colored hue when properly stained. The diagnosis of amyloidosis is subsequently confirmed by the apple-green birefringence demonstration. Nevertheless, this two-step approach still has poor repeatability, sensitivity, and specificity and is largely dependent on the interpretation of pathologists with extensive training. For example, even though the stained material contains amyloid, negative birefringence on a positive Congo red stain test may produce a false-negative result, in addition to the inherent sampling error. By turning the slide table, one can get past this "polarization shadow" and possibly find more trace amounts of amyloid protein. The washing step has a major impact on the stain intensity as well, which reduces reproducibility and necessitates the use of positive control tissue. Congo red further complicates interpretation by staining collagen, elastin, and even non-fibrillary materials like eosinophils.

Additional filters, such as a fluorescein isothiocyanate (FITC) or Texas red filter, can be used to get around the limitations of Congo red stain. By enhancing the weak signal from Congo red into red fluorescence, these filters can significantly increase the sensitivity of detection. It is possible to enlist the aid of additional fluorochrome dyes, such as thioflavin T. Only when the stain is bound to amyloid does it become highly fluorescent, giving it a yellow-green fluorescence when viewed under fluorescence microscopy. Fluorescence filters and dyes should be used in conjunction with Congo red stain as a supplement because they are not totally specific to amyloid. In summary, the on-off signal is only one factor in the light microscopic diagnosis of amyloidosis; other factors include staining methods, specimen alignment in polarized light, fluorescence microscopy, and the pathologist's experience.

Summary

- A generalized, acquired, and typically progressive impairment of cognitive function is called dementia.
- The most common causes of dementia in its most common presentation—a gradual decline in cognitive function in an elderly patient (≥65 years of age)—are Parkinson's disease, Lewy body disease, Alzheimer's disease, and vascular dementia.
- The synthesis of misfolded proteins and their combination to form insoluble aggregates seem to be important pathophysiological factors in several neurodegenerative diseases.
- Early-stage Alzheimer's disease can mimic other conditions like depression or isolated memory problems like Korsakoff amnestic syndrome.
- A group of dementing disorders known as frontotemporal dementia (FTD) are genetically and clinically heterogeneous; they cause degeneration of the frontal and temporal lobes and have a preferential effect on behavior and language.
- Steele-Richardson-Olszewski syndrome, also known as progressive supranuclear palsy (PSP), is an idiopathic degenerative disease that mainly affects the cerebral cortex, subcortical gray matter, and brainstem.
- An autosomal dominant neurodegenerative disease called Huntington's disease is typified by dementia, chorea, and mental symptoms.

References

1. Alzheimer's Association. (2013). 2013 Alzheimer's disease facts and figures. *Alzheimer's & Dementia, 9*, 208–245.
2. Amici, S. (2012). Memory dysfunction. *Frontiers in Neurology and Neuroscience, 30*, 54–56.
3. Asztely, F., & Kumlien, E. (2012). The diagnosis and treatment of limbic encephalitis. *Acta Neurologica Scandinavica, 126*, 365–375.
4. Baskys, A., & Cheng, J. -X. (2012). Pharmacological prevention and treatment of vascular dementia: approaches and perspectives. *Experimental Gerontology, 47*, 887–891.
5. Bruns, M. B., & Josephs, K. A. (2013). Neuropsychiatry of corticobasal degeneration and progressive supranuclear palsy. *International Review of Psychiatry, 25*, 197–209.
6. Bruns, M. B., & Josephs, K. A. (2013). Neuropsychiatry of corticobasal degeneration and progressive supranuclear palsy. *International Review of Psychiatry, 25*, 197–209.
7. Budson, A. E., & Solomon, P. R. (2012). New criteria for Alzheimer's disease and mild cognitive impairment: implications for the practicing clinician. *The Neurologist, 18*, 356–363.
8. Calabrese LH, Molloy E, Berger J. Sorting out the risks in progressive multifocal leukoencephalopathy. *Nat Rev Rheumatol.* (2015) 11:119–23. 10.1038/nrrheum.2014.167
9. Carlesimo, G. A. (2012). Memory disorders in patients with cerebral tumors. *Journal of Neuro-Oncology, 108*, 253–256.
10. Castellani, R. J., & Perry, G. (2014). The complexities of the pathology–pathogenesis relationship in Alzheimer's disease. *Biochemical Pharmacology, 88*, 671–676.

11. Fama, R., Pitel, A. -L., & Sullivan, E. V. (2012). Anterograde episodic memory in Korsakoff syndrome. *Neuropsychology Review, 22*, 93–104.
12. Fugate, J. E., Moore, S. A., Knopman, D. S., et al. (2013). Cognitive outcomes of patients undergoing therapeutic hypothermia after cardiac arrest. *Neurology, 81*, 40–45.
13. Giovagnoli, A. R. (2012). Investigation of cognitive impairments in people with brain tumors. *Journal of Neuro-Oncology, 108*, 277–283.
14. Haeusler, A. R., Donnelly, C. J., Periz, G., et al. (2014). C9orf72 nucleotide repeat structures initiate molecular cascades of disease. *Nature, 507*, 195–200.
15. Iadecola, C. (2013). The pathobiology of vascular dementia. *Neuron, 80*, 844–866.
16. Irani, S. R., Gelfand, J. M., Al-Diwani, A., & Vincent, A. (2014). Cell-surface central nervous system autoantibodies: clinical relevance and emerging paradigms. *Annals of Neurology, 76*, 168–184.
17. Ishii, K., Shioya, A., Fukuda, K., Mori, K., & Tamaoka, A. (2012). Acquired hepatocerebral degeneration with middle cerebellar peduncles lesions: case report and review of the literature. *Clinical Neurology and Neurosurgery, 114*, 1361–1364.
18. Kirshner, H. S. (2014). Frontotemporal dementia and primary progressive aphasia, a review. *Neuropsychiatric Disease and Treatment, 10*, 1045–1055.
19. Kirshner, H. S. (2011). Transient global amnesia: a brief review and update. *Current Neurology and Neuroscience Reports, 11*, 578–582.
20. Kolias, A. G., Chari, A., Santarius, T., & Hutchinson, P. J. (2014). Chronic subdural haematoma: modern management and emerging therapies. *Nature Reviews Neurology, 10*, 570–578.
21. Kuruppu, D. K., & Matthews, B. R. (2013). Young-onset dementia. *Seminars in Neurology, 33*, 365–385.
22. Marshman, L. A., Jakabek, D., Hennessy, M., Quirk, F., & Guazzo, E. P. (2013). Post-traumatic amnesia. *Journal of Clinical Neuroscience, 20*, 1475–1481.
23. McCann, H., Stevens, C. H., Cartwright, H., & Halliday, G. M. (2014). α-Synucleinopathy phenotypes. *Parkinsonism & Related Disorders, 20* (Suppl 1), S62–S67.
24. McKee, A. C., Stein, T. D., Nowinski, C. J., et al. (2013). The spectrum of disease in chronic traumatic encephalopathy. *Brain, 136*, 43–64.
25. Moore, E., Mander, A., Ames, D., et al. (2012). Cognitive impairment and vitamin B12: a review. *International Psychogeriatrics, 24*, 541–556.
26. Naganuma, T., Takemoto, Y., Shoji, T., et al. (2012). Factors associated with cerebral white matter hyperintensities in haemodialysis patients. *Nephrology, 17*, 561–568.
27. Peng, D., Yuan, X., & Zhu, R. (2013). Memantine hydrochloride in the treatment of dementia subtypes. *Journal of Clinical Neuroscience, 20*, 1482–1485.
28. Prusiner, S. B. (2013). Biology and genetics of prions causing neurodegeneration. *Annual Review of Genetics, 47*, 601–623.
29. Reitz, C., & Mayeux, R. (2014). Alzheimer disease: epidemiology, diagnostic criteria, risk factors and biomarkers. *Biochemical Pharmacology, 88*, 640–651.

30. Resta, F., Triggiani, V., Barile, G., et al. (2012). Subclinical hypothyroidism and cognitive dysfunction in the elderly. *Endocrine, Metabolic & Immune Disorders Drug Targets, 12*, 260–267.

31. Ridley, N. J., Draper, B., & Withall, A. (2013). Alcohol-related dementia: an update of the evidence. *Alzheimer's Research & Therapy, 5*, 3.

32. Singer, C. S. (2012). Comprehensive treatment of Huntington's disease and other choreic disorders. *Cleveland Clinic Journal of Medicine, 79* (Suppl 2), S30–S34.

33. Taylor, W. D. (2014). Depression in the elderly. *New England Journal of Medicine, 371*, 1228–1236.

34. Thal, D. R., Grinberg, L. T., & Attems, J. (2012). Vascular dementia: different forms of vessel disorders contribute to the development of dementia in the elderly brain. *Experimental Gerontology, 47*, 816–824.

35. Toma, A. K., Papadopoulos, M. C., Stapleton, S., Kitchen, N. D., & Watkins, L. D. (2013). Systematic review of the outcome of shunt surgery in idiopathic normal-pressure hydrocephalus. *Acta Neurochirurgica, 155*, 1977–1980.

36. Weiss, K. H., & Stremmel, W. (2012). Evolving perspectives in Wilson disease: diagnosis, treatment and monitoring. *Current Gastroenterology Reports, 14*, 1–7.

37. Yokoyama, J. S., Sirkis, D. W., & Miller, B. L. (2014). C9ORF72 hexanucleotide repeats in behavioral and motor neuron disease: clinical heterogeneity and pathological diversity. *American Journal of Neurodegenerative Disease, 3*, 1–18.

38. Zhang, H. L., Lin, L. R., Liu, G. L., et al. (2013). Clinical spectrum of neurosyphilis among HIV-negative patients in the modern era. *Dermatology, 226*, 148–156.

39. Zhou, L., & Saksena, N. K. (2013). HIV associated neurocognitive disorders. *Infection Disease Reports, 5*(Suppl 1), 38–50.

Chapter 6

HEADACHE AND FACIAL PAIN

Contents

Introduction

Headache affects people of all ages and has many different causes. It accounts for 1% to 2% of evaluations in emergency departments and up to 4% of visits to medical offices (Table 6.1). New-onset headaches are usually benign, but they can be the first or main sign of a serious systemic or intracranial disease, so they need to be thoroughly and methodically evaluated. This is especially true when the headaches are chronic and recurrent.

Understanding the pathophysiology of head pain, gathering a medical history and characterizing the pain as acute, subacute, or chronic, doing a thorough physical examination, and developing a differential diagnosis are the foundations of an etiologic diagnosis of headache.

Orientation and Directional Terms

Term	Definition	Illustration
Subacute	Subacute means having a tapered but not sharp point, or falling between acute and chronic in character.	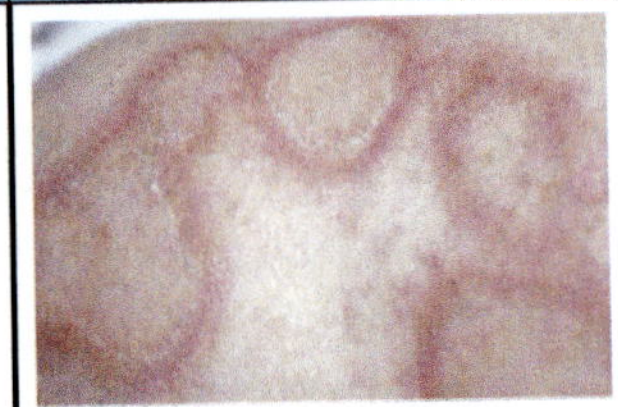
Dermatomes	Dermatomes are areas of skin that receive sensory innervation from a single spinal nerve dorsal root.	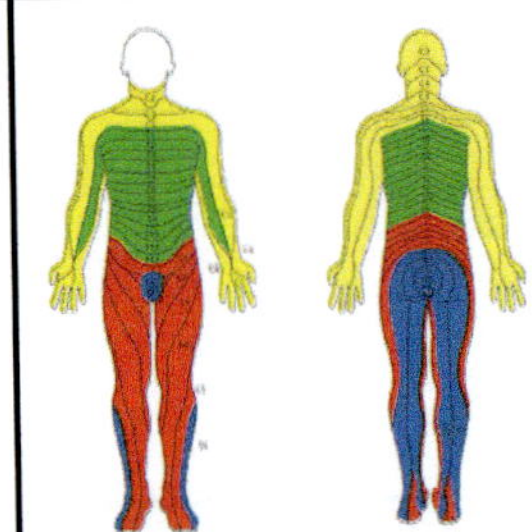
Tic douloureux	Tic douloureux, also known as trigeminal neuralgia (TN), is a chronic pain condition that causes sudden, severe facial pain that feels like an electric shock .	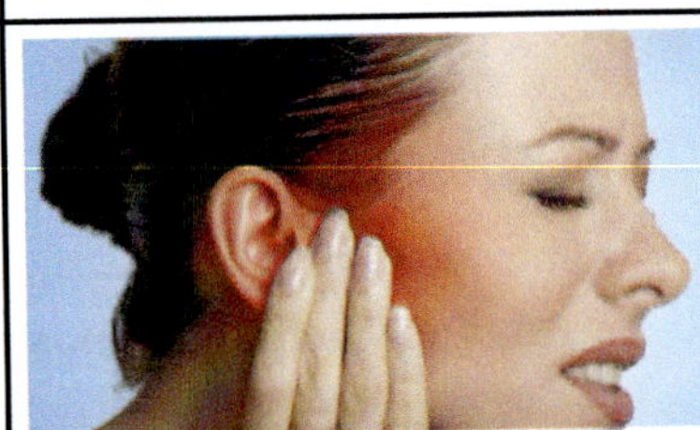
Retro-orbital inflammation	Retro-orbital inflammation is a condition where inflammatory tissue in the orbit extends into the retro-orbital structures through foramina, such as the optic canal, superior orbital fissure, and inferior orbital fissure.	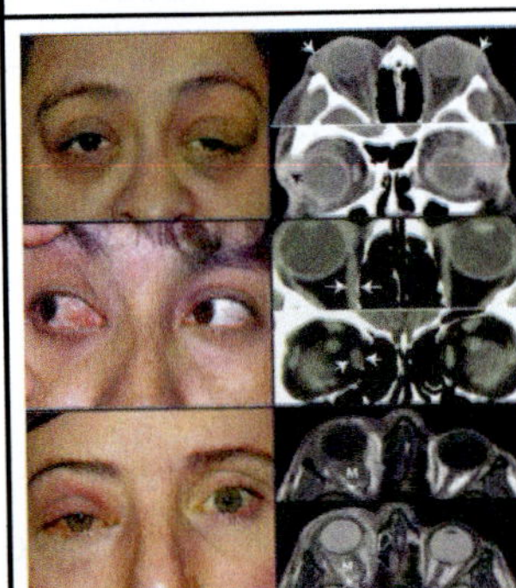
Hypercapnia	Hypercapnia also known as hypercarbia and CO2 retention, is a condition of abnormally elevated carbon dioxide (CO2) levels in the blood.	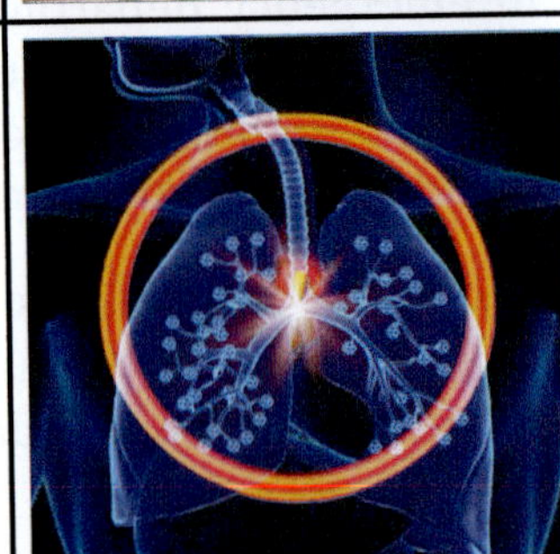

6.1. Approach to Diagnosis

6.1.1. Pathophysiology of Headache and Facial Pain

6.1.1.1. Pain-Sensitive Structures

Traction, displacement, inflammation, or distention of the pain-sensitive structures in the head or neck can result in headaches. Pain is not elicited by isolated involvement of the bony skull, most of the dura, or most brain parenchyma regions.

Table 6.1. Causes of Headache and Facial Pain

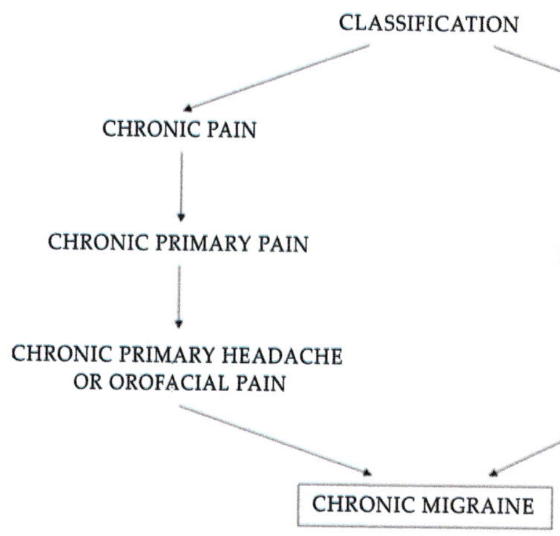

Source: Szok D, Csáti A, Vécsei L, Tajti J. Chronic Migraine as a Primary Chronic Pain Syndrome and Recommended Prophylactic Therapeutic Options: A Literature Review. *Life*. 2023; 13(3):665. https://doi.org/10.3390/life13030665.

- **Pain-Sensitive Structures Within the Cranial Vault:** These include the proximal sections of the internal carotid artery and its branches near the circle of Willis; brainstem periaqueductal gray matter; venous sinuses (e.g., sagittal sinus); anterior and middle meningeal arteries; dura at the base of the skull; trigeminal (V), glossopharyngeal (IX), and vagus (X) nerves; and sensory nuclei of the thalamus.
- **Extracranial Pain-Sensitive Structures:** These comprise the periosteum of the skull, the skin, the arteries, muscles, and subcutaneous tissues; the neck muscles; the second (C2) and third (C3) cervical nerves; the eyes, ears, teeth, sinuses, and oropharynx; and the nasal cavity's mucous membranes.

6.1.1.2. Radiation or Projection of Pain

- The trigeminal (V) nerve carries sensation from intracranial structures in the anterior and middle fossae of the skull (above the cerebellar tentorium). Discrete intracranial lesions in these locations can produce pain that radiates in the trigeminal nerve distribution (Figure 6.1).
- The glossopharyngeal (IX) and vagus (X) nerves convey sensation from part of the

posterior fossa; pain originating in this area may also be referred to the ear or throat, as in glossopharyngeal neuralgia.

- The upper cervical (C2-C3) nerves transmit stimuli from infratentorial and cervical structures; therefore, pain from posterior fossa lesions often projects to the second and third cervical dermatomes (Figure 6.1).

6.1.2. History

6.1.2.1. Classification and Approach to the Differential Diagnosis

- **Acute Headache and Facial Pain:** When a patient experiences a headache that is new or noticeably different from any headaches they have had in the past, it is usually an indication of a serious illness and needs to be evaluated right away. Notable instances include the abrupt onset of "the worst headache I've ever had in my life," which is typically caused by a subarachnoid hemorrhage; diffuse headache accompanied by fever and stiff neck (meningitis); and head pain that is focused in one eye (acute glaucoma). More manageable conditions like systemic viral infections or other feverish illnesses can also cause acute headaches.
- **Subacute Headache and Facial Pain:** Headaches lasting weeks or months are classified as subacute. These types of headaches can also indicate more serious medical conditions, particularly if they worsen over time or affect older patients. Questions about focal neurologic abnormalities or weight loss (primary or metastatic brain tumor), visual changes (giant cell arteritis, idiopathic intracranial hypertension), recent head trauma (subdural hematoma or postconcussive syndrome), malaise, fever, or neck stiffness (subacute meningitis), and medications predisposing to headache (nitrates) should be asked of patients with subacute headache.

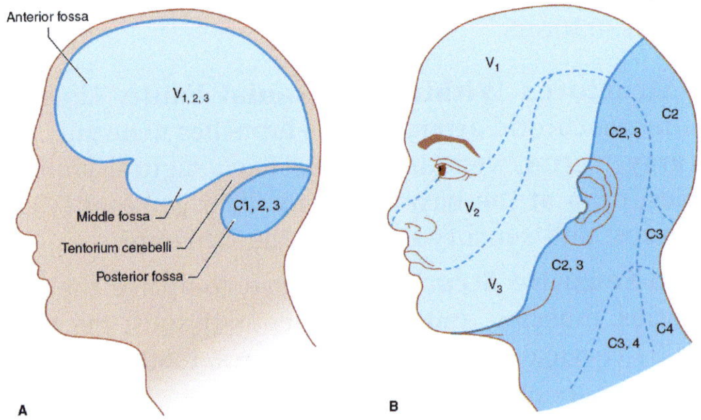

Figure 6.1. Innervation of pain-sensitive intracranial compartments (A) and corresponding extracranial sites of pain radiation (B). The trigeminal (V) nerve, especially its ophthalmic (V1) division, innervates the anterior and middle cranial fossae; lesions in these areas can produce frontal headache. The upper cervical nerve roots (especially C2) innervate the posterior fossa; lesions here can cause occipital headache.

Source: https://dl.mehrsys.ir/pdf-books/Clinical%20Neurology%209%20Edition%20(www.myuptodate.com).pdf.

- **Chronic Headache and Facial Pain:** Recurrent headaches (such as tension or migraine headaches) typically have a benign cause, even though each acute attack can be extremely incapacitating. When treating these patients, it's critical to ascertain whether the current headache is new and thus indicative of a distinct process, or if it's similar to past headaches.

6.1.2.2. Precipitating Factors

The presence of precipitating factors can help identify the headache's etiology. Dental surgery, an acute flare-up of long-term sinusitis or hay fever, a systemic viral infection, psychological tension, emotional stress, or exhaustion, menstruation, hunger, eating ice cream or foods high in nitrite (such as hot dogs, salami, ham, and most sausage), phenylethylamine (found in chocolate), or tyramine (found in cheddar cheese), as well as exposure to bright lights are some examples of these factors. Alcohol-induced headache precipitation is particularly common in cluster headaches. Eating and chewing frequently cause pain linked to tic douloureux and glossopharyngeal neuralgia; jaw claudication is linked to temporomandibular joint dysfunction or giant cell arteritis. Oral contraceptives and nitrates have the potential to cause or worsen migraine. Moreover, coughing or sneezing can cause headaches, particularly in those who have posterior fossa structural lesions.

6.1.2.3. Prodromal Symptoms (Auras)

In addition to being common in patients with migraine, prodromal symptoms or auras, such as scintillating scotomas or other visual abnormalities, can also occur in patients with seizure disorders and postictal headaches.

6.1.2.4. Characteristics of Pain

There are several ways to define a headache or facial pain. Although throbbing or pulsating pain is commonly associated with migraines, tension-type headache patients may also experience it. Constant tightness or pressure is a common symptom of tension-type headaches. Intracerebral mass lesions usually cause dull, constant pain. Trigeminal neuralgia is one example of a neuritic cause of sharp, lancinating (stabbing) pain. Patients with giant cell arteritis, migraine, or cluster headaches may also describe experiencing pain that feels like an ice pick.

Patients with migraines or brain tumors may experience headaches of various descriptions, so the type of pain alone is not a reliable indicator of the cause.

6.1.2.5. Location of Pain

- Unilateral headache is an invariable feature of cluster headache and occurs in the majority of migraine attacks; most patients with tension-type headaches report bilateral pain.
- Ocular or retroorbital pain suggests a primary ophthalmic disorder such as acute iritis or glaucoma, optic (II) nerve disease (e.g., optic neuritis), or retroorbital inflammation (e.g., Tolosa–Hunt syndrome). It is also common in migraine or cluster headaches.
- Paranasal pain localized to one or several sinuses, often associated with tenderness of the overlying periosteum and skin, occurs with an acute sinus infection or outlet obstruction.
- Focal headache may result from intracranial mass lesions, but even in such cases, it is replaced by bioccipital and bifrontal pain when the intracranial pressure becomes elevated.

- Bandlike or occipital discomfort is commonly associated with tension-type headaches. Occipital localization can also occur with meningeal irritation from infection or hemorrhage and with disorders of the joints, muscles, or ligaments of the upper cervical spine.
- Pain within the first (V1) division of the trigeminal nerve, characteristically described as burning in quality, is a common feature of postherpetic neuralgia.
- Lancinating pain localized to the second (V2) or third (V3) division of the trigeminal (V) nerve suggests trigeminal neuralgia (tic douloureux).
- The pharynx and external auditory meatus are the most frequent sites of pain caused by glossopharyngeal neuralgia.

6.1.2.6. Associated Symptoms

Manifestations of underlying systemic disease can aid in the etiologic diagnosis of headache and should always be sought.

- Recent weight loss may accompany cancer, giant cell arteritis, or depression.
- Fever or chills may indicate systemic infection or meningitis.
- Dyspnea or other symptoms of heart disease raise the possibility of subacute infective endocarditis and resultant brain abscess.
- Visual disturbances suggest an ocular disorder (eg, glaucoma), migraine, or an intracranial process involving the optic nerve (optic neuritis) or tract or central visual pathways.
- Nausea and vomiting are common in migraine and post-traumatic headaches and can also be seen with intracranial mass lesions. Some patients with migraine report that diarrhea or other gastrointestinal symptoms accompany attacks.
- Photophobia may be prominent in migraine, acute meningitis, or subarachnoid hemorrhage.
- Myalgias often accompany tension-type headaches, systemic viral infections, and giant cell arteritis.
- Ipsilateral rhinorrhea and lacrimation during attacks typify cluster headaches.
- Transient loss of consciousness may be seen in both migraine (basilar migraine) and glossopharyngeal neuralgia.
- **Other Features of Headache**
  - **Temporal Pattern of Headache:** Both sinus headaches and headaches from mass lesions typically peak right after awakening. However, the intensity of headaches caused by mass lesions increases with time. Patients with cluster headaches often wake up from sleep, and they often recur at the same time every day or night. Every stressful event can cause tension-type headaches, which are most common towards the end of the workday. Periods of menstruation may exacerbate episodic migraine headaches (Figure 6.2).

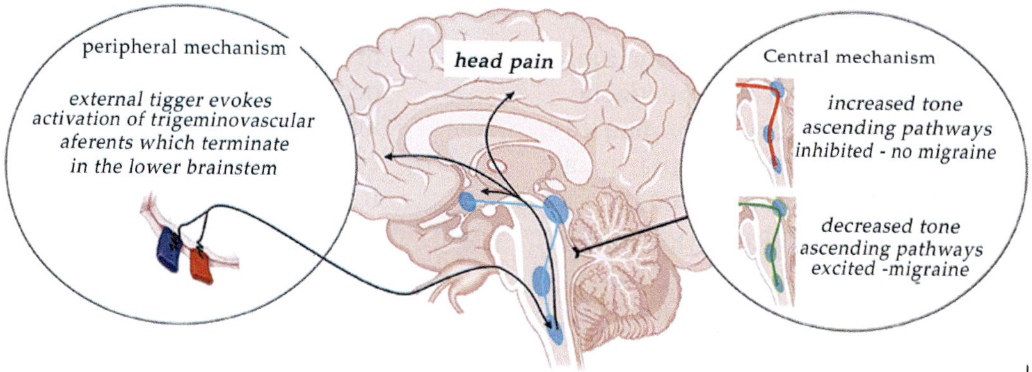

Figure 6.2. Temporal patterns of headache. Migraine headaches are episodic and may occur at varying intervals. Tension-type headaches may be present every day. Cluster headache occurs in bouts separated by symptom-free periods. Headache caused by brain tumors often increases in severity with time.

Source: Mungoven TJ, Henderson LA and Meylakh N (2021) Chronic Migraine Pathophysiology and Treatment: A Review of Current Perspectives. Front. Pain Res. 2:705276. doi: 10.3389/fpain.2021.705276.

- **Conditions Relieving Headache:** Migraine headaches may become less frequent during pregnancy and are often relieved by darkness, sleep, vomiting, or applying pressure to the ipsilateral temporal artery. Headaches resulting from intracranial mass lesions may be less severe when the patient is standing, but post-lumbar puncture and low-pressure headaches are usually relieved by recumbency.
- **Conditions Exacerbating Headache:** A headache or an intracranial mass is frequently linked to discomfort made worse by sudden changes in head position or by situations that momentarily increase intracranial pressure, like sneezing or coughing. Anger, excitement, or irritation can either initiate or exacerbate tension-type headaches and migraines. Sinusitis pain is typically worsened by stooping, bending forward, sneezing, or blowing one's nose. Low cerebral spinal fluid (CSF) pressure from a lumbar puncture, head injury, or spontaneous spinal fluid leak is the cause of postural headache, which is maximal when standing and almost nonexistent when lying down. Subdural hematomas are known to cause headaches that fluctuate in intensity and duration without a clear cause, especially when accompanied by comparable changes in mental state.

6.1.3. Physical Examination

Given that many systemic disorders have headaches as a nonspecific accompaniment, a general physical examination is required. When the patient is experiencing a headache or facial pain, it is best to watch them.

6.1.3.1. Vital Signs

- **Temperature:** Fever is indicative of a viral syndrome, meningitis, encephalitis, or brain abscess; however, these conditions can also cause headaches in the absence of fever. Furthermore, a headache is often a side effect of systemic infections.

- **Pulse:** Tachycardia may accompany any severe pain or occur in a tense, anxious patient with a tension-type headache. A paroxysmal headache accompanied by sweating and tachycardia is a hallmark of pheochromocytoma.
- **Blood Pressure:** Unless the blood pressure elevation is severe, as in the case of pheochromocytoma, or extremely high, as in the case of early hypertensive encephalopathy, headaches are rarely caused by hypertension per se. However, the main risk factor for ischemic or hemorrhagic stroke, which can be linked to an acute headache, is chronic hypertension. After a subarachnoid hemorrhage, blood pressure usually rises sharply and suddenly.
- **Respiration:** Any cause of respiratory insufficiency that results in hypercapnia can raise intracranial pressure and cause headaches.

6.1.3.2. General Physical Examination

- **Weight Loss:** Weight loss or cachexia in a patient with a headache may indicate the presence of cancer or chronic infection. Weight loss can also occur in conditions such as polymyalgia rheumatica and giant cell arteritis.
- **Skin:** Cellulitis, or focal inflammation of the face or skull covering, is indicative of a localized infection that could be the cause of venous sinus thrombosis or an intracranial abscess. Other cutaneous anomalies could indicate endocarditis, cancer, or vasculitis (including meningococcemia). Benign or malignant intracranial tumors that can cause headaches are linked to the neurofibromas, also known as café-au-lait spots, of von Recklinghausen disease (neurofibromatosis). Arteriovenous malformations (AVMs) of the central nervous system are occasionally accompanied by cutaneous angiomas. These AVMs may cause chronic headaches, or acute headaches if they bleed. Face and head herpes zoster typically affects the eye and the skin surrounding the periorbital tissue, resulting in facial pain.
- **Scalp, Face, and Head:** Giant cell arteritis, postherpetic neuralgia, subdural hematomas, and migraine headaches are all characterized by tenderness in the scalp. Giant cell arteritis is suggested by nodularity, erythema, or tenderness over the temporal artery. Along with acute migraine, there may also be localized superficial temporal artery tenderness. A localized tender spot may result from a mass lesion or recent head trauma. Characteristic ecchymosis results from trauma.

Pain in the head that is dull in nature and accompanied by tenderness in the skull can be caused by metastatic cancer of the skull, myeloma, or Paget disease. The scalp may feel warm in Paget disease due to arteriovenous shunting within the bone.

Headaches can be caused by issues with the teeth, ears, or vision. Periodontal abscess may be discovered by tooth percussion. Pain in the sinuses could be a sign of sinusitis. An intracranial AVM, carotid artery–cavernous sinus fistula, aneurysm, or meningioma are all possible causes of a bruit over the orbit or skull. An increased risk of postictal headache is associated with tongue lacerations. Cluster headache is associated with ipsilateral conjunctival injection, lacrimation, Horner syndrome, and rhinorrhea. The symptoms of temporomandibular joint disease include crepitus over the joint and localized tenderness.

- **Neck:** Cervical spine injuries, meningitis, cervical arthritis, and tension-type and migraine headaches can all cause cervical muscle spasms. Cerebrovascular disease may be linked to carotid bruits.

Meningeal signs need to be carefully looked for, particularly if the headache just started. While cervical spine disorders limit movement in all directions, meningeal irritation primarily causes nuchal (neck) stiffness in the anteroposterior direction. Meningeal irritation is indicated by discomfort or hip and knee flexion during neck flexion (Brudzinski sign). In the initial hours following a subarachnoid hemorrhage, in patients in a comatose state, and in the early stages of subacute meningitis (such as tuberculous meningitis), meningeal signs may be absent or challenging to demonstrate.

- Heart and Lungs: Heart murmurs or cyanosis are signs of congenital heart disease, which can be connected to brain abscesses. Brain abscesses can also originate from lung abscesses.

6.1.4. Neurologic Examination

- **Mental Status Examination:** Patients experiencing an acute headache, as is frequently the case with subarachnoid hemorrhage and meningitis, may exhibit confusion during the mental status examination. An intracranial tumor, especially one that has spread throughout the corpus callosum or is located in the frontal lobe, may be the cause of a headache accompanied by dementia.
- **Cranial Nerve Examination:** An intracranial tumor or other mass lesion may be suggested and localized by abnormalities of the cranial nerve. Pseudotumor cerebri, hypertensive encephalopathy, carotid artery–cavernous sinus fistula, and space-occupying intracranial lesions can all cause papilledema, the classic sign of elevated intracranial pressure. Adult subarachnoid hemorrhage is characterized by superficial retinal hemorrhages, also known as subhyaloid hemorrhages (Figure 6.3). Vasculitis patients may experience ischemic retinopathy.

Progressive oculomotor (III) nerve palsy may indicate an expanding posterior communicating artery aneurysm, particularly when it causes pupillary dilation. On the other hand, it may also indicate rising intracranial pressure and a developing brain herniation. Optic neuritis causes decreased pupillary reactivity to light. Tolosa-Hunt syndrome is characterized by extraocular muscle palsies. Proptosis indicates a carotid artery–cavernous sinus fistula or an orbital mass lesion.

Postherpetic neuralgia is characterized by decreased sensation over the site of facial pain, which is typically the first (V1) division of the trigeminal (V) nerve. Face and pharynx trigger points indicate trigeminal and glossopharyngeal neuralgia, respectively.

- **Motor Examination:** In order to rule out intracranial mass lesions, asymmetric motor function or gait ataxia in a patient with a history of subacute headache requires thorough evaluation.
- **Sensory Examination:** There is compelling evidence to rule out a benign cause of pain in cases of focal or segmental sensory impairment or diminished corneal sensation (corneal reflex).

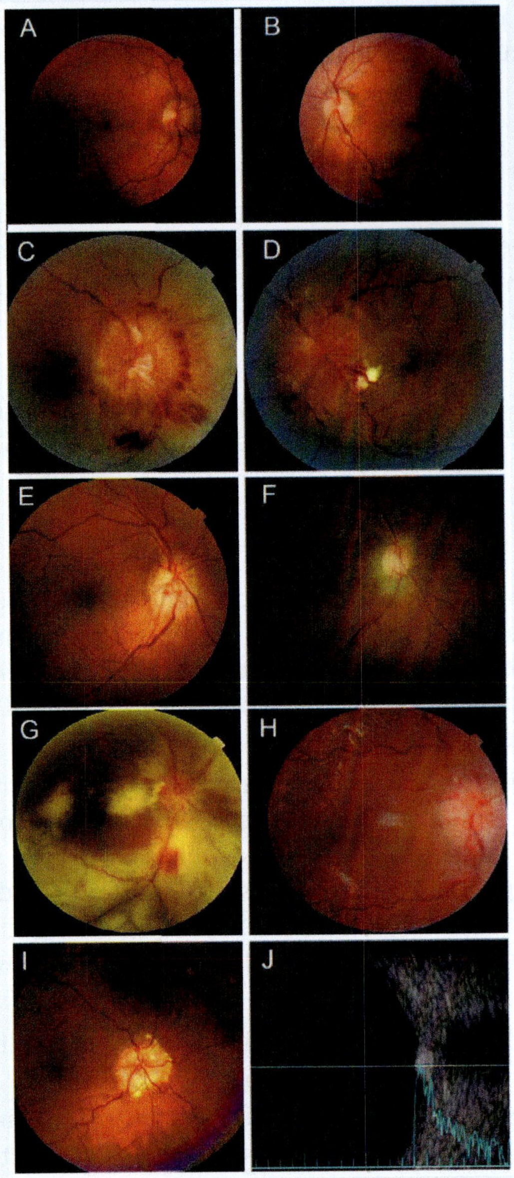

Figure 6.3. Disc edema and a large peripapillary subhyaloid hemorrhage in the right eye of a patient with aneurysmal rupture and subarachnoid hemorrhage.

Source: Yousef YA, Sid Ahmed IM, Kanj Ahmad D, Mohammad M, Makahleh H, AlJabari R, Alkhatib F, Toro MD, Rejdak R, Mehyar M, et al. Optic Disc Swelling in Cancer Patients: Etiology and Implications. *Journal of Clinical Medicine*. 2023; 12(22):7140. https://doi.org/10.3390/jcm12227140.

6.2. Acute Headache

A new headache that appears out of the blue needs to be thoroughly and quickly investigated because it could be a sign of a serious intracranial or systemic disease.

6.2.1. Subarachnoid Hemorrhage

Bleeding into the subarachnoid space that occurs spontaneously (non-traumatically) is typically caused by an AVM or a burst cerebral artery aneurysm.

With an annual incidence of 6 per 100,000, rupture of a saccular (berry) aneurysm is thought to be responsible for approximately 75% of cases of subarachnoid hemorrhage. While some are familial, the majority are sporadic. Every member of a family with two or more affected individuals needs to be screened. There are two types of inheritance patterns: recessive and autosomal.

The fifth and sixth decades are the most common times for rupture, with roughly equal sex distribution. About 5% of autopsied people have cerebral aneurysms; the majority of these patients have never had symptoms. The risk of rupture for an intracranial aneurysm depends on the patient's age, the location, and the size of the aneurysm. Although it hasn't been proven beyond a shadow of a doubt that hypertension makes people more likely to develop aneurysms, sudden spikes in blood pressure, like those experienced during an orgasm, maybe the cause of the rupture.

A cerebral artery trunk's circumferential dilatation causes fusiform aneurysms. They affect the vertebrobasilar system preferentially, are thought to be caused by atherosclerosis or dissection as opposed to saccular aneurysms, and can present with symptoms from ischemia or mass effect in addition to rupture.

AVMs in the brain, a less common cause of subarachnoid hemorrhage (10%), are twice as common in men than in women. They typically bleed in the second or fourth decades of life, though a notable incidence can occur well into the sixties. Other causes of blood in the subarachnoid space include trauma, embolic stroke, and intracerebral hemorrhage.

6.2.1.1. Pathology

The majority of cerebral arterial aneurysms are congenital and are caused by the vessel wall becoming weaker during development, particularly at the locations where it branches. They usually occur in two percent of patients, are multiple in about 20% of cases, and originate from intracranial arteries around the circle of Willis at the base of the brain (Figure 6.4). Berries may also be linked to other congenital anomalies like coarctation of the aorta or polycystic kidney disease.

Mycotic aneurysms, which account for 2–3% of aneurysmal ruptures, are occasionally caused by systemic infections like infective endocarditis that spread to a cerebral artery. Generally speaking, mycotic aneurysms are located further along the cerebral artery's course than berry aneurysms.

AVMs are characterized by anomalous vascular connections that allow arterial blood to enter the venous system without going via a capillary bed. The distribution of the middle cerebral arteries is where they are most prevalent.

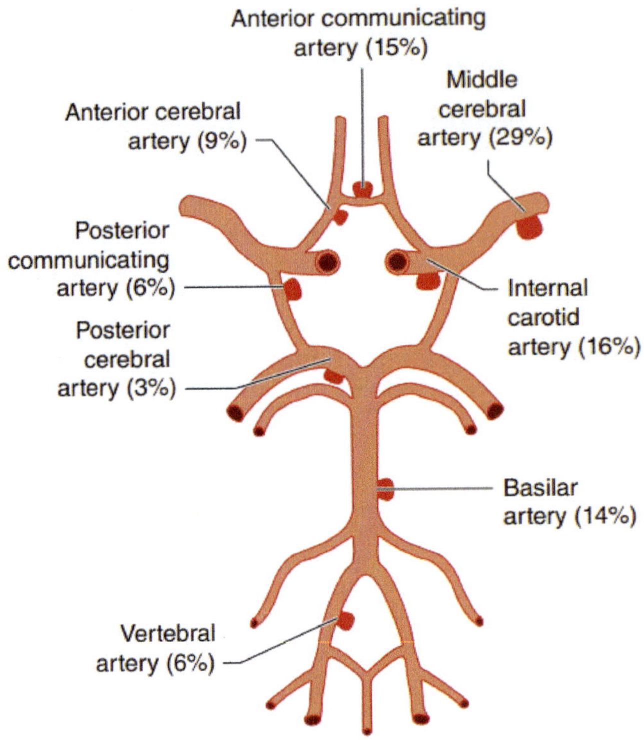

Figure 6.4. Frequency distribution of intracranial aneurysms.

Source: https://dl.mehrsys.ir/pdf-books/Clinical%20Neurology%209%20Edition%20(www.myuptodate.com).pdf.

6.2.1.2. Pathophysiology

An intracranial artery rupture causes headaches by increasing intracranial pressure and causing pain-sensitive structures to be distorted. In addition to the concussive effect of the rupture, intracranial pressure may reach systemic perfusion pressure and sharply reduce cerebral blood flow; this is assumed to be the cause of the initial loss of consciousness that affects about 50% of patients. Subhyaloid retinal hemorrhages can also result from abruptly raising intracranial pressure (Figure 6.3).

6.2.1.3. Clinical Findings

- **Symptoms and Signs:** Subarachnoid hemorrhage typically manifests as a sudden, extremely severe generalized headache that the patient describes as the worst headache they have ever had. However, this is not always the case. Nonetheless, only 8–10% of patients who arrive with an unexpectedly severe headache will experience subarachnoid hemorrhage. The diagnosis is essentially ruled out in the absence of a headache. Only headaches account for one-third of patient presentations. In the remaining, vomiting and stiff neck are common initial symptoms, as is loss of consciousness. Any time of day and during either rest or activity can cause symptoms to appear.

The primary characteristic of the headache is its recent onset. Sentinel headaches, which are milder but otherwise similar headaches, are likely the result of small prodromal hemorrhages or aneurysmal stretch that happened in the weeks before the acute event.

Particularly when the bleeding is from a ruptured AVM rather than an aneurysm, the headache may not always be very bad. Even though the bleeding stops quickly, the headache's intensity might stay the same for a few days before gradually decreasing over two weeks. A relapse in headache symptoms typically indicates rebleeding.

The hemorrhage frequently causes blood pressure to rise suddenly. For the first two weeks, meningeal irritation can cause temperature elevations as high as 39°C (102.2°F). Oftentimes, stupor, coma, or confusion are present. It is not uncommon for nuchal rigidity and other signs of meningeal irritation to appear several hours after the headache first appears. The most suggestive of the diagnosis are preretinal globular subhyaloid hemorrhages, which are present in 20–40% of cases (Figure 6.3).

Instead of the brain parenchyma, bleeding mostly happens in the subarachnoid space when an aneurysmal rupture occurs. Consequently, prominent focal neurologic signs are rare, and even when they do occur, they might not be related to the aneurysm site. Oculomotor (III) nerve palsy resulting from ipsilateral nerve compression due to a posterior communicating artery aneurysm is an exception. Increased intracranial pressure frequently causes nonlocalizing signs such as bilateral extensor plantar responses and abducens (VI) nerve palsy.

Because ruptured AVMs typically occur within brain tissue, they can cause focal neurologic symptoms like hemiparesis, aphasia, or abnormalities in the visual field.

- **Laboratory Findings:** Computed tomography (CT) scanning is the initial diagnostic method used on patients who present with subarachnoid hemorrhage (Figure 6.5). In over 90% of cases of aneurysmal rupture, a CT scan confirms the presence of hemorrhage and can assist in locating a focal source. The test is most sensitive in patients who have altered consciousness and on the day that bleeding occurs. It is also possible to identify complications such as infarction, hydrocephalus, and intracerebral or intraventricular blood extension. While aneurysms may not always be visible on CT scans, most AVMs are visible following the injection of contrast material. When it comes to identifying tiny AVMs in the brainstem that are difficult to see on a CT scan, magnetic resonance imaging (MRI) is particularly helpful.

Some authorities believe that a normal CT scan performed within 6 hours of the onset of symptoms can rule out subarachnoid hemorrhage in patients with a normal neurologic examination. Lumbar punctures are required for CT scans that are technically insufficient, take too long, or otherwise are unable to confirm the diagnosis of subarachnoid hemorrhage.

In subarachnoid hemorrhage, the CSF typically has a markedly elevated opening pressure and is extremely bloody, with1–100,000million red blood cells per microliter. Within 12 hours after the bleeding, the supernatant of the centrifuged CSF turns yellow-tinged (xanthochromic) as the heme from these cells is broken down, first by heme oxygenase to the green pigment biliverdin and then by biliverdin reductase to the yellow pigment bilirubin. Spectrophotometric detection of the pigment is possible. Initially, the CSF contains white blood cells in the same ratio to red blood cells as peripheral blood. Nevertheless, pleocytosis of several thousand white blood cells during the first 48 hours and a decrease in CSF glucose 4 to 8 days after bleeding are possible symptoms of chemical meningitis caused by blood in the subarachnoid space. Following subarachnoid hemorrhage, CSF glucose is normal in the absence of pleocytosis. Peripheral white blood cell counts are frequently slightly elevated and infrequently surpass 15,000/μL.

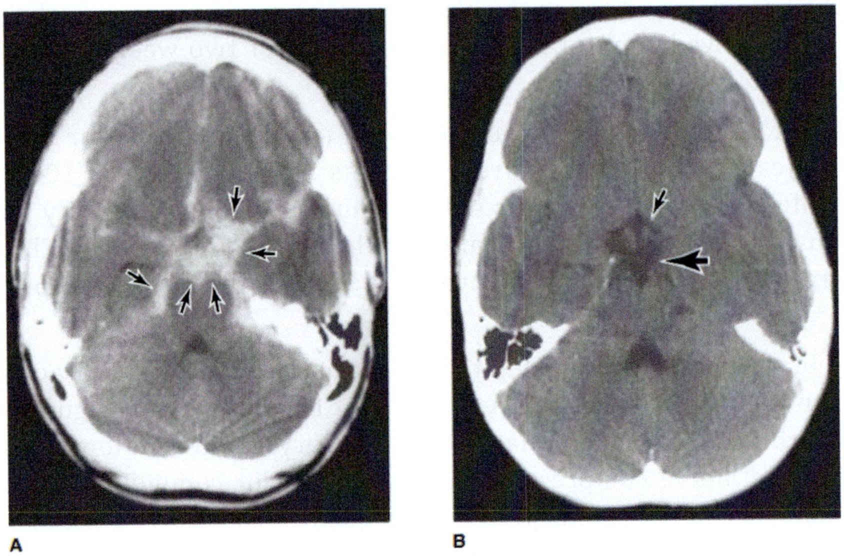

Figure 6.5. (A) Nonenhanced brain CT scan from a patient with an acute aneurysmal subarachnoid hemorrhage. Areas of high density (arrows) represent blood in the subarachnoid space at the base of the brain (most aneurysms occur in this region about the circle of Willis; see figure 6.4). (B) A normal nonenhanced brain CT scan of the same region. Interpeduncular cistern, large arrow; suprasellar cistern, small arrow.

Source: (Used with permission from C. Jungreis.).

The electrocardiogram (ECG) can show a number of abnormalities, such as tall U waves, short PR intervals, or peaked or deeply inverted T waves.

Four-vessel cerebral arteriography is performed if the diagnosis of subarachnoid hemorrhage is verified by lumbar puncture or CT scan. Studies of the carotid and vertebral arteries are necessary to visualize the entire cerebral vascular anatomy because 20% of patients have multiple aneurysms and because AVMs are often supplied by multiple vessels. When an emergency study is needed in the middle of the night, it is usually best to perform the angiography as soon as it is convenient for the radiology department staff. Angiography is not required for patients who are not surgical candidates, such as those who are profoundly unconscious, as it is a requirement for the logical planning of surgical treatment. The sensitivity of traditional catheter angiography is being approached by CT and magnetic resonance angiography.

6.2.1.4. Differential Diagnosis

Subarachnoid hemorrhage is highly specific for the abrupt onset of severe headache, along with bloody spinal fluid, nuchal rigidity, absence of focal neurologic deficits, and confusion or obtundation. While obtundation and bloody spinal fluid are also symptoms of other disorders, these can be identified by other findings, such as signs of endocarditis (ruptured mycotic aneurysm) or prominent focal neurologic deficits (hypertensive intracerebral hemorrhage).

By comparing the numbers of red blood cells in the first and last tubes of CSF obtained and examining the centrifuged CSF specimen, traumatic lumbar puncture can be ruled out as the cause of bloody CSF. After a traumatizing tap, blood drains as the fluid is removed, but not when there is a subarachnoid hemorrhage. Centrifugation of the specimen yields a colorless supernatant because the blood introduced by traumatic lumbar puncture does not have time to undergo enzymatic breakdown to bilirubin.

Bacterial meningitis is excluded by the presence of blood in the CSF or on a CT scan.

6.2.1.5. Complications and Sequelae

- **Recurrence of Hemorrhage:** About 20% of patients experience aneurysmal hemorrhage again within a span of 10 to 14 days. It is the primary acute complication and causes the death rate to nearly double. Acute hemorrhage from an AVM recurrence is less frequent.
- **Intraparenchymal Extension of Hemorrhage:** While aneurysmal hemorrhage is much less common than hemorrhages from an AVM, both frequently involve the brain parenchyma. However, if an aneurysm in the middle or anterior cerebral arteries bursts, blood may shoot into the brain, causing an intracerebral hematoma that can cause transtentorial herniation, hemiparesis, and aphasia.
- **Arterial Vasospasm:** More than one-third of cases of delayed arterial narrowing, or vasospasm, which happens in vessels surrounded by subarachnoid blood, are linked to ischemic neurologic deficits. Clinical ischemia usually doesn't show up until day 4 following the bleeding, peaks between days 7 and 8, and then goes away on its own. Cerebral angiography or transcranial Doppler can verify the diagnosis. Vasospasm is less common when there is less blood present, such as following a traumatic subarachnoid hemorrhage or rupture of an AVM. The severity of vasospasm is correlated with the amount of subarachnoid blood present. Given that one-third of patients with delayed ischemia do not exhibit clinically significant vasospasm, vasospasm appears to be only one factor contributing to the development of delayed ischemic neurologic deficits after subarachnoid hemorrhage.
- **Acute or Subacute Hydrocephalus:** The first three days or even weeks may see the development of acute or subacute hydrocephalus due to poor CSF absorption in the subarachnoid space. The diagnosis should be suggested by progressive somnolence, nonfocal findings, and impaired upgaze as a result of downward pressure on the midbrain.
- **Seizures:** Less than 10% of patients experience seizures, and they only happen when the cerebral cortex is harmed. Acute decerebrate or decorticate posturing is common and can be confused with seizures.

6.2.1.6. Treatment

- **Medical Treatment:** The goal of medical treatment is to avoid raising intracranial or arterial pressure to the point where the aneurysm or AVM might burst again. Typical treatments include mild sedation, analgesics for headaches, and complete bed rest with the head of the bed raised 15 to 20 degrees (antiplatelet drugs should be avoided). Reducing blood pressure (to roughly 160/100 mm Hg) is prudent because patients who are hypertensive upon admission have a higher mortality rate; however, bed rest and mild sedation are frequently sufficient in this regard.

To guarantee proper cerebral perfusion, hypotension should be avoided; however, intravenous fluids should be isosmotic (normal saline) and should be given carefully because overhydration can worsen cerebral swelling. Hydration restriction is not the best way to treat hyponatremia, which is more commonly treated with intravenous three percent normal saline or oral administration of NaCl.

Vasospasm can be treated by induced hypertension with phenylephrine or dopamine after the ruptured aneurysm has been surgically treated definitively and there are no other aneurysms. Through neuroprotective mechanisms rather than a direct effect on vasospasm, the calcium channel antagonist nimodipine, 60 mg orally (or by nasogastric tube) every 4 hours for 21 days, reduces delayed ischemic neurologic deficits in patients with a ruptured aneurysm. After aneurysmal rupture, seizures are rare, but the risk of re-rupture is increased by the hypertension that follows an acute seizure. That being said, administering an anticonvulsant (e.g., phenytoin, 300 mg/d) is advised during the recovery phase before being stopped.

- **Surgical Treatment**
  - **Aneurysm:** Definitive surgical therapy of a ruptured aneurysm consists of clipping the neck of the aneurysm or endovascular placement of a coil to induce clotting.

Table 6.2. Clinical Grading of Patients with Aneurysmal Subarachnoid Hemorrhage

Grade	Level of Consciousness	Associated Clinical Features	Surgical Candidate
I	Normal	None or mild headache and stiff neck	Yes
II	Normal	Moderate headache and stiff neck; minimal neurologic deficit (eg, cranial nerve palsy) in some cases	Yes
III	Confusional state	Focal neurologic deficits in some cases	Yes
IV	Stupor	Focal neurologic deficits in some cases	No
V	Coma	Decerebrate posturing in some cases	No

Source: https://dl.mehrsys.ir/pdf-books/Clinical%20Neurology%209%20Edition%20(www.myuptodate.com).pdf.

The patient's surgical candidacy is evaluated based on the results of the neurologic examination (Table 6.2). Surgery has been demonstrated to improve the clinical outcome in fully alert patients (Hunt and Hess grades I and II) or only mildly confused (grade III). Patients who are comatose (grade V) or stuporous (grade IV), however, do not seem to benefit.

The first 24 hours after aneurysmal rupture are when rebleeding peaks, so early surgical intervention is advised. By using volume expansion and pharmacologic blood pressure elevation, this method shortens the time that patients are at risk of bleeding again and enables aggressive treatment of vasospasm.

Individualized care is provided for associated unruptured aneurysms. Young age, prior rupture, a family history of aneurysmal rupture, aneurysm growth noted, and low operative risk all favor surgery. Conservative management is preferred for small (<7-mm diameter) asymptomatic aneurysms due to their decreased life expectancy.

- o **AVM:** Surgically accessible AVMs may be removed by en-bloc resection or obliterated by ligation of feeding vessels or by embolization with a local intra-arterial catheter. Because the risk of an early second hemorrhage is much less with AVMs than with aneurysms, surgical treatment can be undertaken electively at a convenient time after the bleeding episode.

6.2.1.7. Prognosis

Aneurysmal subarachnoid hemorrhage has a high death rate. 20% of patients pass away before they get to the hospital, 20% pass away later from the original hemorrhage or its complications, and 20% pass away from rebleeding before surgery is performed. The majority of deaths happen in the initial days following the bleeding.

The likelihood of survival following aneurysmal rupture is contingent upon the patient's level of consciousness and the amount of time that has passed since the rupture. Patients without symptoms have a 60% chance of surviving on day 1, while somnolent patients have a 30% chance; after one month, these groups' chances of surviving are 60% and 90%, respectively. About 50% of aneurysmal subarachnoid hemorrhage survivors have irreversible brain damage.

6.2.2. Other Cerebrovascular Disorders

- **Intracerebral Hemorrhage:** Focal neurologic deficits, headache, vomiting, and altered consciousness are typical symptoms of intracerebral hemorrhage. In this case, the hematoma compresses pain-sensitive structures, causing headaches. Although hypertension is the most frequent cause of nontraumatic intracerebral hemorrhage, bleeding into tumors and AVMs can also present similarly. A hematoma, which is typically found in the thalamus, cerebellum, pons, basal ganglia, or subcortical white matter, is visible on the CT scan.
- **Cerebral Ischemia:** In one-third of cases, headaches start at the time of a stroke or transient ischemic attack and last for several hours to several days. The etiology of the stroke (thrombotic, embolic, or lacunar), the severity of the stroke, or hypertension are not related to the headache association. Younger age, female gender, cerebellar location, and migraine history are associated with a higher prevalence of headaches.

The headaches that accompany ischemic stroke are usually not throbbing and range in intensity from mild to moderate. Their location is usually, but not always, ipsilateral to the ischemic hemisphere and is dictated by the pain projection sites of the involved arteries. Whereas posterior fossa strokes typically manifest as occipital headaches, carotid lesions typically cause frontal (trigeminal distribution) pain. Due to the accompanying visual impairment, headaches associated with posterior cerebral artery spasm, occlusion, or retinal artery embolism may be mistakenly diagnosed as migraines.

Following a carotid endarterectomy, headache is also a part of the cerebral hyperperfusion syndrome, which can also include hypertension, focal sensory or motor signs, seizures, and altered consciousness. This syndrome usually manifests as a severe throbbing anterior headache on the operated side, often accompanied by nausea, on the second or third postoperative day. Impaired cerebral blood flow autoregulation is considered to be the cause. Analgesics may be necessary for cerebral infarction-related headaches to relieve symptoms.

6.2.3. Meningitis or Encephalitis

Meningitis, an infection of the meningeal covering of the brain, is diagnosed in patients who exhibit fever (77%), altered mental state (69%), new headaches (87%), and stiff necks (83%). Similar symptoms such as headache (81%) fever (90%) and altered consciousness (97%) are present in cases of infection involving the brain parenchyma (encephalitis); however, seizures are more common (67% in encephalitis and only 5% in meningitis).

When the brain (encephalitis) or its meningeal coverings (meningitis) becomes inflamed due to bacterial, viral, or other infections, granulomatous processes, neoplasms, or chemical irritants, headache is a common symptom. Inflammation of intracranial pain sensitive structures, such as blood vessels at the base of the brain, is the cause of the pain.

The headache is usually bilateral, throbbing, and centered in the occipital or nuchal region. Sitting up straight, moving the head, compressing the jugular vein, and other actions (like coughing or sneezing) that momentarily raise intracranial pressure can all make it more severe. Phobias could be quite noticeable. The headache rarely appears all at once; instead, it usually takes hours or days to manifest.

It is important to seek out symptoms of meningeal irritation carefully, as they may not be evident in the early stages of encephalitis or neck stiffness. Lethargy or confusion along with a fever are common, though not always noticeable symptoms.

Most cases of bacterial meningitis, but not many cases of aseptic meningitis, are accompanied by abnormal mental status. Rapid changes are possible, ranging in intensity from mild disorientation to a coma. In about half of cases of bacterial meningitis, they last less than 24 hours at the time of presentation.

A CSF examination that reveals low glucose concentration (hypoglycorrhachia) and an increased white blood cell count (pleocytosis) suggests the diagnosis of bacterial meningitis. Various methods such as CSF glucose, Gram stain, acid-fast stain, India ink preparation, cryptococcal antibody assays, Venereal Disease Research Laboratory (VDRL), and cultures can be used to differentiate between bacterial, syphilitic, tuberculous, viral, fungal, and parasitic infections.

6.2.4. Brain Abscess

Contiguous or hematogenous encapsulated pus causes an expanding mass that can cause fever, focal neurologic defects, headaches, and changes in mental status. Twenty to 25% of cases present with seizures. Although headaches are the most common presentation, less than 20% of cases have the classic triad of headache, fever, and focal neurologic signs. With a mean delay of 8 +/- 3 days between symptom onset and hospital admission, the progression is rapid.

6.2.5. Other Causes of Acute Headache

- **Seizures:** Only postictal headaches

are common; they can occur after seizures of both simple and complex partial phenomenology, but they are most frequently associated with generalized tonic-clonic seizures. Migraine symptoms, such as throbbing, nausea, vomiting, photophobia, and phonophobia, are common and resemble non-ictal headaches in patients. Distinguishing these headaches from those caused by meningitis or a subarachnoid hemorrhage may be crucial. Should uncertainty persist regarding the reason, a lumbar puncture ought to be conducted: seizures might result in a mild CSF pleocytosis (up to roughly 10 cells/μL following a single seizure or up to roughly 100 cells/μL following status epilepticus); however, the CSF glucose level remains normal.

- **Lumbar Puncture:** A history of a dural puncture (such as a spinal tap or spinal anesthesia) is required for the diagnosis of post-lumbar puncture headache, which is characterized as a postural headache with a marked increase in pain when upright and relief when in a recumbent position. Usually occipital, the pain lasts for one to two days and appears 48 to 72 hours after the procedure. There could be vomiting and nausea. Chronic CSF leakage from the spinal subarachnoid space pulls on pain-sensitive brain structures, which is what causes headaches.

By making the puncture with a small-gauge needle (22 gauge or smaller), the chance of this consequence can be decreased. Any amount of time spent lying flat does not reduce the risk. Low-pressure headache syndromes typically go away on their own. If this isn't the case, they might benefit from receiving 500 mg of intravenous caffeine sodium benzoate; if the headache doesn't go away or comes back when standing, this treatment can be repeated after 45 minutes. A skilled anesthesiologist is needed to inject autologous blood into the epidural space at the puncture site to seal the subarachnoid rent in severe cases.

The headache that results from spontaneous intracranial hypotension can resemble the headache that is caused by lumbar puncture. Smooth enhancement of the pachymeninges and a "sagging brain" may be seen on a T1-weighted, gadolinium-enhanced MRI (Figure 6.6); the enhancement may be mistaken for that linked to meningitis. When there is no headache, low CSF pressure can still result in the same MRI image. An autologous blood patch injection could result in relief right away.

- **Hypertensive Encephalopathy:** Headache can be brought on by a sharp rise in blood pressure from pheochromocytoma, sexual activity, monoamine oxidase inhibitors plus foods high in tyramine, like cheddar cheese, or—most importantly—malignant hypertension. Malignant hypertension is characterized by blood pressures of 250/150 mm Hg or higher, which cause cerebral edema and displace pain-sensitive structures. It is said that the induced pain is excruciating and throbbing. Lethargy, hemiparesis, and focal seizures are among the additional symptoms of diffuse or focal central nervous system dysfunction that may be observed; posterior white matter abnormalities on CT or MRI may also be observed. Antihypertensive medications are used as a form of treatment; however, hypotension must be avoided as this can result in cerebral ischemia and stroke.

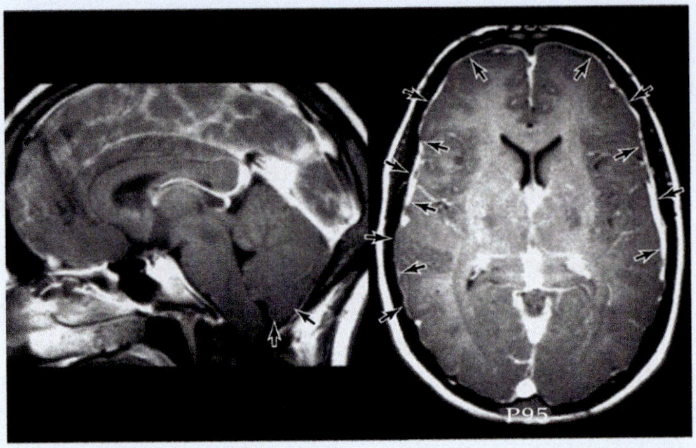

Figure 6.6. Spontaneous intracranial hypotension in a 27-year-old woman presenting with severe postural headaches. Sagittal and axial T1-weighted images obtained after gadolinium injections show features of "sagging brain": downward displacement of the cerebellar tonsils into the foramen magnum (arrows, left image), effacement of the brainstem cisterns (left image; compare with normal sagittal MRI in Figure 2.3), and diffuse dural enhancement (arrows, right image). MRI abnormalities and symptoms reversed following an epidural blood patch.

Source: Used with permission from H.A. Rowley.

- **Coitus:** Coital headaches are generally benign. Males are impacted more frequently than females. Either a dull, bilateral pain during sexual excitement or a severe, sudden headache during the orgasm, likely due to a marked rise in systemic blood pressure, can be experienced. It has also been reported that low opening pressures at the lumbar puncture are linked to a persistent headache that worsens in an upright position following an orgasm. This headache is similar to post-lumbar puncture headache. These headaches are all benign and go away in a matter of minutes to days.

  Individuals who experience intense headaches along with orgasms ought to be assessed for potential subarachnoid hemorrhage (refer to the previous conversation). If no bleeding is discovered, taking 50–100 mg of indomethacin orally 30–60 minutes before sexual activity may be beneficial as a preventative measure.

- **Ophthalmic Disorders:** Pain surrounding the eyes can be a symptom of glaucoma, iritis, and migraines. It can also occur in cluster headaches. Acute iritis causes severe photophobia and eye pain. Slit-lamp examination is used to confirm the diagnosis, and medication-assisted pupil dilatation is the acute management strategy. Pain from angle-closure glaucoma radiates to the forehead from the globe. Such a pain syndrome should prompt diagnostic tonometry when it manifests after middle age.

6.3. Subacute Headache

6.3.1. Giant Cell Arteritis

Giant cell arteritis, sometimes called temporal arteritis, is a type of systemic vasculitis that primarily affects the branches of the external carotid artery and other medium- and large-sized arteries.

Subacute granulomatous inflammation, which includes neutrophils, lymphocytes, and giant cells, is its pathological hallmark. Headache is caused by inflammation of the pain-sensitive arterial wall, and ischemia is caused by arterial stenosis.

Giant cell arteritis predominantly affects Caucasians, with women being affected twice as often as men, and is rarely seen in individuals under 60 years of age. Common symptoms include malaise, myalgia, weight loss, arthralgia, and fever, known as the polymyalgia rheumatica complex, due to inflammation around the joints. The most common indicator is a new, vague headache that can be one-sided or on both sides, typically severe and dull, mainly focused on the scalp, especially over the temporal arteries. Scalp tenderness may be noticeable when resting the head or brushing the hair. Pain or stiffness in the jaw while eating (jaw claudication) is a significant sign of giant cell arteritis, caused by reduced blood flow in the muscles of mastication. Ocular symptoms may include temporary vision impairment in one or both eyes lasting minutes to hours, as well as double vision from nerve or muscle ischemia. Anterior ischemic optic neuropathy, marked by pale swelling of the optic disc in one or both eyes, can result in permanent vision loss. Sudden vision loss may occur if the ophthalmic artery is affected.

Though not always, the erythrocyte sedimentation rate (ESR) is raised. In giant cell arteritis (range, 29–144 mm/h) and polymyalgia rheumatica (range, 58–160 mm/h), the mean Westergren ESR is roughly 100 mm/h; the upper limit of the Westergren ESR in elderly patients is reported to be as high as 40 mm/h. The diagnosis is more likely in cases of elevated ESR, thrombocytosis (>400,000 platelets/μL), and C-reactive protein level >2.45 mg/dL.

The affected temporal artery, which is thickened, nonpulsatile, dilated, and tender, is biopsied to make the diagnosis. Histologic vasculitis may be demonstrated by serial sections if the arteries are affected patchily.

Early evaluation is necessary to prevent vision loss in potential cases of giant cell arteritis. The decision to start therapy should not wait for biopsy results and should be continued even if the biopsy is negative but the diagnosis is certain clinically. The initial treatment is typically prednisone administered orally at a dosage of 60 to 100 mg per day. The dose can be reduced after 1 to 2 months based on the patient's response. Another option is to begin with intravenous methylprednisolone for 2 days, followed by prednisone. Prednisone helps reduce the sedimentation rate quickly and should be maintained within normal levels while tapering the dose over 1 to 2 years. While headaches may improve soon after starting treatment, vision loss is often permanent.

6.3.2. Intracranial Mass

A mass lesion, such as a brain tumor (Table 6.3), subdural hematoma, or brain abscess, should always be suspected when headaches suddenly appear in middle or late life. These lesions may or may not cause headaches, depending on how close they are to pain-sensitive intracranial structures. Table 6.4 shows that only roughly 50% of patients with brain tumors report headaches, though the symptoms do vary somewhat depending on the type of tumor.

The majority of the time, headaches linked to brain tumors are dull, steady, sporadic, nonspecific, and mild to moderate in intensity. Coughing, sneezing, and straining at stool are examples of actions that increase intracranial pressure. The pain is ipsilateral, bifrontal, and exacerbates with positional changes. Typically, the headache peaks when one wakes up in the morning and is linked to nausea and vomiting.

Table 6.3. Relative Incidence of Primary Central Nervous System Tumors

Tumor Type	Incidence (%)
Meningioma	34.4
Glioblastoma	16.7
Pituitary	13.1
Nerve sheath[1]	8.6
Astrocytoma	7.0
Other neuroepithelial	5.1
Lymphoma	2.4
Oligodendroglioma	2.0
Ependymoma	1.8
Embryonal[2]	1.0
Craniopharyngioma	0.7
Germ cell tumor	0.5
Other	6.6

[1]Includes acoustic neuroma.

[2]Includes medulloblastoma.

Source: Data for 2004–2007 from Central Brain Tumor Registry of the United States (www.cbtrus.org).

Table 6.4. Symptoms of Brain Tumors

Symptom	Percent With Symptom		
	Low-Grade Glioma	Malignant Glioma	Meningioma (Benign)
Headache	40	50	36
Seizure	65-95	15-25	40
Hemiparesis	5-15	30-50	22
Altered mental status	10	40–60	21

Source: Data from De Angelis LM. Brain tumors. N Engl J Med. 2001; 344:114.

Since subdural hematomas are large and more likely to impinge upon pain-sensitive structures, they often present with a noticeable headache.

A rare kind of headache that may indicate a brain tumor is characterized by an abrupt onset of intense pain that intensifies to its maximum in a matter of seconds, lasts for minutes to hours, and then quickly fades. This could be connected to "drop attacks" or altered consciousness. These paroxysmal headaches are typically linked to third ventricular colloid cysts, but they can also be caused by tumors at various other intracranial locations.

When there is a suspicion of an intracranial mass lesion, an MRI or CT scan must be performed right away. A normal brain MRI with contrast enhancement rules out brain tumors. Treatment for tumors varies according to the histologic type (primary or metastatic, benign or malignant, pathologic grade), but it may involve radiation, chemotherapy, and surgical excision. The prognosis is also affected by age, gene polymorphisms, biomarkers, and tumor characteristics.

6.3.3. Idiopathic Intracranial Hypertension

Diffuse intracranial hypertension, also known as pseudotumor cerebri, is caused by an increase in intracranial pressure that can cause papilledema, pulsatile tinnitus, visual loss, and diplopia (due to abducens [VI] nerve palsy), among other symptoms. It's possible that pathogenesis involves impaired CSF absorption. A number of illnesses can also present as symptoms of intracranial hypertension (Table 6.5), though these are less frequent than the idiopathic kind.

With a peak incidence in the third decade, women experience the condition far more frequently than men do. Obese patients make up the majority. The presenting symptom of diffuse headache is nearly always present. In most situations, there are also brief (duration of a few seconds) visual obscurations and blurring. At presentation, most patients have normal visual acuity, but nearly all have moderate to severe papilledema. Increased intracranial pressure can cause optic (II) nerve atrophy, which can result in visual loss. Similar to visual loss resulting from glaucoma, visual fields associated with idiopathic intracranial hypertension gradually narrow and eventually lose central acuity.

Table 6.5. Disorders Associated with Intracranial Hypertension

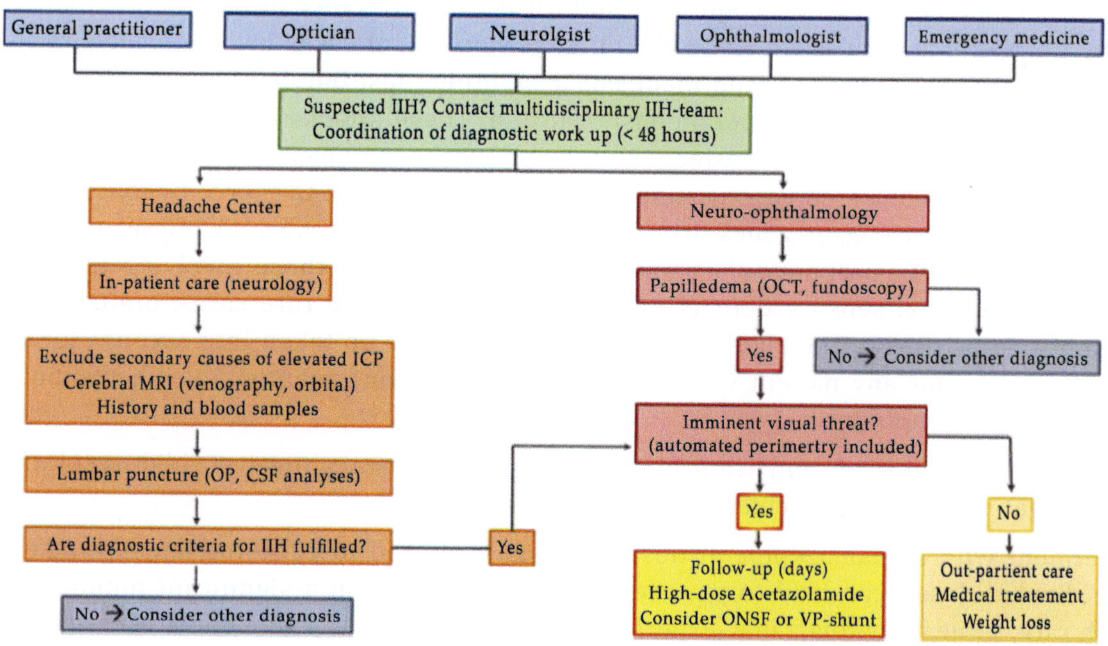

Source: Jensen RH, Vukovic-Cvetkovic V, Korsbaek JJ, Wegener M, Hamann S, Beier D. Awareness, Diagnosis and Management of Idiopathic Intracranial Hypertension. *Life*. 2021; 11(7):718. https://doi.org/10.3390/life11070718.

Symptoms of idiopathic intracranial hypertension typically improve over time, but elevated CSF pressure may persist for years and recurrent episodes can occur in 10% of cases. Diagnosis of this condition requires imaging tests such as MRI or CT scans, as well as lumbar puncture and lab studies to rule out other potential causes. Imaging may reveal small ventricles and an empty sella turcica in a majority of cases. Dilated optic nerve sheaths and flattened back of the globe are also common findings. Treatment may involve the removal of CSF to temporarily relieve symptoms, but it's important to note that high CSF pressure can also occur in obese individuals without this condition. The CSF analysis typically shows normal cell count, glucose, and protein levels.

If a cause is found (refer to Table 6.5), a particular course of action needs to be taken. Acetazolamide (1–2 g/d) is the recommended treatment for idiopathic cases; topiramate may also be useful. Although corticosteroids are useful, they come with unwanted side effects, and stopping them tends to make papilledema worse. Patients who are obese ought to be motivated to shed pounds. To preserve vision and reduce headaches in cases that do not respond to medical treatment, lumboperitoneal or ventriculoperitoneal shunting, or optic nerve sheath fenestration, may be necessary.

6.3.4. Trigeminal Neuralgia

Trigeminal neuralgia, also known as tic douloureux, is a facial pain condition that typically occurs in women during middle to late adulthood. The disorder is thought to be caused by microvascular compression near the trigeminal (V) nerve roots, leading to demyelination and the development of the syndrome.

The trigeminal (V) nerve's second (V2) and third (V3) divisions supply the area where pain is usually unilateral and localized (Figure 6.7). Less than 5% of cases involve involvement of the first division or bilateral disease. Pain manifests as lightning-fast bursts of intense agony that last longer than a second and then spontaneously subside. These attacks are typical for a particular patient. Occurs rarely while you're asleep. Minutes to weeks may pass during pain-free intervals, but long-term spontaneous remission is uncommon. The pain can be triggered by touch, cold, wind, talking, or chewing on trigger zones around the mouth, nose, or cheek. A physical examination reveals no abnormalities; abnormal trigeminal reflexes (such as those involving the cornea or jaw jerk) or trigeminal sensory deficits rule out the diagnosis. In rare cases, brainstem tumors or multiple sclerosis may cause pain akin to this. This should be taken into account for younger patients as well as for any patient who exhibits neurologic abnormalities during examination or who has bilateral symptoms.

Arteriography, CT scan, and traditional MRI are all normal; however, high-resolution MRI methods might reveal microvascular nerve compression.

Treatment with carbamazepine at doses ranging from 400 to 1200 mg per day, taken orally in three divided doses, can lead to pain relief within 24 hours in a significant number of cases. Although rare, some individuals may experience blood dyscrasia as a side effect of carbamazepine. Alternatively, oxcarbazepine can be used at doses of 600–1800 mg per day in two divided doses, with similar effectiveness and no risk of blood dyscrasia. In cases of acute attacks, intravenous phenytoin at a dose of 250 mg can be administered to abort the attack, while oral phenytoin at doses of 200–400 mg per day can be effective either alone or in combination with carbamazepine if additional treatment is needed. Lamotrigine at a dose of 400 mg per day or baclofen at doses ranging from 10 mg three times daily to 20 mg four times daily can be considered for cases that are refractory to other treatments. For patients who do not respond to medication, posterior fossa microvascular decompression surgery may be recommended.

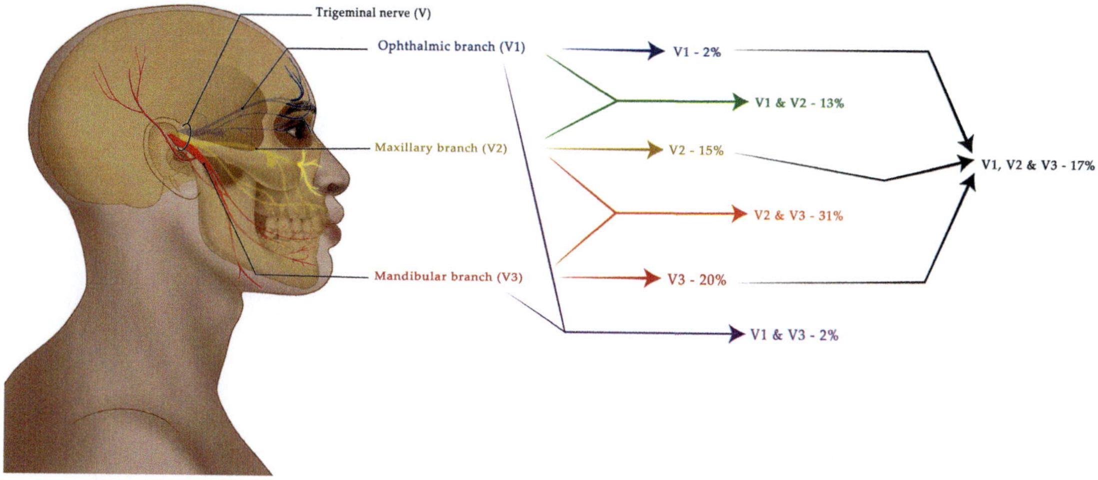

Figure 6.7. Distribution of symptoms in trigeminal neuralgia.

Source: Jarrahi A, Cantrell R, Norris C, Dhandapani K, Barrett J, Vender J. Trigeminal Neuralgia Treatment Outcomes Following Gamma Knife Stereotactic Radiosurgery. *International Journal of Translational Medicine*. 2022; 2(4):543–554. https://doi.org/10.3390/ijtm2040041.

6.3.5. Glossopharyngeal Neuralgia

Unilateral pain that is restricted to the base of the tongue, tonsillar pillars, auditory meatus, or oropharynx is the hallmark of the uncommon syndrome known as glossopharyngeal neuralgia. Pain can be more persistent and burning or aching, or it can be paroxysmal, similar to the trigeminal neuralgia described in the section above. Rarely, the pain is accompanied by bradyarrhythmic cardiac syncope. Talking or swallowing can cause symptoms to start because trigger areas are often located near the tonsillar pillars. Pain paroxysms can happen frequently throughout the day.

Both men and women are affected at similar rates, with symptoms typically starting at a younger age compared to trigeminal neuralgia. The diagnosis is confirmed through patient history and reproducing pain by stimulating peritonsillar trigger zones. There are no abnormal neurological signs present. If bilateral symptoms, abnormal signs, or other unusual features are present, further investigation is necessary to rule out disorders that may mimic glossopharyngeal neuralgia, including multiple sclerosis, cerebellopontine angle tumors, and nasopharyngeal carcinoma.

Conventional imaging methods reveal no abnormalities, similar to trigeminal neuralgia; however, high-resolution MRI methods might reveal microvascular compression of the glossopharyngeal (IX) nerve. Applying a local anesthetic to the trigger area, such as 10% lidocaine, may prevent the pain reaction. For trigeminal neuralgia, carbamazepine or phenytoin (as previously mentioned) typically results in significant relief; in drug-resistant cases, microvascular decompression has been employed.

6.3.6. Postherpetic Neuralgia

Herpes zoster, also known as shingles, is a vesicular skin eruption in the trigeminal (V) nerve distribution that is accompanied by pain and tenderness. It is caused by the varicella-zoster virus reactivating in the trigeminal, or Gasserian, ganglion. Most patients experience a resolution of their symptoms in one to two months, but some develop postherpetic neuralgia, which causes pain to last for months or years. The syndrome does not manifest before the age of fifty, and as people age, it becomes more prevalent. Patients with leukemia or lymphoma, as well as those with compromised immune systems, also exhibit it.

The hallmark of postherpetic neuralgia is persistent, intense dysesthetic pain that stabs or burns. Pain is typically localized to one side of the forehead because the first division (V1) of the trigeminal (V) nerve is most frequently affected in the head (Figure 6.8). There could be some scarring. Decreased cutaneous sensitivity to pinprick is revealed by careful testing of the painful area. Reduced corneal sensation and an impaired blink reflex are the other main herpes zoster complications in the trigeminal distribution. These conditions can result in corneal abrasion, scarring, and eventually blindness.

Treatment with acyclovir (800 mg five times daily), famciclovir, or valacyclovir for seven to ten days can lessen the severity and duration of the cutaneous eruption and the acute pain associated with herpes zoster; however, there is no evidence that this treatment reduces the risk of postherpetic neuralgia. Corticosteroids also lessen the incidence of acute herpetic pain when taken orally for two weeks during an acute herpetic eruption (60 mg/d prednisone, with rapid tapering). However, their impact on postherpetic pain is unknown.

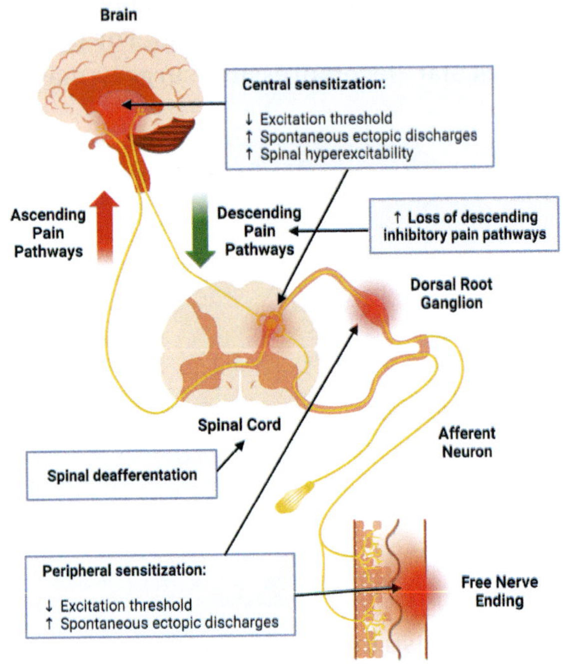

Figure 6.8. Distribution of symptoms and signs in postherpetic neuralgia.

Source: Huerta MÁ, Garcia MM, García-Parra B, Serrano-Afonso A, Paniagua N. Investigational Drugs for the Treatment of Postherpetic Neuralgia: Systematic Review of Randomized Controlled Trials. *International Journal of Molecular Sciences*. 2023; 24(16):12987. https://doi.org/10.3390/ijms241612987.

Tricyclic antidepressants, such as amitriptyline, 25 to 150 mg/d orally, have proven to be the most effective treatment for postherpetic pain syndrome once it has been diagnosed. This is because these drugs are believed to act directly on central nervous system pain integration pathways, rather than through an antidepressant effect; desipramine or nortriptyline may be more tolerable. Combining tricyclic antidepressants with phenothiazine may increase their efficacy. Pregabalin (600 mg/d) and gabapentin (1,800–3,600 mg/d) are two anticonvulsants that have demonstrated some benefit.

An efficient topical treatment is lidocaine (five percent gel or cutaneous patch) or lidocaine-prilocaine (two percent cream). Topical capsaicin (0.075% cream or 8% patch) can be beneficial as well, although it may irritate nearby skin. By acting as an antagonist of the transient receptor potential cation channel (TRPV1), capsaicin reduces the amount of substance P, also known as calcitonin gene-related peptide, which mediates pain, in peripheral sensory neurons. Weekly intrathecal methylprednisolone administration has been shown to alleviate pain in otherwise incurable cases.

6.3.7. Persistent Idiopathic Facial Pain

Persistent idiopathic or atypical facial pain is characterized by constant, dull pain in the lower face with no identifiable cause. It differs from trigeminal neuralgia as it is not limited to the trigeminal nerve and is not sudden in onset. Neurological examination is typically normal. This condition must be distinguished from pain syndromes associated with certain cancers or infections. Treatment typically involves oral medications such as amitriptyline or phenelzine, with phenytoin being an alternative option for those who cannot tolerate tricyclic antidepressants.

6.4. Chronic Headache

6.4.1. Migraine

Migraine is a prevalent condition, affecting 12% of the population. It is characterized by recurring headaches that are often one-sided and pulsating, accompanied by symptoms such as nausea, vomiting, sensitivity to light and sound, and fatigue. Many patients experience warning signs that can affect mood, appetite, or cognition. Some people may also have visual or sensory symptoms before the headache begins, while others do not. Migraine affects both males and females before puberty, but after puberty, it is more common in women. The condition usually starts early in life, with 25% of cases beginning in the first decade, 55% by age 20, and over 90% before age 40.

6.4.2. Genetics

Genes play a major role in migraine susceptibility. Most cases have a family history of migraine in at least one first-degree relative, and twin studies show that both genetic and environmental factors are involved. Numerous well-known syndromes, such as cerebral autosomal dominant arteriopathy with subcortical infarcts (CADASIL) and familial hemiplegic migraine, are associated with autosomal dominant inheritance of migraine (Table 6.6).

6.4.3. Structural Features

Increases in white matter lesions identified by MRI, infarct-like lesions, and volumetric alterations in the cerebral gray and white matter are linked to migraine. Both patients with and without aura experience the same effects. There is no conclusive evidence linking headache frequency to this. There have been no findings regarding cognitive consequences, so the clinical significance of these findings is unknown.

Table 6.6. Autosomal Dominant and Hereditary Disorders Associated with Migraine

Gene	Protein	Disease	Features
CACNA1A	α_1 subunit of neuronal $Ca_v2.1$ (P/Q-type) voltage-gated calcium channel	Familial hemiplegic migraine (FHM1); (50% of identified families have *CACNA1A* mutations)	Hemiplegic migraine, cerebellar ataxia, seizures
ATP1A2	α_2 subunit of sodium-potassium pump	Familial hemiplegic migraine (FHM2); (20% of identified families have *ATP1A2* mutations)	Hemiplegic migraine, seizures
SCN1A	α subunit of $Na_v1.1$ voltage-gated sodium channel	Familial hemiplegic migraine (FHM3)	Hemiplegic migraine, seizures
MTTL1	mtDNA A-to-G transition at nucleotide 3243	Mitochondrial encephalopathy with lactic acidosis and stroke-like episodes (MELAS)	Migraine, seizures, hemiparesis, hemianopsia, cortical blindness, and episodic vomiting
NOTCH3	Notch3 (transmembrane receptor)	Cerebral autosomal dominant arteriopathy with subcortical infarcts (CADASIL)	Migraine with aura, stroke, dementia
TREX1	3′ repair exonuclease 1 (DNA repair enzyme)	Retinal vasculopathy with cerebral leukodystrophy (RVCL)	Migraine, blindness, stroke, dementia, Raynaud phenomenon, nephropathy, cirrhosis

Source: https://dl.mehrsys.ir/pdf-books/Clinical%20Neurology%209%20Edition%20(www.myuptodate.com).pdf.

6.4.3.1. Pathogenesis

It has long been believed that the causes of the aura and headache phases of migraine are, respectively, extracranial vasodilation and intracranial vasoconstriction. The ability of vasodilators like amyl nitrite to eliminate the migraine aura and the vasoconstrictive ergot alkaloids (such as ergotamine) to stop an acute migraine attack provided evidence in favor of this theory. Current research presents a more nuanced picture, indicating that the headache and aura phases may be caused by a primary disruption of central neuronal activity.

Migraine attacks in numerous patients are preceded by symptoms such as fatigue, cognitive issues, mood disturbances, or gastrointestinal problems, which can persist for a day. The cause of these early warning signs is not fully understood, but it may be linked to changes in hypothalamic or brainstem functions.

During the aura phase of a migraine, there is a decrease in cerebral blood flow starting in the occipital cortex and moving towards the front of the brain along cytoarchitectural boundaries rather than vascular ones. This decrease in blood flow mirrors the phenomenon of spreading depression, where depolarization of neurons and glial cells slows down blood flow and inhibits neuronal function. This reduction in blood flow does not align with the specific areas of the brain responsible for the aura, and the decrease is not enough to cause symptoms of lack of oxygen (ischemia). In some cases, blood flow remains low even after the aura has passed and the headache has started. It has been observed that inhibiting spreading depression can prevent the aura, but not the headache that follows. These findings suggest that changes in neuronal activity, rather than lack of oxygen, are responsible for the aura. However, the exact cause of spreading depression and its connection to the premonitory phase of a migraine remain poorly understood (Figure 6.9).

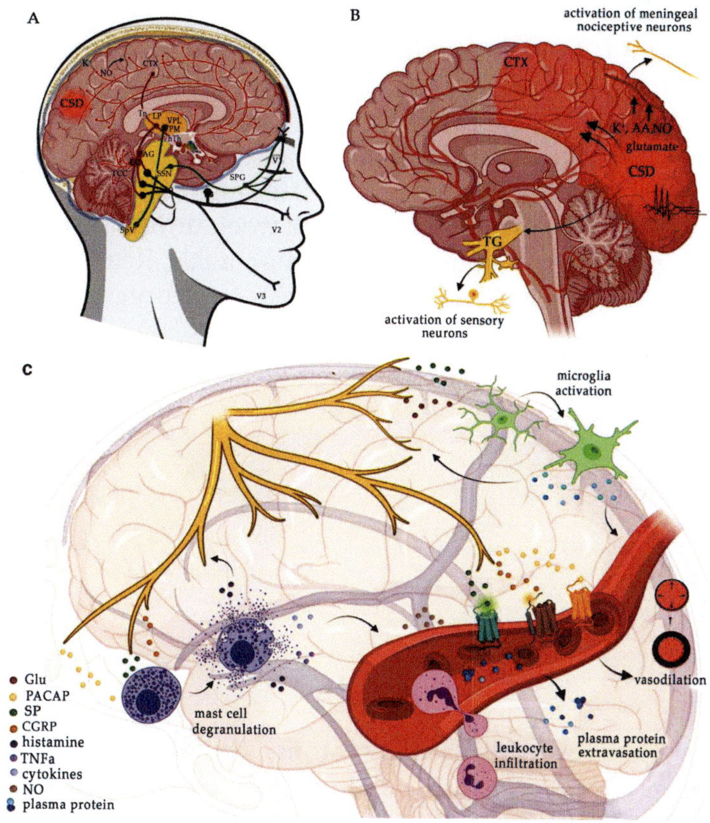

Figure 6.9. Central and peripheral nervous system sites proposed to be involved in migraine pathogenesis. During the aura phase, a reduction in cortical blood flow spreads anteriorly from the occipital cortex (large arrow), which is thought to be due to spreading depression. During the headache phase, sterile inflammation in the meninges may activate trigeminal (V) nerve sensory fibers that project to the nucleus caudalis, periaqueductal gray, sensory thalamic nuclei, and primary somatosensory cortex (small arrows). Alternatively, this central sensory pathway may convey normal afferent signals that are interpreted as noxious.

Source: Spekker E, Nagy-Grócz G, Vécsei L. Ion Channel Disturbances in Migraine Headache: Exploring the Potential Role of the Kynurenine System in the Context of the Trigeminovascular System. *International Journal of Molecular Sciences*. 2023; 24(23):16574. https://doi.org/10.3390/ijms242316574.

There are two main theories that have been put forth to explain the headache phase. One theory states that pain is possibly caused by sterile inflammation and is triggered peripherally in primary sensory trigeminal neurons that innervate the meninges and blood vessels. These neurons project to the periaqueductal gray, sensory thalamic nuclei, and somatosensory cortex from the nucleus caudalis in the brainstem. According to a different theory, there is a primary disruption of the central pain pathways, which results in allodynia—the misinterpretation of normally harmless sensory input as pain signals.

6.4.3.2. Clinical Findings

- **Migraine With Aura (Classic Migraine):** 30% of migraineurs experience brief neurologic symptoms (aura) prior to headache. Visual abnormalities, especially hemianopic field defects and scotomas (blind spots) and scintillations (flickerings) that enlarge and spread peripherally are the most common types of auras (Figure 6.10). This is followed by a throbbing unilateral headache (Figure 6.11). Although the frequency of headaches varies, over 50% of patients only have one attack per week or less. For the majority of patients, episodes last longer than two hours and less than a day. Remissions are typical following menopause and in the second and third trimesters of pregnancy.

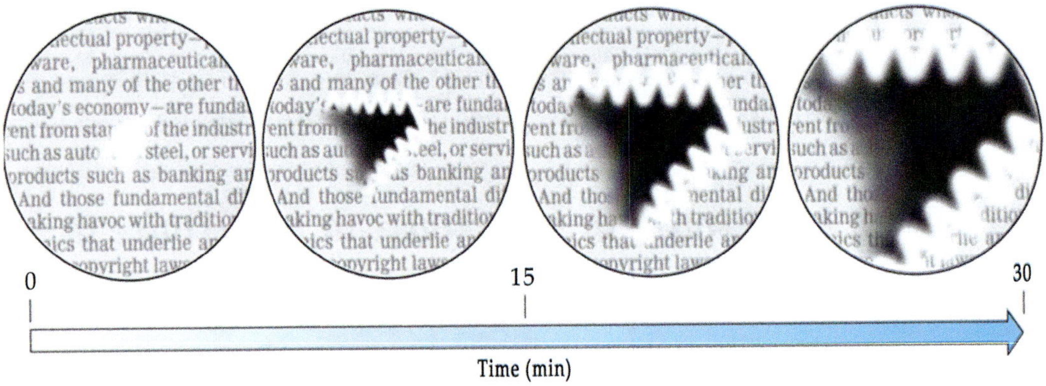

Figure 6.10. Successive maps of scintillating scotoma (blind spot) to show the evolution of fortification figures (jagged edges) and associated scotoma in a patient with classic migraine. As the fortification moves laterally, a region of transient blindness remains.

Source: https://dl.mehrsys.ir/pdf-books/Clinical%20Neurology%209%20Edition%20(www.myuptodate.com).pdf.

Bilateral headaches are also possible, even though hemicranial pain is the classic migraine's defining feature. They may also be occipital in location, which is a feature that is frequently connected to headaches of the tension variety.

During the headache, photophobia, phonophobia, lassitude, nausea, vomiting, and irritability are commonly associated symptoms. Autonomic and vasomotor symptoms are also frequent. Basilar migraine differs from stroke in that symptoms appear gradually ("migrainous march") and go away on their own. Lightheadedness, vertigo, ataxia, or altered consciousness are possible symptoms. Hemiplegic migraine is one type of migraine that can occasionally result in neurologic deficits that last into or past the pain phase. Stroke is another rare side effect of migraine.

The aura (late-life equivalents of migraines) may occur without a headache, especially after the age of fifty. The symptoms, which typically last for 15 to 60 minutes, include visual disturbance, hemiparesis, hemisensory loss, dysarthria, or aphasia.

- **Migraine without Aura (Common Migraine):** Headache caused by migraine without aura is typically bilateral and periorbital in location, and it is far more common than migraine with aura. One could characterize the pain as throbbing, especially in more severe cases. Photophobia, vomiting, and nausea are frequent. Complications from associated cervical muscle contraction may worsen the pain as long as it lasts. During the episode, there is frequently tenderness in the scalp. If left untreated, a headache typically lasts between four and seventy-two hours and is sometimes relieved by vomiting. Compressing the ipsilateral carotid or superficial temporal artery during a migraine attack can lessen the intensity of both common and classic migraines.

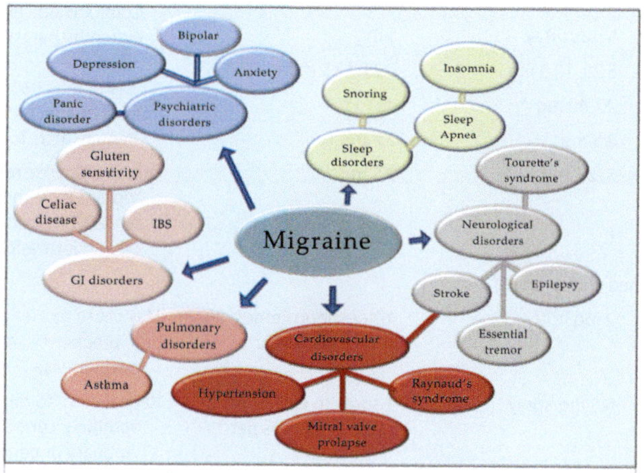

Migraine Comorbidities

Figure 6.11. *Migraine comorbidies.*

Source: By 7mike5000 – Own work, CC BY-SA 3.0, https://commons.wikimedia.org/w/index.php?curid=23724426

- **Chronic (Transformed) Migraine and Medication Overuse Headache:** Over the course of months or years, episodic migraine can transform into a chronic headache syndrome with almost constant pain. Frequently, the headache loses its characteristic migrainous qualities. Risk factors include prior headache frequency, obesity, and caffeine use. Headache from overusing medications is a common subgroup of chronic migraine.

Table 6.7. Acute (Abortive) Treatment of Migraine Headache

Drug	Route[1]	Strength	Recommended Dose	Comments
Simple analgesics				
Aspirin	PO	325 mg	650 mg q4h	May cause gastric pain or bleeding and rebound headache if used frequently.
Naproxen sodium	PO	250, 375, 500 mg	500–1,000 mg at onset, then 250–500 prn after 1 hour	
Ibuprofen	PO	200, 400, 600, 800 mg	800-1,200 mg at onset, then 600-800 mg q4–8h	
Ketoprofen	PO	25, 50, 75, 100, 150, 200 mg	75-150 mg q6h	
Acetaminophen	PO PR	325, 500 mg	650-1,000 mg at onset, then q4h	Acetaminophen/isometheptene/dichloralphenazone is marketed as Midrin.
(If analgesics ineffective, switch to triptans for next headache.)				

Triptans				
Sumatriptan**	NS	20 mg/spray	20 mg	May repeat once after 2 hours for partial response. May cause nausea and vomiting; contraindicated by pregnancy, coronary or peripheral vascular disease, concurrent treatment with monoamine oxidase inhibitors, and possibly hemiplegic or basilar migraine. Common side effects: chest tightness, extremity parasthesias
	PO	25, 50, 100 mg	50-100 mg	
	SC	6 mg	6 mg	
Rizatriptan*	PO	5, 10 mg	10 mg	
Zolmitriptan**	PO	2.5, 5 mg	2.5-5 mg	
	NS	5 mg/spray	5 mg	
Almotriptan**	PO	6.25, 12.5 mg	6.25-12.5 mg	*Onset of effect 30 minutes **Onset of effect 45-60 minutes *** Require 4 hrs for effect but are long acting
Eletriptan*	PO	20, 40 mg	40 mg	
Frovatriptan***	PO	2.5 mg	2.5 mg	
Naratriptan***	PO	1, 2.5 mg	2.5 mg	Triptan response rate 60-80%. Faster-acting triptans have more frequent headache recurrence which can be attenuated by NSAID co-administration.
Ergot alkaloids (not to be combined with triptans)				
Ergotamine/caffeine (Cafergot)	PR	2 mg/100 mg	1/4-2 suppositories, up to 5 per week	May cause nausea and vomiting; contraindicated in pregnancy and coronary or peripheral vascular disease.
Dihydroergotamine (DHE)	NS	0.5 mg/spray	1 spray to each nostril, up to 5 times per week	Repeat after 15 minutes. May cause nausea and vomiting; contraindicated in pregnancy and coronary or peripheral vascular disease.
	SC	1 mg/mL	1-2 mg	Repeat 1 mg q12h, up to 6 mg
	IV		0.75-1.25 mg IV	
Narcotic analgesics				
Codeine/aspirin	PO	15, 30, 60/325 mg	30-120 mg codeine	
Meperidine	PO IM	50, 100 mg	50-200 mg	
Butorphanol	NS	10 mg/mL (1 mg/spray)	1 spray every 3-4 hours as needed	
Antiemetics				
Prochlorperazine	PO	5, 10, 15 mg	25 mg q6h	Adjunctive treatment to reduce nausea and improve enteric absorption of antimigraine drugs. Extrapyramidal side effects may occur.
	PR	2.5, 5, 25 mg	25 mg q12h	
	IM, IV	5 mg/mL	10 mg (with 10 mg diphenhydramine)	
Chlorpromazine	IM	25 mg/mL	50 mg	
	IV	25 mg/mL	0.1 mg/kg drip over 20 minutes	
Promethazine	PO, PR	12.5, 25, 50 mg	25-50 mg q6h	
Metoclopramide	PO	5, 10 mg	5-20 mg tid	

[1]bid, twice daily; hs, at bedtime; IM, intramuscular; IV, intravenous; NS, nasal spray; PO, oral; PR, rectal; prn, as needed; q, every; qd, every day; qod, every other day; SC, subcutaneous; tid, three times daily

Source: https://dl.mehrsys.ir/pdf-books/Clinical%20Neurology%209%20Edition%20(www.myuptodate.com).pdf.

Chronic daily headache syndrome can result from the overuse of medications intended to treat migraine or other types of headaches. Patients with other types of headaches and those on different drug classes are also susceptible, but the majority of patients have migraine as their underlying condition and have overused simple analgesics or triptans. Women make up the majority of patients. A headache typically lasts for at least three months, occurring at least fifteen days a month. The course of treatment entails starting preventative therapy and reducing or stopping the offending medications (Table 6.8). Corticosteroids may be helpful in "bridge therapy," which lessens the intensity of headaches caused by drug withdrawal.

6.4.4. Precipitating Factors

Certain foods (tyramine-containing cheeses; meat with nitrite preservatives, such as hot dogs or bacon; chocolate that contains phenylethylamine but not chocolate alone) and food additives, like monosodium glutamate, a frequently used flavor enhancer, can trigger migraine attacks. Attacks can also be triggered by menstruation, fasting, emotions, medications (particularly oral contraceptives and vasodilators like nitroglycerin), and bright lights.

6.4.4.1. Treatment

The migraine treatment options are compiled in Tables 6.7 and 6.8, where they are categorized into two categories: preventive measures and abortive measures.

Simple analgesics, or ergot alkaloids (e.g., dihydroergotamine) or serotonin 5-HT1B/D receptor agonists (triptans), are often effective in treating acute migraine attacks. Calcitonin gene-related peptide receptor antagonists, such as telcagepant and olcegepant, are a novel class of antimigraine medications that may also be helpful in this regard. For maximum effectiveness, medications for acute (abortive) treatment (Table 6.7) must be taken as soon as symptoms appear. Parenteral formulations that absorb quickly are preferable to oral ones. As a common side effect of some antimigraine medications is nausea, which is a prominent feature of migraine, it may be necessary to administer the medication by a method other than oral administration or to concurrently administer an antiemetic (Table 6.8). Combining ergot alkaloids and triptans is not advised for individuals with hypertension or other cardiovascular conditions.

Patients who experience two or more headaches per week or for whom abortive treatment is insufficient should receive preventive care. Unless prescribed otherwise by Table 6.8, tricyclic antidepressants, β-blockers, anticonvulsants, and calcium channel blockers can be tried in that order.

In pregnancy, sumatriptan is safe to use during the first trimester, but narcotic analgesics are the only effective treatment for migraine. While some antimigraine medications may be teratogenic or cause pregnancy difficulties, acetaminophen is occasionally beneficial. Avoiding precipitating factors is advised.

Table 6.8. Prophylactic Treatment of Migraine Headache

Drug	Route[1]	Strength	Recommended Dose	Comments
Anti-inflammatory agents				
Aspirin	PO	325 mg	325 mg qod	May cause gastric pain or bleeding
Naproxen sodium	PO	275, 550 mg	550-825 mg bid	
Tricyclic antidepressants				
Amitriptyline	PO	10, 25, 50, 75, 100, 150 mg	10-300 mg hs	May cause dry mouth or urinary retention. Begin with lowest dose and increase slowly. Adding an anticonvulsant may increase efficacy.
Nortriptyline	PO	10, 25, 50, 75 mg	10-150 mg hs	
Desipramine	PO	10, 25, 50, 75, 100 mh	25-300 mg qhs	
Protriptyline	PO	5, 10 mg	15-40 md/d in 3-4 doses	Protriptyline is less sedating than other tricyclics but dry mouth and constipation may be problematic
β-Receptor antagonists				
Propranolol*	PO	10, 20, 40, 60, 80, 90 mg	20-120 mg bid	Listed in descending order of efficacy. Symptomatic bradycardia may occur at high doses. Contraindicated in asthma and congestive heart failure and in patients on calcium channel blockers. To discontinue, taper over 1-2 weeks.* most effective
	PO (long acting)	60, 80, 120, 160 mg	60-320 mg qd	
Timolol*	PO	10, 20 mg	10-30 mg qd	
Metoprolol*	PO	50, 100 mg	100-200 mg qd	
Nadolol	PO	40, 80, 120, 160 mg	40-240 mg qd	
Atenolol	PO	50, 100 mg	50-200 mg qd	
Anticonvulsants				
Valproic acid	PO	125, 250, 500 mg; 500 mg extended release	250-500 mg bid or 1,000 mg qhs as single dose with extended release	Begin with lowest dose. Contraindicated in women of childbearing age.
Topiramate	PO	25, 50, 100, 200 mg	25-200 mg qd	Start 25 mg hs and increase by 25 mg/d every 7 days as tolerated. Optimal dose 100 mg/d. Paresthesias in 50%. Altered mental state may require lowering dose. Rare: nephrolithiasis, angle-closure glaucoma.
Gabapentin	PO	100, 300, 400, 600, 800 mg	1800-2,400 mg qd	Less effective than other anticonvulsants. Sedating.
Calcium channel antagonists				
Verapamil	PO	40, 80, 120 mg	80-160 mg tid	Contraindicated by severe left ventricular dysfunction, hypotension, sick sinus syndrome without artificial pacemaker, second- or third-degree AV nodal block, and in patients on β-blockers. Constipation is most common side effect. Verapamil ineffective in migraine without aura.
Flunarizine	PO (long acting)	240 mg	240 mg qd-bid	
	PO	5, 10 mg	5-15 mg/day	
Other agents[2]				
Riboflavin (vitamin B2)	PO	Various	400 mg/d	May require 4-8 weeks for onset and increased effect over 3-6 months. Urine turns dark.
Onabotulinum toxin A	IM	100 units/vial	100-250 units	Not effective in episodic but very effective in chronic migraine. Injected into head and neck muscles.

[1] bid, twice daily; hs, at bedtime; IM, intramuscular; IV, intravenous; NS, nasal spray; PO, oral; PR, rectal; prn, as needed; q, every; qd, every day; qod, every other day; SC, subcutaneous; tid, three times daily.

[2] Other agents reported as effective include magnesium 200–1200 mg/d, coenzyme Q10 150 mg tid, feverfew 6.25 mg tid, butterbur 75 mg bid, and memantine 5–20 mg tid.

Source: https://dl.mehrsys.ir/pdf-books/Clinical%20Neurology%209%20Edition%20(www.myuptodate.com).pdf.

6.4.5. Cluster Headache and Trigeminal Autonomic Cephalalgias

6.4.5.1. Clinical Findings

Cluster headaches manifest as brief, intense, unilateral, continuous, non-throbbing headaches that occur in clusters and last anywhere from 15 minutes to 3 hours. Cluster headaches are always unilateral and typically recur on the same side in any given patient, in contrast to migraine headaches. They usually wake the patient up at night and repeat every day, sometimes at almost the same time (circadian periodicity), for a few months to a few weeks at a time. During an attack, patients may pace erratically. The patient may experience months or even years without headaches in between clusters. Although the cause is unknown, functional MRI during an attack has revealed activation of the hypothalamus.

Compared to migraine, cluster headaches are much more common in men than in women and usually start later in life (mean onset at 25 years old). Rarely does one have a family history.

The headache can start as a burning feeling on the side of the nose or as pressure behind the eye. The pain can be thumping, sharp, or stabbing. Other symptoms that are often linked to the attack include redness of the conjunctiva on the same side, tearing of the eye, stuffy nose, and Horner syndrome. Episodes may be triggered by alcohol or drugs that widen blood vessels, particularly if used during a cluster headache episode.

6.4.5.2. Treatment

Treatment for a cluster of headaches includes taking steps to stop the acute attack as soon as it starts as well as to avoid more.

- **Acute Treatment:** Sumatriptan (6 mg, repeated once per attack if necessary) administered subcutaneously can provide immediate pain relief, as can breathing 100% oxygen (7–12 L/min for 15–20 minutes) (Table 6.7). Other abortive treatments include subcutaneous octreotide; intravenous, intramuscular, subcutaneous, or intranasal dihydroergotamine; oral zolmitriptan; and intranasal sumatriptan, zolmitriptan, or lidocaine.
- **Maintenance Prophylaxis:** A number of medications used to treat migraines (refer to Table 6.8) can also be helpful in maintaining prophylaxis, or preventing recurrent cluster headache symptoms while the condition is active. Verapamil (80 mg three times daily or sustained-release 240 mg/d; doses of 720 mg/d may be necessary) is the most commonly used medication. Second-line medications include anticonvulsants like topiramate (50–200 mg/d), gabapentin (300–3,600 mg/d), and valproic acid (500–2,000 mg/d). Moreover, melatonin (10 mg/d) may be beneficial. When a cluster comes to an end, medications used for maintenance prophylaxis are stopped (Figure 6.12).

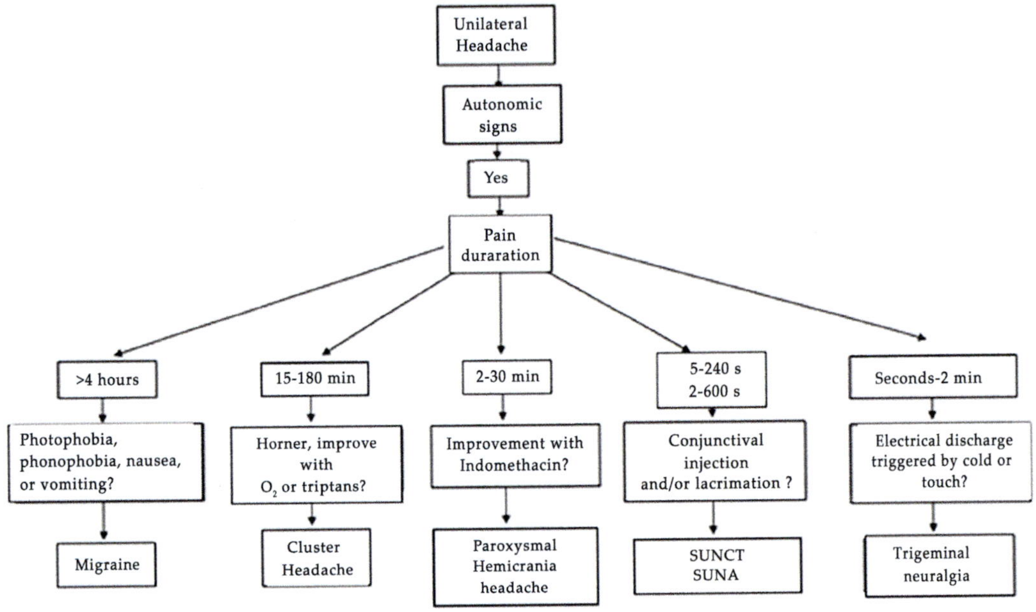

Figure 6.12. Distribution of symptoms and signs in cluster headache.

Source: San-Juan D, Velez-Jimenez K, Hoffmann J, Martínez-Mayorga AP, Melo-Carrillo A, Rodríguez-Leyva I, García S, Collado-Ortiz MÁ, Chiquete E, Gudiño-Castelazo M, Juárez-Jimenez H, Martínez-Gurrola M, Marfil A, Nader-Kawachi JA, Uribe-Jaimes PD, Darío-Vargas R and Villareal-Careaga J (2024) Cluster headache: an update on clinical features, epidemiology, pathophysiology, diagnosis, and treatment. Front. Pain Res. 5:1373528. doi: 10.3389/fpain.2024.1373528.

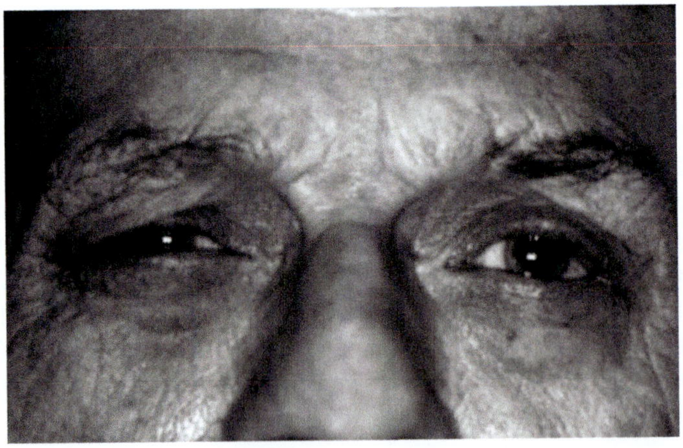

Figure 6.13. Ptosis of the right eye during acute cluster headache. Other components of Horner syndrome (pupillary miosis, and regional anhydrosis) may also occur.

Source: https://dl.mehrsys.ir/pdf-books/Clinical%20Neurology%209%20Edition%20(www.myuptodate.com).pdf.

- **Transitional Prophylaxis:** When prednisone is administered orally at a dose of 40 to 80 mg/d for one week at the start of a cluster cycle, it can be stopped by gradually reducing the dosage over the course of the next week. Dihydroergotamine or intravenous methylprednisolone may also be helpful.
- **Cluster Headache Variants:** Cluster headaches may be chronic in nature as opposed to episodic. Hypnic headache is a bilateral variant that affects the elderly and does not have the autonomic components of cluster headache. Paroxysmal hemicrania is the term used to describe recurrent, multiple, short-duration (10–20 minute) episodes of pain lasting roughly five days. These are more typical in females. The administration of indomethacin 25 to 50 mg three times a day significantly improves each of these syndromes (Figure 6.13).
- **Invasive Treatment:** Patients who do not respond to medicine may be treated with invasive procedures such as radiofrequency trigeminal ganglion ablation, trigeminal rhizotomy, and greater occipital nerve block.

6.4.6. Tension-Type Headache

The term "tension-type headache" refers to persistent or recurrent headaches without a clear cause that do not exhibit the symptoms of a migraine or other headache syndromes. It is unclear what the underlying pathophysiologic mechanism is, but "tension" is not likely to be the main culprit. Electromyography has not shown the contraction of the muscles in the neck and scalp, and if it is, it is most likely a secondary phenomenon.

Tension-type headaches, in their classic form (Figure 6.14), are chronic headaches that usually start after the age of twenty. It is typified by bilateral, non-throbbing occipital headache attacks that are not accompanied by prodromal visual disturbance, nausea, or vomiting. Headaches can last for hours or even days. There are times when the pain is compared to a tight band around the head.

Compared to men, women are more frequently impacted. Many patients experience headaches that share characteristics with migraine and tension-type headaches, despite the fact that these two conditions are traditionally seen as separate conditions. Thus, throbbing headaches, unilateral head pain, or nausea with attacks are experienced by some patients who are diagnosed with tension-type headaches. Therefore, it might be more accurate to think of migraine and tension-type headaches as the two extremes of a single clinical spectrum.

Many of the medications used to treat migraines are also used to treat tension-type headaches (Tables 6.7 and 6.8). Acetaminophen, aspirin, and other nonsteroidal anti-inflammatory medications may be effective in treating acute attacks. Triptans may be effective for migraineurs with tension-type headaches. Propranolol may be helpful in certain situations, but amitriptyline, nortriptyline, or imipramine are frequently the most effective medications for preventive care. Serotonin reuptake inhibitors that are selective are less efficient. Most botulinum toxin trials indicate that the substance is ineffective. In certain situations, massage, physical therapy, and relaxation methods can be especially beneficial.

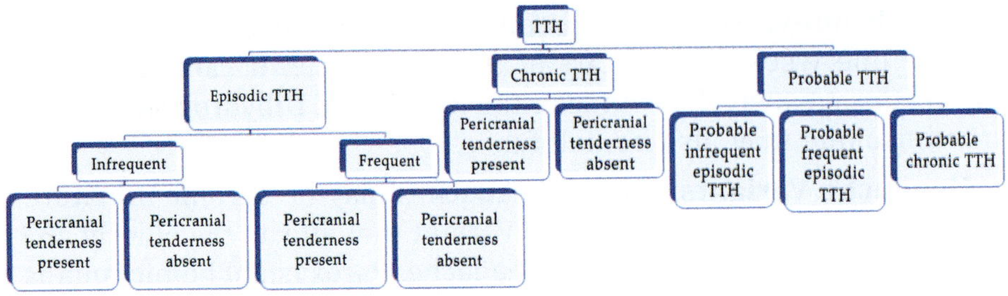

Figure 6.14. Distribution of symptoms and signs in tension-type headache.

Source: By Ucfmed2019 - Own work, CC BY-SA 4.0, https://commons.wikimedia.org/w/index.php?curid=75786854.

6.4.7. Icepick-Like Pain

"Icepick-like pain" refers to extremely brief, sharp, intense pain that is felt in the scalp but is not related to the trigeminal nerve. Pain paroxysms can be solitary, repetitive, or clustered, and they can happen all over the scalp or just at one location. Pain is felt as an electric-like jab that resolves quickly, reaches its peak intensity in less than a second, and is severe enough to make one flinch uncontrollably. Although it can happen to people without headaches in general, icepick-like pain is more common in those who have migraine or cluster headaches. Because the pain is so severe, patients frequently seek medical attention. If the pain episodes are frequent, medical intervention might be necessary. Indomethacin (25–50 mg three times a day) is effective in treating the syndrome; gabapentin (400 mg twice a day) and melatonin (3–12 mg before bed) have also been found to be beneficial.

6.4.8. Cervical Spine Disease

Occipital or orbital pain may be a result of upper neck trauma or degenerative disease processes. Irritation of the second cervical (C2) nerve root is the main cause of discomfort. Pain is referred to the ipsilateral arm or shoulder rather than the head by disk disease or abnormalities of the articular processes affecting the lower cervical spine, though cervical muscle spasms may also occur. Analgesic or anti-inflammatory medications combined with cervical immobilization (such as wearing a soft collar) are used to treat acute pain of cervical origin.

6.4.9. Sinusitis

Localized pain and tenderness in the frontal or maxillary sinuses can be a sign of acute sinusitis. A sharp pain in the midline behind the nose is caused by inflammation in the sphenoidal or ethmoidal sinuses. Bending forward and sneezing or coughing aggravate sinusitis. Tenderness and an intensification of pain are the results of percussion applied to the frontal or maxillary area.

Vasoconstrictor nose drops (e.g., phenylephrine, 0.25%, administered every two to three hours), antihistamines, and antibiotics are used to treat sinusitis. Surgical sinus drainage may be required in refractory cases. Individuals who report having a persistent "sinus" headache are much more likely to have a primary headache syndrome than recurrent sinus inflammation.

6.4.10. Dental Disease

A poorly defined syndrome known as temporomandibular joint dysfunction is typified by preauricular facial pain, restricted jaw movement, soreness in the masticatory muscles, and "clicking" of the jaw when moving. The symptoms can be caused by a spasm of the masticatory muscles and are frequently linked to malocclusion, bruxism, or clenching of the teeth. Applying heat locally, doing jaw exercises, using a bite guard at night, or taking nonsteroidal anti-inflammatory medications are beneficial for certain patients.

Pain that is characteristically constant, unilateral, and aching or burning can also result from infected tooth extraction sites. A local anesthetic injected at the extraction site relieves the symptoms, even if radiologic studies show nothing abnormal. Antibiotics and jawbone curettage are used as treatments.

A Closer Look

Tic Douloureux

Tic douloureux or trigeminal neuralgia is a severe, stabbing pain to one side of the face. It stems from one or more branches of the nerve that supply sensation to the face, the trigeminal nerve. It is considered one of the most painful conditions to affect people.

The pain usually lasts from a few seconds to a few minutes. It may be so intense that you wince involuntarily, hence the term tic. There is usually no pain or numbness between attacks and no dysfunction of the muscles of the face. Most people feel the pain in their jaw, cheek, or lip on one side of the face only. Pain is usually triggered by a light touch of the face or mouth on the same side as the pain. The pain is so severe that people can become afraid to talk, eat, or move during periods of attacks.

Although a flurry of attacks can last for weeks or months, there are usually periods of months or even years that are symptom-free. The pain of tic douloureux is usually controlled with medications or surgery. Tic douloureux is generally a disease of middle age or later life. Women are affected more often than men. People with multiple sclerosis are affected much more frequently than the general population. The cause of tic douloureux is unknown. There are several theories as to why the trigeminal nerve is affected.

The most commonly accepted theory is compression of the trigeminal nerve, usually by a blood vessel, causing it to become irritated. This irritation causes the outer covering of the nerve (the myelin sheath) to erode over time. The irritated nerve then becomes more excitable and erratically fires pain impulses.

Tumors and bony abnormalities of the skull may also press on and irritate the trigeminal nerve. In addition, trauma, infections, and multiple sclerosis can also damage the trigeminal nerve.

The main symptom of tic douloureux is a sudden, severe, stabbing, sharp, shooting, electric-shock-like pain on one side of the face. Because the second and third divisions of the trigeminal nerve are the most commonly affected, the pain is usually felt in the lower half of the face.

The pain comes in intermittent episodes that last from a few seconds to a few minutes. There may be many episodes of pain each day. There is usually no pain between episodes.

The flurry of pain episodes may last from a few weeks to a few months, followed by pain-free periods of months to even years. Generally, the episodes become more frequent and more resistant to treatment with medications over time. The attacks of pain are often initiated by physical stimulation of a trigger point on the same side of the face as the pain. Trigger points can be anywhere on the face or in the mouth or nose. They are generally not in the same place as the pain. Stimuli that can initiate the pain include talking, eating, brushing the teeth, or even cool air on the face. There is no loss of taste, hearing, or sensation in someone suffering from tic douloureux.

Summary

- The trigeminal (V) nerve carries sensation from intracranial structures in the anterior and middle fossae of the skull (above the cerebellar tentorium).
- Recurrent headaches (such as tension or migraine headaches) typically have a benign cause, even though each acute attack can be extremely incapacitating.
- Unilateral headache is an invariable feature of cluster headache and occurs in the majority of migraine attacks; most patients with tension-type headache report bilateral pain.
- Migraine headaches may become less frequent during pregnancy and are often relieved by darkness, sleep, vomiting, or applying pressure to the ipsilateral temporal artery.
- Patients experiencing an acute headache, as is frequently the case with subarachnoid hemorrhage and meningitis, may exhibit confusion during the mental status examination.
- Bleeding into the subarachnoid space that occurs spontaneously (nontraumatically) is typically caused by an AVM or a burst cerebral artery aneurysm.
- Subarachnoid hemorrhage typically manifests as a sudden, extremely severe generalized headache that the patient describes as the worst headache they have ever had.
- Subarachnoid hemorrhage is highly specific for the abrupt onset of severe headache, along with bloody spinal fluid, nuchal rigidity, absence of focal neurologic deficits, and confusion or obtundation.
- Meningitis, an infection of the meningeal covering of the brain, is diagnosed in patients who exhibit fever (77%), altered mental state (69%), new headaches (87%), and stiff necks (83%).

References

1. Backes, D., Rinkel, G. J., Kemperman, H., Linn, F. H., & Vergouwen, M. D. (2012). Time-dependent test characteristics of head computed tomography in patients suspected of nontraumatic subarachnoid hemorrhage. *Stroke, 43*, 2115–2119.
2. Bashir, A., Lipton, R. B., Ashina, S., & Ashina, M. (2013). Migraine and structural changes in the brain: A systematic review and meta-analysis. *Neurology, 81*, 1260–1268.
3. Bennetto, L., Patel, N. K., & Fuller, G. (2007). Trigeminal neuralgia and its management. *BMJ, 334*, 201–205.
4. Bezov, D., Ashina, S., & Lipton, R. B. (2010). Post-dural puncture headache: Part II. Prevention, management, and prognosis. *Headache, 50*, 1482–1498.
5. Bezov, D., Lipton, R. B., & Ashina, S. (2010). Post-dural puncture headache: Part I. Diagnosis, epidemiology, etiology, and pathophysiology. *Headache, 50*, 1144–1152.
6. Blumenfeld, A., & Nikolskaya, G. (2013). Glossopharyngeal neuralgia. *Curr. Pain. Headache Rep., 17*, 343–350.
7. Bo, S. H., Davidsen, E. M., Gulbrandsen, P., & Dietrichs, E. (2008). Acute headache: A prospective diagnostic work-up of patients admitted to a general hospital. *Eur. J. Neurol., 15*, 1293–1299.

8. Bogduk, N., & Govind, J. (2009). Cervicogenic headache: An assessment of the evidence on clinical diagnosis, invasive tests, and treatment. *Lancet Neurol., 8*, 959–968.
9. Brouwer, M. C., Tunkel, A. R., McKhann, G. M., & van de Beek, D. (2014). Brain abscess. *N. Engl. J. Med., 371*, 447–456.
10. Brown, S. C., Brew, S., & Madigan, J. (2011). Investigating suspected subarachnoid haemorrhage in adults. *BMJ, 342*, d2644.
11. Cady, R. K., Dodick, D. W., Levine, H. L., et al. (2005). Sinus headache: A neurology, otolaryngology, allergy, and primary care consensus on diagnosis and treatment. *Mayo. Clin. Proc., 80*, 908–916.
12. Danesh-Meyer, H. V., & Savino, P. J. (2007). Giant cell arteritis. *Curr. Opin. Ophthalmol., 18*, 443–449.
13. Diringer, M. N. (2009). Management of aneurysmal subarachnoid hemorrhage. *Crit. Care. Med., 37*, 432–440.
14. Dodick, D. W. (2006). Chronic daily headache. *N. Engl. J. Med., 354*, 158–165.
15. Dodick, D. W. (2004). Indomethacin-responsive headache syndromes. *Curr. Pain Headache Rep., 8*, 19–26.
16. Edlow, J. A., & Caplan, L. R. (2000). Avoiding pitfalls in the diagnosis of subarachnoid hemorrhage. *N. Engl. J. Med., 342*, 29–36.
17. Ekstein, D., & Schachter, S. C. (2010). Postictal headache. *Epilepsy Behav., 19*, 151–155.
18. Ezeonyeji, A. N., Borg, F. A., & Dasgupta, B. (2011). Delays in recognition and management of giant cell arteritis: Results from a retrospective audit. *Clin. Rheumatol., 30*, 259–262.
19. Francis, G. J., Becker, W. J., & Pringsheim, T. M. (2010). Acute and preventive pharmacologic treatment of cluster headache. *Neurology, 75*, 463–473.
20. Friedman, D. I. (2014). The pseudotumor cerebri syndrome. *Neurol. Clin., 32*, 363–396.
21. Fumal, A., & Schoenen, J. (2008). Tension-type headache: Current research and clinical management. *Lancet Neurol., 7*, 70–83.
22. Gladstone, J., & Bigal, M. E. (2010). Headaches attributable to infectious diseases. *Curr. Pain Headache Rep., 14*, 299–308.
23. Goadsby, P. J., Goldberg, J., & Silberstein, S. D. (2008). Migraine in pregnancy. *BMJ, 336*, 1502–1504.
24. Goadsby, P. J., & Sprenger, T. (2010). Current practice and future directions in the prevention and acute management of migraine. *Lancet Neurol., 9*, 285–298.
25. Johnson, R. W., & Rice, A. S. C. (2014). Postherpetic neuralgia. *N. Engl. J. Med., 371*, 1526–1533.
26. Kruit, M. C., van Buchem, M. A., Launer, L. J., Terwindt, G. M., & Ferrari, M. D. (2010). Migraine is associated with an increased risk of deep white matter lesions, subclinical posterior circulation infarcts and brain iron accumulation: The population-based MRI CAMERA study. *Cephalalgia, 30*, 129–136.
27. Loder, E., & Rizzoli, P. (2008). Tension-type headache. *BMJ, 336*, 88–92.
28. Nappi, G., & Moskowitz, M. A. (Eds.). (2011). Headache. *Handbook of Clinical Neurology, Vol 97*. Amsterdam: Elsevier.

29. Robbins, M. S., Grosberg, B. M., & Lipton, R. B. (Eds.). (2013). Headache. Chichester, UK: Wiley Blackwell.

30. Rodriguez, M. A., Kumar, S. K., & De Caro, M. (2010). Hypertensive crisis. *Cardiol. Rev., 18*, 102–107.

31. Scrivani, S. J., Keith, D. A., & Kaban, L. B. (2008). Temporomandibular disorders. *N. Engl. J. Med., 359*, 2693–2705.

32. Tentschert, S., Wimmer, R., Greisenegger, S., Lang, W., & Lalouschek, W. (2005). Headache at stroke onset in 2196 patients with ischemic stroke or transient ischemic attack. *Stroke, 36*, e1–e3.

33. Van de Beek, D., de Gans, J., Spanjaard, L., et al. (2004). Clinical features and prognostic factors in adults with bacterial meningitis. *N. Engl. J. Med., 351*, 1849–1859.

34. Van de Beek, D., de Gans, J., Tunkel, A. R., & Wijdicks, E. F. (2006). Community-acquired bacterial meningitis in adults. *N. Engl. J. Med., 354*, 44–53.

35. Worthington, I., Pringsheim, T., Gawel, M. J., et al. (2013). Canadian Headache Society Guideline: Acute drug therapy for migraine headache. *Can. J. Neurol. Sci., 40*(suppl 3), S1–S80.

36. Yeh, Y. C., Fuh, J. L., Chen, S. P., & Wang, S. J. (2010). Clinical features, imaging findings and outcomes of headache associated with sexual activity. *Cephalalgia, 30*, 1329–1335.

Chapter 7

NEURO-OPHTHALMIC DISORDERS

Contents

Introduction

The term "neuro-ophthalmologic disease" refers to a broad range of visual issues that are associated with the optic nerve, eye movements, and the visual-related brain regions. Many of these problems aren't so much related to the eyes as they are to the connections that the eyes and brain, as well as the brain and the eye muscles, make.

The optic nerve is the crucial "cable" that transmits data from the retina and eye to the brain. Numerous illnesses can have an impact on the optic nerve. In certain cases, diagnosing potentially fatal conditions and preventing irreversible vision loss depend greatly on the ability to recognize optic nerve disease.

Orientation and Directional Terms

Term	Definition	Illustration
Occipital lobes	The occipital lobes are the smallest lobes of the brain, located at the rear and under the parietal lobe, and above the temporal lobe.	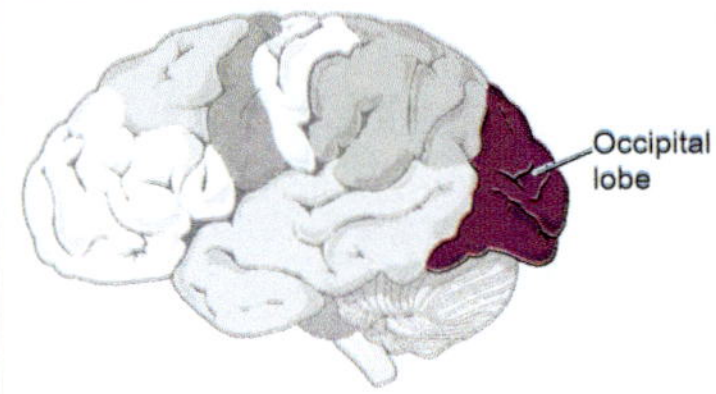
Vascular disease	Vascular disease, also known as vasculopathy, is a group of diseases that affect the body's circulatory system, including blood vessels and lymphatic vessels.	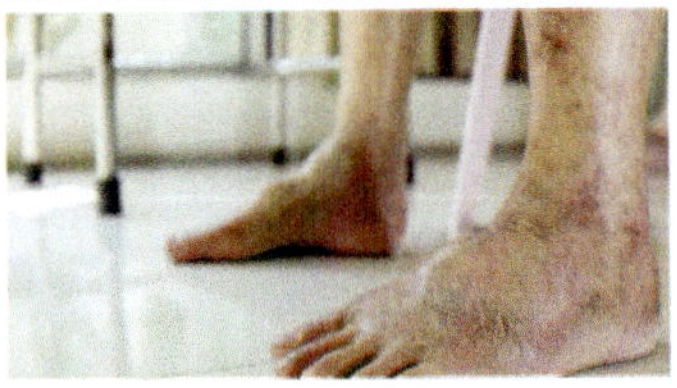
Ophthalmoplegia	Ophthalmoplegia is the paralysis or weakness of the eye muscles that control eye movement. It can affect one or more of the six muscles that hold the eye in place.	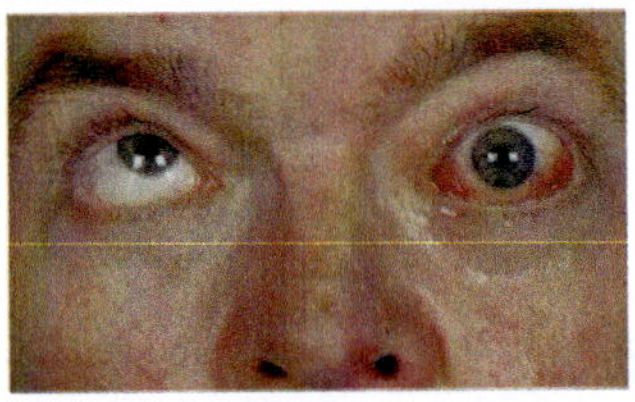
Myasthenia gravis	Myasthenia gravis (MG) is a chronic autoimmune disorder in which antibodies destroy the communication between nerves and muscle, resulting in weakness of the skeletal muscles.	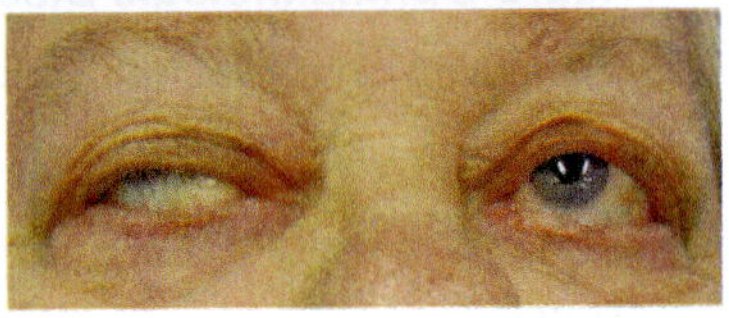
Ophthalmoscopy	Ophthalmoscopy, also known as fundoscopy, is an eye exam that allows a doctor to see the back of the eye, or fundus , and other structures using a magnifying lens and light.	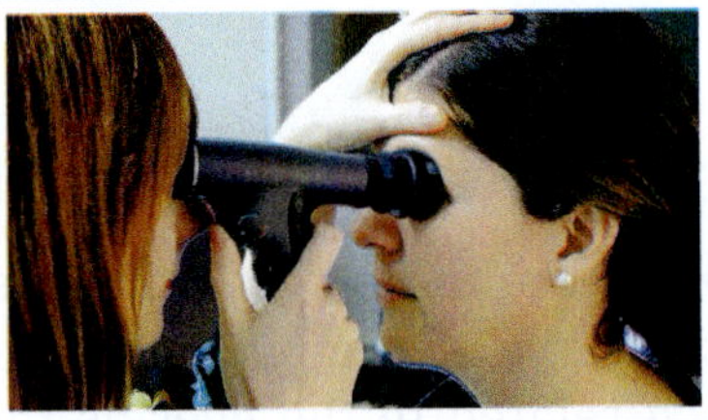

7.1. Neuro-Ophthalmologic Disease Approach to Diagnosis

A wide range of neuro-ophthalmic disturbances are caused by disorders affecting the ocular muscles, ocular motor (III, IV, and VI) cranial nerves, or visual or ocular motor pathways in the brain. The visual and ocular motor systems' anatomic pathways pass through significant areas of the cerebral hemispheres and brainstem, making neuro-ophthalmic symptoms and signs useful for locating and diagnosing neurologic diseases.

7.1.1. Functional Anatomy of the Visual Sys

- **Visual Input:** When light is focused and refracted by the lens to produce an image on the retina at the back of the eye, visual information is transferred to the nervous system (Figure 7.1). This image is inverted in both the horizontal and vertical planes due to the lens's action. As a result, the temporal (lateral) and nasal (medial) fields are inverted, and the superior part of the visual image rests on the inferior retina and vice versa (Figure 7.2). The fovea, where the retina's perceptual sensitivity is highest, is the focus of the visual field. Photoreceptor cells (rods and cones) in the retina convert incident light into neuronal impulses, which are then sent to the optic (II) nerve by retinal neurons. The topographic relations of the visual field are maintained at this level as well as all subsequent levels of the visual system.
- **Peripheral Visual Pathways:** Though the nasal (medial) fibers, which carry information from the temporal (lateral) visual fields, cross in the optic chiasm, each optic nerve carries fibers from one eye (Figure 7.2). As a result, fibers from one-half of the visual fields, not just one eye, are present in each optic tract. This arrangement causes defects in the contralateral half of both eyes' visual fields when retrochiasmal lesions occur, and vision impairments in the ipsilateral eye when prechiasmal lesions occur.
- **Central Visual Pathways:** The lateral geniculate nuclei is where the optic tracts end. From there, they synapse on neurons that project through the optic radiations to the visual association areas (areas 18 and 19) and primary visual or calcarine cortex (area 17), which are situated close to the posterior poles of the occipital lobes. The visual image is depicted in this instance as well, maintaining the topographic organization (Figure 7.3). The inferior and superior portions of the visual field—the superior and inferior retina—are represented above and below the calcarine fissure, respectively, while the central region of the field—the macula—is represented in the most posterior part of the visual cortex.
- **Vascular Supply of Visual Pathways:** The ophthalmic, middle cerebral, and posterior cerebral arteries supply the vascular supply of the visual system (Figure 7.4). Visual field defects can result from ischemia or infarction within the territory of any of these vessels.
    - **Retina:** The central retinal artery, a branch of the ophthalmic artery, which is a branch of the internal carotid artery, supplies blood to the retina. Vascular disease of the retina typically results in altitudinal (i.e., superior or inferior) visual field deficits because the central retinal artery subsequently splits into superior and inferior retinal branches.
    - **Optic Nerve:** The ophthalmic artery and its branches are the main sources of arterial blood supply to the optic nerve.

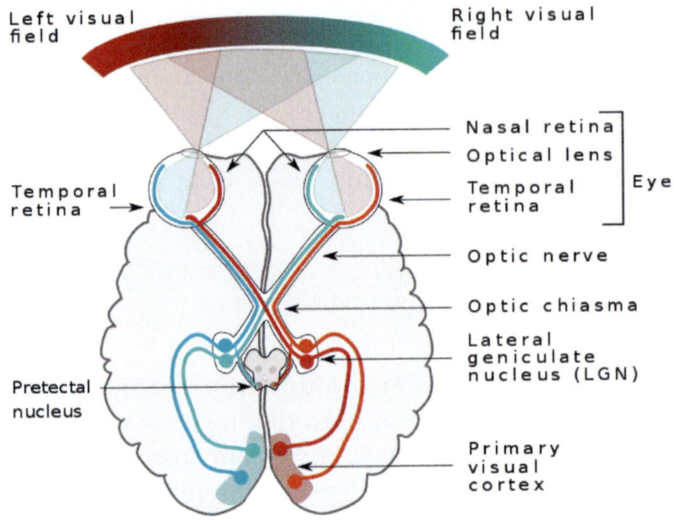

Figure 7.1. Representation of the visual field at the level of the retina. The point of fixation is focused on the fovea, the physiologic blind spot on the optic disk, the temporal half of the visual field on the nasal side of the retina, and the nasal half of the visual field on the temporal side of the retina.

Source: By <a href="//commons.wikimedia.org/wiki/User: Perellonieto" title="User: Perellonieto">Miquel Perello Nieto</a> – <span class="int-own-work" lang="en">Own work</span>, <a href="https://creativecommons.org/licenses/by-sa/4.0" title="Creative Commons Attribution-Share Alike 4.0">CC BY-SA 4.0</a>, <a href="https://commons.wikimedia.org/w/index.php?curid=37868501">Link</a>.

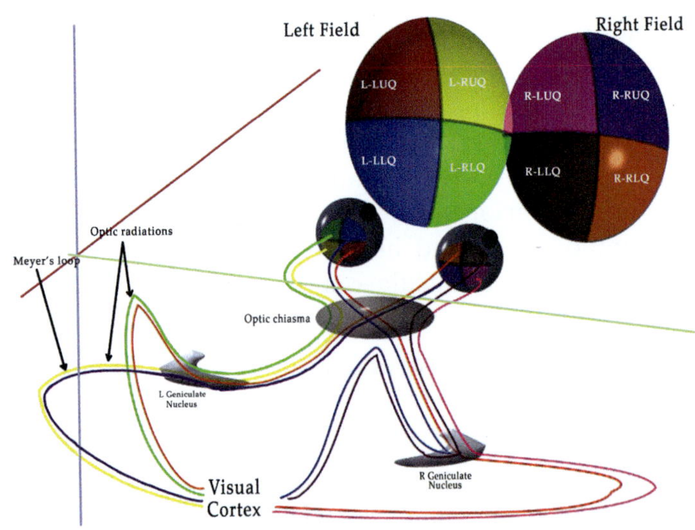

Figure 7.2. Representation of the visual field at the level of the optic nerve, chiasm, and tract. Quadrants of the visual field are designated ST (superior temporal), IT (inferior temporal), SN (superior nasal), and IN (inferior nasal).

Source: By Ratznium at en.wikipedia, CC BY 2.5, https://commons.wikimedia.org/w/index.php?curid=3199004.

- **Optic Radiations:** The optic radiations are supplied by branches of the middle cerebral artery as they travel backward toward the visual cortex. In the contralateral visual field, loss of vision may result from ischemia or infarction in the middle cerebral artery distribution.
- **Primary Visual Cortex:** The posterior cerebral artery provides the majority of the blood supply to the primary visual cortex. While the dual (middle and posterior cerebral) artery supply to the macular region of the visual cortex may preserve central (macular) vision, occlusion of one posterior cerebral artery results in blindness in the contralateral visual field. Since the basilar artery is the source of the posterior cerebral arteries, blockage at the basilar artery's tip can result in bilateral occipital infarction and total cortical blindness, though macular vision may occasionally be preserved.

7.1.2. Functional Anatomy of the Ocular Motor Sys

- **Extraocular Muscle:** Six muscles attached to each globe are responsible for movable eyes (Figure 7.5). Each of the six cardinal positions of gaze is achieved by the action of these muscles on the eye. When these six muscles are at rest, they act in an equal and opposite manner, positioning the eye in the mid- or primary position, which is to look straight ahead. Ophthalmoplegia is the inability of the eye to move in the direction of the affected extraocular muscle's action; as a result, unopposed action by other extraocular muscles may cause the eye to deviate in the opposite direction. A different area of each retina receives visual images of perceived objects when the eyes are misaligned, giving the appearance of double vision, or diplopia.
- **Cranial Nerve:** The oculomotor (III), trochlear (IV), and abducens (VI) nerves innervate the extraocular muscles. Ocular muscles have differential innervation, which makes it possible to differentiate between disorders of the ocular muscles and disorders affecting cranial nerves based on the pattern of their involvement in pathologic conditions. The cranial nerves responsible for regulating eye movement travel great distances from the brainstem to the eye, making them susceptible to damage from a range of pathological conditions.
  - **Oculomotor (III) Nerve:** The oculomotor nerve sends fibers to the levator palpebrae, which raises the eyelid, as well as the medial rectus, superior and inferior rectus, and inferior oblique muscles. Additionally, it provides the parasympathetic fibers that constrict the pupils. A complete nerve III lesion causes the pupil to be nonreactive, the eyelid to droop (ptosis), the eye to be partially abducted and unable to be raised or depressed.
  - **Trochlear (IV) nerve:** The superior oblique muscle is innervated by the trochlear nerve. Defective depression of the adducted eye is the outcome of lesions to this nerve.
  - **Abducens (VI) Nerve:** Lateral rectus palsy results from lesions to the abducens nerve, which impairs the affected eye's ability to abduct.
- **Cranial Nerve Nuclei:** The abducens (VI) nerve nucleus is situated in the pons in a similarly dorsal and periventricular position to that of the oculomotor (III) and trochlear (IV) nerve nuclei, which are situated in the dorsal midbrain, ventral to the cerebral aqueduct (of Sylvius). When these nuclei are affected by a lesion, the resulting clinical abnormalities are comparable to when the corresponding cranial nerves are involved; in certain situations, it is possible to distinguish between nuclear and nerve lesions.

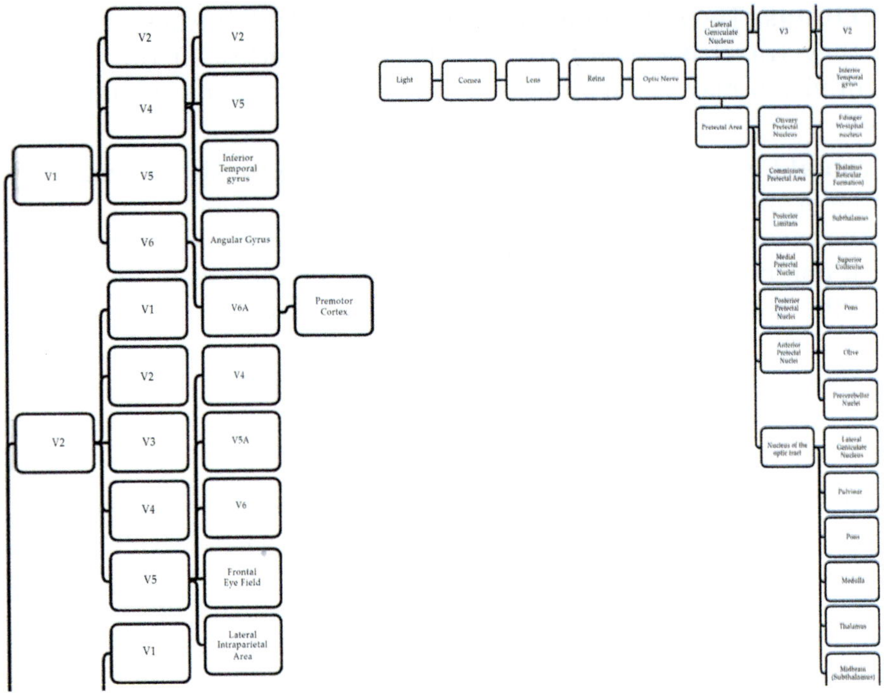

Figure 7.3. Representation of the relevant brain structures.

Source: By XenusG – Own work, CC BY-SA 4.0, https://commons.wikimedia.org/w/index.php?curid=47829942.

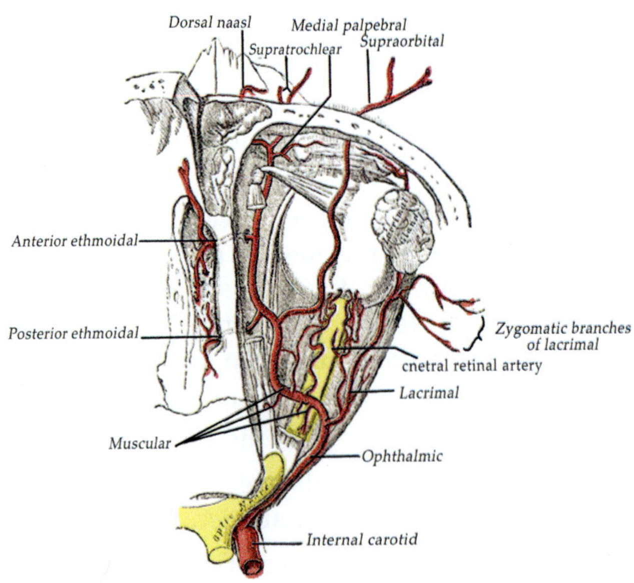

Figure 7.4. Arteries of the visual system.

Source: By Henry Vandyke Carter – Henry Gray (1918) Anatomy of the Human Body (See "Book" section below)Bartleby.com: Gray's Anatomy, Plate 514, Public Domain, https://commons.wikimedia.org/w/index.php?curid=2945440.

- o **Oculomotor (III) Nerve Nucleus**: Although each oculomotor nerve supplies muscles of the ipsilateral eye only, fibers to the superior rectus originate in the contralateral oculomotor nerve nucleus, and the levator palpebrae receives bilateral nuclear innervation. Thus ophthalmoplegia affecting only one eye with ipsilateral ptosis or superior rectus palsy suggests oculomotor nerve disease, whereas ophthalmoplegia with by bilateral ptosis or a contralateral superior rectus palsy is probably due to a nuclear lesion.
- o **Trochlear (IV) Nerve Nucleus**: It is not possible to distinguish clinically between lesions of the trochlear nerve (see earlier) and those of its nucleus.
- o **Abducens (VI) Nerve Nucleus**: In disorders affecting the abducens nerve nucleus (rather than the nerve itself), lateral rectus paresis is often associated with facial weakness, paresis of ipsilateral conjugate gaze, or a depressed level of consciousness. This is because of the proximity of the abducens nerve nucleus to the facial (VII) nerve fasciculus, pontine lateral gaze center, and ascending reticular activating system, respectively. When a Horner syndrome (miosis of the pupil, ptosis, and sometimes segmental anhidrosis) accompanies an abducens nerve palsy, the lesion is in the cavernous sinus.

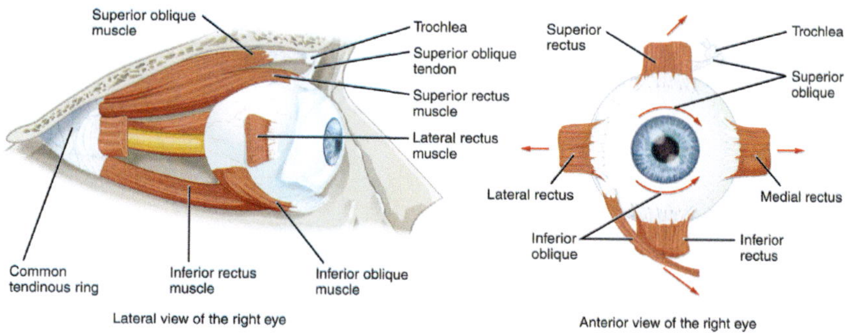

Figure 7.5. Anatomy and function of extraocular muscles. With the eye directed to the right, the superior and inferior rectus muscles can now be examined as pure elevators and depressors of the globe (right image), and with the eye deviated to the left, the oblique muscles can now be examined as pure elevators and depressors of the globe the eye is adducted by the medial rectus and abducted by the lateral rectus. The adducted eye is elevated by the inferior oblique and depressed by the superior oblique; the abducted eye is elevated by the superior rectus and depressed by the inferior rectus.

- **Supranuclear Control of Eye Movements:** The two eyes can work together to produce vergence (convergence and divergence) or version (conjugate gaze) movements thanks to supranuclear control of eye movements.
- o **Brainstem Gaze Centers:** The cerebral cortex sends descending inputs to the pons and pretectal region of the midbrain, respectively, to the centers that govern horizontal (lateral) and vertical gaze (Figure 7.6). These inputs enable voluntary control of gaze. Through its connections to the contralateral oculomotor (III) and ipsilateral abducens (VI) nerve nuclei, each lateral gaze center, situated in the paramedian pontine reticular formation (PPRF) next to the abducens nerve nucleus, mediates ipsilateral, conjugate, horizontal

gaze. Therefore, a lesion in the pons that affects the PPRF causes a gaze preference toward the side of any associated hemiparesis and away from the lesion's side, if any. A mass lesion, such as a pineal tumor (Parinaud syndrome), that applies downward pressure to the dorsal midbrain can cause disorders of vertical gaze, most commonly impaired upgaze.

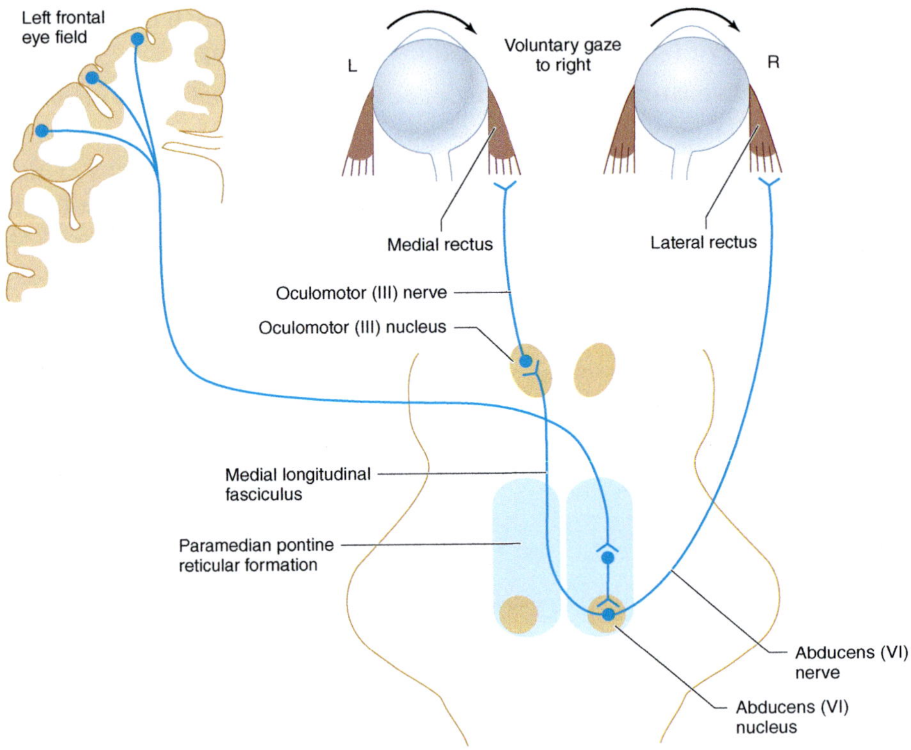

Figure 7.6. Neuronal pathways involved in horizontal gaze.

Source: https://dl.mehrsys.ir/pdf-books/Clinical%20Neurology%209%20Edition%20(www.myuptodate.com).pdf.

- o **Cortical Input:** The ipsilateral parietooccipital lobe, which controls slow eye movements (pursuits), and the contralateral frontal lobe, which controls rapid eye movements (saccades), both provide cortical input to the PPRF. Thus, a frontal cortex-related destructive lesion disrupts the contralateral horizontal gaze mechanism and may lead to a preference for looking to the lesion's side (and away from the side of associated hemiparesis). On the other hand, gaze may shift away from the side of a frontal lobe focus that is irritative (seizure-related).

7.1.3. History

- **Nature of Complaint:** Getting a detailed description of the complaint is the first step. Patients may only report nebulous symptoms, like blurred vision, which don't really tell us much about the condition. As a result, it's critical to ascertain whether the patient is referring to diplopia, an unstable visual image, decreased visual acuity in one or both eyes, loss of vision in a portion of the visual field, pain in or around the eye, or another issue.

- **Temporal Pattern of Symptom:** After determining the complaint's nature, questions about its temporal pattern can reveal information about the underlying pathologic process.
  - **Sudden Onset:** Vascular disorders that affect the eye or its connections in the brain tend to produce symptoms of sudden onset.
  - **Slow Onset:** With inflammatory or neoplastic disease, symptoms usually evolve over a longer period.
  - **Transient, Recurrent Symptoms**: Transient and recurrent symptoms suggest a select group of pathologic processes, including intermittent ischemia, multiple sclerosis, and myasthenia gravis.
- **Associated Neurologic Abnormalities:** Localizing the site of involvement can be aided by the characteristics of any concomitant neurologic abnormalities, such as weakness, aphasia, impaired facial sensation, or ataxia.
- **Medical History:** Carefully examining the patient's past should reveal any conditions that may have predisposed them to neuro-ophthalmic issues.
  - Multiple sclerosis often involves the optic nerve or brainstem, leading to a variety of neuro-ophthalmic disorders. A history of disturbances that also involve other parts of the central nervous system should suggest this diagnosis.
  - Atherosclerosis, hypertension, and diabetes can be complicated by vascular disorders of the eye, cranial nerves, or visual or ocular motor pathways in the brain.
  - Endocrine disorders (e.g., hyperthyroidism) can cause ocular myopathy.
  - Connective tissue disease and systemic cancer can affect the visual and ocular motor systems at a variety of sites in the brain or subarachnoid space.
  - Nutritional deficiencies may present with neuro-ophthalmic symptoms, as in the amblyopia (decreased visual acuity) associated with malnutrition and the ophthalmoplegia of Wernicke encephalopathy (thiamine deficiency).
  - Drugs (e.g., ethambutol, isoniazid, digitalis, clioquinol) may be toxic to the visual system, and others (sedative drugs, anticonvulsants) commonly produce ocular motor disorders.

7.1.4. Neuro-Ophthalmic Examination

7.1.4.1. Visual Acuity

- **Assessment:** Refractive errors should be removed from vision tests in order to detect neuro-ophthalmic issues. As a result, patients should be evaluated while wearing their glasses (if the customary corrective lenses are not available at the time of testing, a pinhole can be used in their place). Each eye's visual acuity needs to be evaluated independently. The patient is placed 6 meters (20 feet) away from a Snellen eye chart to test their distant vision. A Rosenbaum pocket eye chart is used to test near vision, and it is held about 36 cm (14 in) away from the patient. The smallest legible line of print in each instance is noted.
- **Recording:** A fraction is used to express visual acuity, such as 20/20, 20/40, or 20/200.

The distance (in feet) at which the examination is conducted in relation to the test figures is the numerator, and the distance (in feet) at which people with normal vision can correctly identify figures of a given size is the denominator. The visual acuity is recorded as 20/40, for instance, if a patient standing 20 feet away from the eye chart is unable to identify figures that are typically visible from that distance but can identify the larger figures that would be visible 40 feet away with normal acuity. Acuity may be recorded as 20/40–1, for example, meaning that all but one letter on the 20/40 line were correctly identified if the patient can read most of a line but makes some mistakes. When a patient's visual acuity is significantly diminished, it can still be measured, albeit with less accuracy, by how far they can count fingers (CF), recognize hand movements (HM), or perceive light. No light perception (NLP) will be found during the examination if an eye is completely blind.

- **Red–Green Color Vision:** Color vision plates or colored pens or hatpins can be used to test red-green color vision, which is frequently disproportionately impaired in optic nerve lesions.

7.1.4.2. Visual Fields

If done aimlessly, evaluating the visual fields can be a drawn-out and difficult process. Understanding the most prevalent kinds of visual field impairments is crucial for testing to proceed fairly quickly and produce meaningful results. Figure 7.7 shows the most prevalent abnormalities of the visual field.

- **Extent of Visual Fields:** An angle of roughly 160 degrees in the horizontal plane and 135 degrees in the vertical plane is subtended by the normal monocular visual field. The horizontal field of vision when using binoculars is greater than 180 degrees.
- **Physiologic Blind Spot:** There is a 5-degree blind area in each eye's normal field of vision, which corresponds to the optic disk's absence of receptor cells. The blind spot in each eye is situated 15 degrees temporally from fixation.
- **Measurement Techniques:** Like visual acuity, the visual field must be examined separately for each eye.

o For visual field testing, confrontation (Figure 7.8) is the most straightforward approach. Both the patient's and the examiner's eyes are in the same horizontal plane as they stand approximately an arm's length apart. The patient wears an eye patch or covers the eye that isn't being tested. The patient is told to focus on the examiner's open eye while the examiner closes the eye across from the covered one. The examiner's and patient's monocular fields are now superimposed, enabling a comparison between the patient's field and the examiner's likely normal field. The examiner locates the patient's field of view by using the index fingers of both hands, slowly moving them in all directions inward from the periphery until the patient recognizes them. Then, by identifying the furthest peripheral sites at which the patient can detect minute movements of the fingertips or the white head of a pin, the boundaries are precisely defined. A pin with a white head as the target can be used to compare the sizes of the patient's and examiner's blind spots, which can be found in the same area. After that, the process is carried out for the other eye.

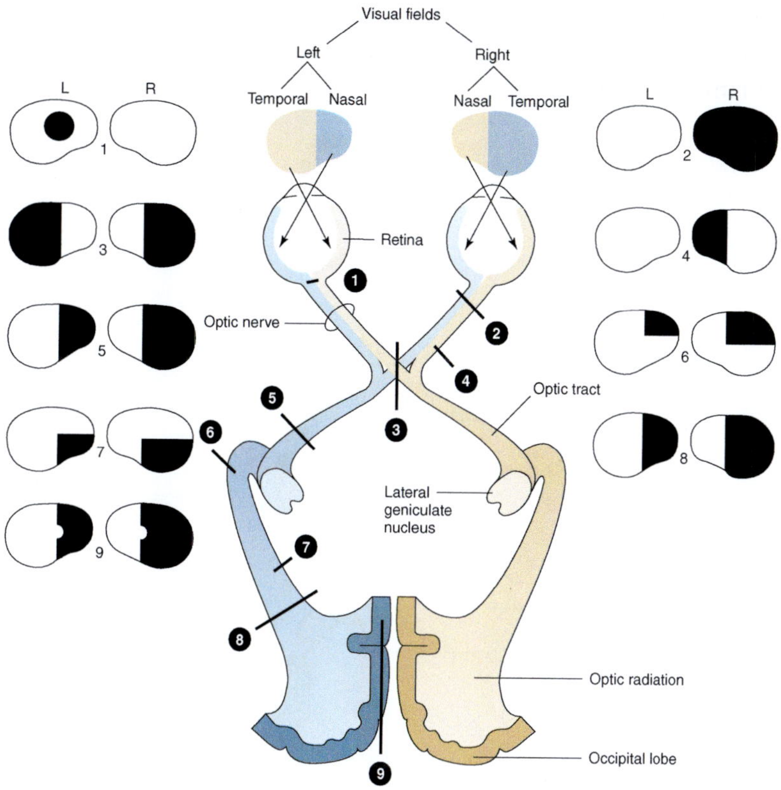

Figure 7.7. Common visual field defects and their anatomic bases. 1. Central scotoma caused by inflammation of the optic disk (optic neuritis) or optic nerve (retrobulbar neuritis). 2. Total blindness of the right eye from a complete lesion of the right optic nerve. 3. Bitemporal hemianopia caused by pressure exerted on the optic chiasm by a pituitary tumor. 4. Right nasal hemianopia caused by a perichiasmal lesion (e.g., calcified internal carotid artery). 5. Right homonymous hemianopia from a lesion of the left optic tract. 6. Right homonymous superior quadrantanopia caused by partial involvement of the optic radiation by a lesion in the left temporal lobe (Meyer loop). 7. Right homonymous inferior quadrantanopia caused by partial involvement of the optic radiation by a lesion in the left parietal lobe. 8. Right homonymous hemianopia from a complete lesion of the left optic radiation. (A similar defect may also result from lesion 9.) 9. Right homonymous hemianopia (with macular sparing) resulting from posterior cerebral artery occlusion.

Source: By As eo, , https://commons.wikimedia.org/w/index.php?curid=91096349.

- o A pin with a red head used as the target can be used to measure the fields or ask the patient to compare the brightness of colored objects presented at various locations in the field to identify subtle field defects.
- o In young children, the fields may be assessed by standing behind the child and bringing an attention-getting object, such as a toy, forward around the child's head in various directions until it is first noticed.
- o A gross indication of visual field abnormalities may be obtained in obtunded patients by determining whether they blink in response to a visual threat—typically the examiner's finger—brought toward the patient's eye in various regions of the field.

- Although many visual field deficits are detectable by these screening procedures, more precise mapping of the fields requires the use of standard tangent screen testing or automated perimetry techniques.

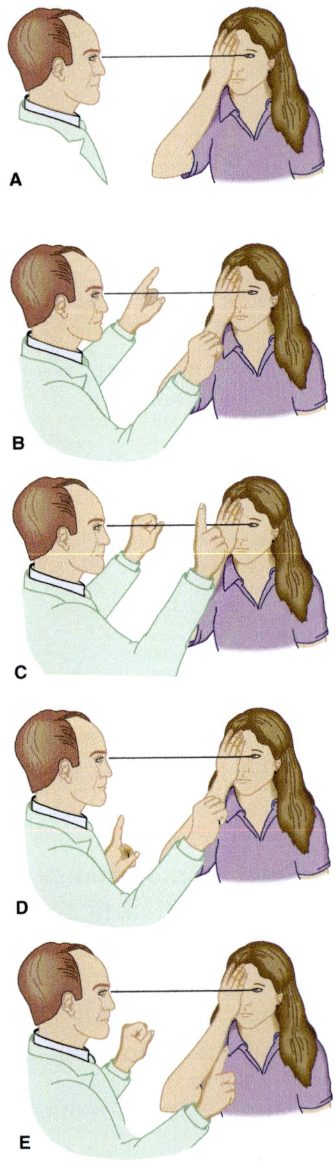

Figure7.8. Confrontation testing of the visual field. (A) The left eye of the patient and the right eye of the examiner are aligned. (B) Testing the superior nasal quadrant. (C) Testing the superior temporal quadrant. (D) Testing the inferior nasal quadrant. (E) Testing the inferior temporal quadrant. The procedure is then repeated for the patient's other eye.

Source: https://dl.mehrsys.ir/pdf-books/Clinical%20Neurology%209%20Edition%20(www.myuptodate.com).pdf.

7.1.4.3. Ophthalmoscopy

Examining patients who may have an increase in intracranial pressure and assessing conditions affecting the retina or optic disk call for the use of an ophthalmoscopy of the optic fundus.

1. **Preparation of the Patient:** Pupils should be dilated for the examination in a dark room; some patients may require the use of mydriatic (sympathomimetic or anticholinergic) eye drops. In the latter instance, before administering the drops, visual acuity and pupillary reflexes should be evaluated. In patients with untreated closed-angle glaucoma and in circumstances where pupillary reactivity plays a crucial role in management—such as a transtentorial herniation that is about to occur or is already occurring—mydriatic agents should be avoided.
2. **Examination of the Fundus:** To recognize abnormalities, one must be familiar with the optic fundus's typical appearance.

i. Optic Disk

- **Normal Appearance**: The optic disk is typically easily identified as a slightly oval, yellowish structure located nasally at the posterior pole of the eye. The disk's temporal side is frequently paler than its nasal side. The nasal and temporal disk margins should be clearly defined, although the nasal edge is often less so. The disk and surrounding retinal tissue normally lie in the same plane. The distinct and pulsating blood vessels that cross the border of the optic disk become obscured when the disk swells.
- **Optic Disk Swelling**: It is important to distinguish between swelling resulting from papilledema-caused optic nerve swelling and swelling resulting from other conditions like ischemic optic neuropathy and localized inflammation (papillitis). Except for the blind spot's enlargement, papailledema is almost always bilateral and does not usually cause eye pain. Disk anomalies like drusen (colloid or hyaline bodies) can mimic papilledema.

  It is believed that papilledema is caused by elevated intracranial pressure, which obstructs axonal transport in the optic nerve. Disorders associated with increased intracranial pressure that also obstruct the subarachnoid space, like meningitis, are less likely to cause papilledema because the subarachnoid space and the optic nerve sheath communicate. The ophthalmoscopic changes associated with papilledema usually take days or weeks to manifest, but they can also show up in a matter of hours following an abrupt spike in intracranial pressure, such as that which occurs following an intracranial hemorrhage. The retinal veins appear enlarged and spontaneous venous pulsations are absent in the early stages of papilledema. There could be linear hemorrhages at the disk's edges and a hyperemic disk.

The disk margins become hazy, starting from the temporal edge and progressing to the other. The optic disk is raised above the retinal plane in fully developed papilledema, and blood vessels that cross the disk's border are hidden.

- **Optic Disk Pallor:** A wide range of disorders affecting the optic nerve, such as inflammatory conditions, nutritional deficiencies, and degenerative diseases, are linked to optic disk pallor accompanied by impaired visual acuity, visual field defects, or loss of pupillary reactivity. A congenital variant of a pale optic disk with normal visual function can also occur, and if a cataract has been removed, the optic disk may appear artificially pale.

ii. **Arteries and Veins:** When the retinal arteries and veins emerge from the disk and cross its borders to reach the retina, their quality should be noted. The presence of spontaneous venous pulsations, which signify normal intracranial pressure, and whether these vessels are readily visible throughout their course are noteworthy features. Examining the remaining portion of the visible retina, any hemorrhages, exudates, or other anomalies are noted.

iii. **Macula:** Approximately two disk diameters temporal to the optic disk's temporal margin is the macula, an area of the retina that is somewhat paler than the rest of the retina. The patient can be quickly made to see it by having them look at the ophthalmoscope's light. Macular holes, age-related macular degeneration, and hereditary cerebromacular degenerations are among the conditions for which ophthalmoscopic examination of the macula can identify abnormalities related to visual loss.

7.1.4.4. Pupils

1. **Size:** The integrity of the neural pathways connecting the optic nerve to the midbrain is reflected in the size and reactivity of the pupils (Figure 7.9). The size of the typical pupil, which is spherical, regular, and centered within the iris, changes with age and with the amount of surrounding light. The diameter of normal pupils in an illuminated room is approximately 3 mm for adults, less than or equal to 5 mm for children, and smaller for the elderly. Up to 20% of individuals may have asymmetric pupil size (physiologic anisocoria), but the difference is always less than or equal to 1 mm. In bright light, symmetrically fast pupil constriction rules out oculomotor (III) nerve compression and indicates normal pupillary function.
2. **Reaction to Light:** The integrity of the pathways depicted in Figure 7.9 is demonstrated by direct (ipsilateral) and consensual (contralateral) pupillary constriction

in response to a bright light shining in one eye. Generally speaking, the consensual response to light is less pronounced and slightly brisker than the direct response.

3. **Reaction to Accommodation:** Normally, the pupils contract when the eyes converge to focus on a closer object or accommodation. The patient is asked to alternately focus on a finger held directly in front of their nose and a faraway object to test their response.

4. Pupillary Abnormalities

   i. **Nonreactive Pupils:** Unilateral disorders of pupillary constriction include optic nerve disorders (optic neuritis, multiple sclerosis), mydriatic agent administration, oculomotor (III) nerve compression (tumor, aneurysm), and local diseases of the iris (trauma, iritis, glaucoma).

   ii. **Light-Near Dissociation:** Light-near dissociation, or impaired pupillary reactivity to light with preserved constriction during accommodation, is typically bilateral and can be caused by tumors compressing the midbrain tectum, neurosyphilis, diabetes, and optic nerve disorders.

   iii. **Argyll Robertson Pupils:** These pupils exhibit light-near dissociation; they are small, poorly responsive to light, frequently irregular in shape, and frequently unequal in size. The traditional cause is neurosyphilis, but other lesions (like multiple sclerosis) in the vicinity of the Edinger-Westphal nucleus are becoming more prevalent (Table 7.1).

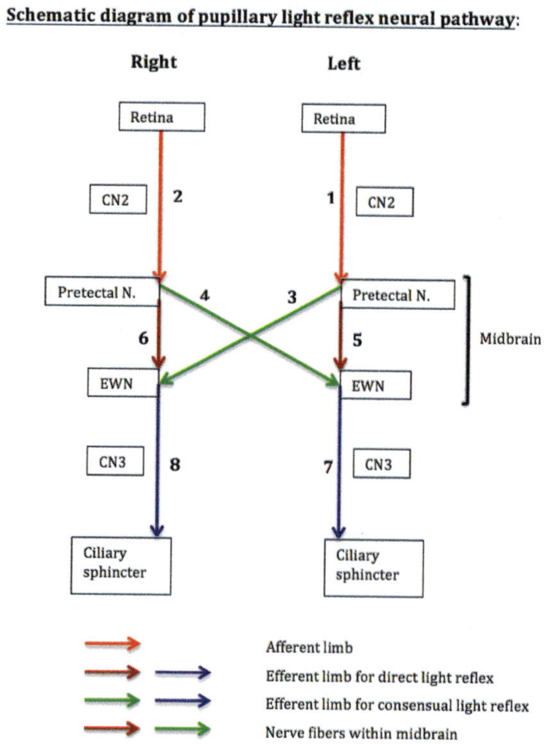

Figure 7.9. Anatomic basis of the pupillary light reflex. The afferent visual pathways from the retina to the pretectal nuclei of the midbrain are represented by dashed lines and the efferent pupilloconstrictor pathways from the midbrain to the pupillary constrictor muscles by solid lines. Note that illumination of one eye results in bilateral pupillary constriction.

Source: By Angusng – Own work, CC BY-SA 4.0, https://commons.wikimedia.org/w/index.php?curid=49805996.

   iv. **Tonic Pupil:** Larger than the unaffected contralateral pupil, the tonic (Adie) pupil (Table 7.1) responds slowly to changes in both illumination and accommodation.

Anisocoria becomes less noticeable during the exam because the tonic pupil does eventually react. Holmes-Adie syndrome, a benign, frequently familial disorder that commonly affects young women, is most commonly responsible for this abnormality. It may also be linked to depressed deep tendon reflexes (particularly in the legs), segmental anhidrosis (localized lack of sweating), orthostatic hypotension, or cardiovascular autonomic instability. Bilateral Adie pupils are possible. Degeneration of the ciliary ganglion and abnormal reinnervation of the pupilloconstrictor muscles may be the cause of the pupillary abnormality.

Table 7.1. Common Pupillary Abnormalities

	Appearance	Response	Differential Diagnosis
Tonic (Adie) pupil	Unilateral (rarely bilateral) dilated pupil	Reacts sluggishly and only to persistent bright light or 0.125% pilocarpine eye drops; accommodation less affected	Holmes-Adie syndrome, ocular trauma, autonomic neuropathy
Horner syndrome	Unilateral small pupil and slight ptosis	Normal response to light and accommodation	Lateral medullary infarcts, cervical cord lesions, pulmonary apical or mediastinal tumors, neck trauma or masses, carotid artery dissection or thrombosis, intrapartum brachial plexus injury, cluster headache
Argyll Robertson pupil	Unequal irregular pupils <3 mm in diameter (usually bilateral)	Poorly reactive to light; more responsive to accommodation	Neurosyphilis; mimicked by diabetes, pineal region tumors, multiple sclerosis

Source: https://dl.mehrsys.ir/pdf-books/Clinical%20Neurology%209%20Edition%20(www.myuptodate.com).pdf.

Table 7.2. Causes of Horner Syndrome

Central (first) neuron Brainstem infarction* Hypothalamic region tumor, hemorrhage or infarction Multiple sclerosis Syrinx Transverse myelopathy	28%
Preganglionic (second) neuron Thoracic or neck tumor (Pancoast tumor, schwannoma, neuroblastoma, thyroid) Trauma or surgery (neck, thorax) Vascular (jugular ectasia, subclavian artery aneurysm)	44%
Postganglionic (third) neuron Base of skull, parasellar, orbital, or cavernous sinus* mass Vascular (fibromuscular dysplasia, carotid dissection*) Cluster headache	28%
Unknown cause	15%

Source: Percentages from from Almog Y, Gepstein R, Kesler A. Diagnostic value of imaging in Horner syndrome in adults. J Neuro-Ophthalmol. 2010;30:7–11. Etiologies from Reede D, Garcon E, Smoker

WRK, Kardon R. Horner's syndrome: clinical and radiographic evaluation. Neuroimag Clin N Am, 2008;18:369–385. (*) Most common.

v. **Horner Syndrome:** Horner syndrome (Tables 7.1 and 7.2) is characterized by a small (miotic) pupil along with mild ptosis (Figure 7.10) and occasionally a loss of sweating (anhidrosis) due to a lesion of the central or peripheral sympathetic nervous system.

a. **Oculosympathetic Pathways**: An uncrossed three-neuron arc makes up the sympathetic pathway that regulates pupillary dilation: postganglionic sympathetic neurons originate in the superior cervical ganglion, ascend in the neck along the internal carotid artery, and enter the orbit with the first (ophthalmic) division of the trigeminal (V) nerve; preganglionic sympathetic neurons project from the spinal cord to the superior cervical ganglion; and hypothalamic neurons, which descend through the brainstem to the intermediolateral column of the spinal cord at the T1 level. Any disruption of these pathways can result in Horner syndrome.

b. **Clinical Features:** Usually, only one pupillary abnormality results from the lesions. In comparison to the normal side, the involved side's pupil diameter is usually reduced by 0.5 to 1 mm. In low light, this disparity is most noticeable. As opposed to the marked ptosis seen with oculomotor nerve lesions, the pupillary abnormality is accompanied by mild to moderate upper lid ptosis (see below), which is frequently linked to elevation of the lower lid (lower lid ptosis). If a person has Horner syndrome from birth, their ipsilateral iris will be lighter and bluer (heterochromia iridis).

Localizing the lesion can be aided by deficiencies in the pattern of sweating, which are most noticeable in acute-onset Horner syndrome. If there is less perspiration on the face and on the whole body, there is a central nervous system lesion. Anhidrosis solely of the face, neck, and arm is caused by cervical lesions. If the lesion is above the carotid artery bifurcation, breathing is unaffected. Table 7.2 presents the differential diagnosis for Horner syndrome.

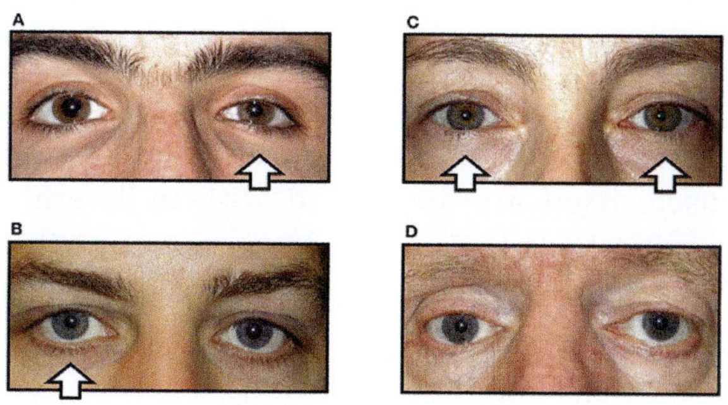

Figure 7.10. (A) Horner syndrome. Athree-neuron pathway projects from the hypothalamus to the intermediolateral column of the spinal cord, then to the superior cervical (sympathetic) ganglion, and finally to the pupil, smooth muscle of the eyelid, and sweat glands of the forehead and face.

Source: Bremner F (2019) Apraclonidine Is Better Than Cocaine for Detection of Horner Syndrome. Front. Neurol. 10:55. doi: 10.3389/fneur.2019.00055.

vi. **Relative Afferent Pupillary Defect (Marcus Gunn Pupil):** In contrast to the contralateral pupil, the involved pupil contracts less noticeably in response to direct illumination, although typically the direct response is larger than the consensual response. The suspected pupil is continuously observed while a bright flashlight is quickly moved back and forth between the eyes to identify any abnormalities (Gunn pupillary test). Disorders of the ipsilateral optic nerve, which interrupt the afferent limb and impact the pupillary light reflex, are frequently linked to relative afferent pupillary defect (Figure 7.9). The affected eye's vision, particularly color vision, is frequently affected by these conditions.

7.1.4.5. Optokinetic Response

Eye movements caused by a patient's sequential fixation on a series of targets that are passing in front of their eyes, like telephone poles seen from a moving train, are known as optokinetic nystagmus. These movements are produced for clinical testing by moving a vertically striped strip of cloth or a revolving drum across the visual field. When something is being tested, there is a slow following phase in the target's direction and a quick return jerk in the opposite direction. Parietooccipital function is tested during the slow (pursuit) phase, and frontal lobe function in the hemisphere that the stimulus is moved toward is tested during the rapid (saccadic) movement. The ability to detect movement or contour is reflected by the presence of an optokinetic response, which can help record visual perception in neonates or in cases of psychogenic blindness. The optokinetic response can be produced with very little visual acuity (20/400, or finger counting at 3 to 5 feet). When targets are shifted in the direction of a parietal lobe lesion, unilateral impairment of the optokinetic response may be observed.

7.1.4.6. Eyelid

The patient should be examined with their eyes open to examine the palpebrae, or eyelids. Although there can occasionally be physiologic asymmetries, the interpalpebral fissure—the space between the upper and lower lids—is normally equal in both eyes and measures around 10 mm. To identify abnormal elevation of the eyelid (lid retraction) or drooping (ptosis), one should record the position of the inferior margin of the upper lid in relation to the superior border of the iris. Normally, 1 to 2 mm of the iris is covered by the upper lid.

Horner syndrome, lesions of the oculomotor (III) nerve or its superior branch, and paralysis of the levator palpebrae muscle itself are associated with unilateral ptosis. Ptosis in the latter condition is usually accompanied by miosis and can be temporarily corrected with forced eye opening.

A condition affecting the neuromuscular junction (such as myasthenia gravis), the muscle (such as myotonic, ocular, or oculopharyngeal dystrophy), or the oculomotor (III) nerve nucleus is suggested by bilateral ptosis.

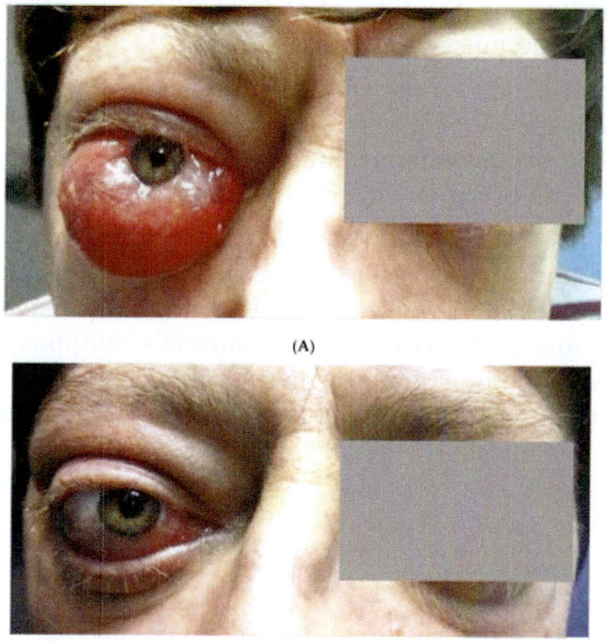

Figure 7.11. Patient included in this series with severe and refractory Graves' orbitopathy at (A) Tocilizumab onset and (B) after five months of Tocilizumab therapy. (Courtesy of Dr. Torre-Salaberri, Basurto Hospital, Bilbao).

Source: Sánchez-Bilbao L, Martínez-López D, Revenga M, López-Vázquez Á, Valls-Pascual E, Atienza-Mateo B, Valls-Espinosa B, Maiz-Alonso O, Blanco A, Torre-Salaberri I, et al. Anti-IL-6 Receptor Tocilizumab in Refractory Graves' Orbitopathy: National Multicenter Observational Study of 48 Patients. *Journal of Clinical Medicine.* 2020; 9(9):2816. https://doi.org/10.3390/jcm9092816.

An abnormal elevation of the upper lid, or lid retraction, is observed in hyperthyroidism and Parinaud syndrome, which are conditions caused by tumors in the pineal region.

7.1.4.7. Exophthalmos

The best way to identify an abnormal protrusion of the eye from the orbit (exophthalmos or proptosis) in a seated patient is to stand behind them and look down at their eyes from above. Causes include orbital tumor or pseudotumor, carotid artery–cavernous sinus fistula, and hyperthyroidism (Graves disease, Figure 7.11). Patients with carotid artery–cavernous sinus fistula or other vascular anomalies may hear a bruit when auscultating over the proptotic eye.

7.1.4.8. Eye Movements

1. **Ocular Excursion and Gaze:** Examining the patient in each of the six cardinal positions will reveal ocular palsies and gaze palsies (Figure 7.5). Reflex eye movements can be induced by doll's head (oculocephalic) or cold-water caloric (oculovestibular) testing if the patient is unable to cooperate with the examination or has impaired voluntary eye movement. If there are any

movement limitations, the type of abnormality is identified using the following scheme, noting the muscles that are affected.

i. **Ocular Palsy:** Nuclear or infranuclear (nerve, neuromuscular junction, or muscle) lesions cause weakness of one or more eye muscles. It is not possible to overcome an ocular palsy by stimulating reflex eye movement with calories. Different patterns of ocular muscle involvement are produced by nerve lesions.

a. **Oculomotor (III) Nerve Palsy:** When the oculomotor nerve is completely damaged, the impacted eye closes due to decreased levator function. The affected eye is laterally deviated when the paralyzed lid is passively raised (Figure 7.12). This is due to the lateral rectus muscle's unopposed action, which is not innervated by the oculomotor nerve. All gaze directions exhibit diplopia, except for lateral gaze toward the side of involvement. Pupil function might be compromised or normal (pupillary sparing).

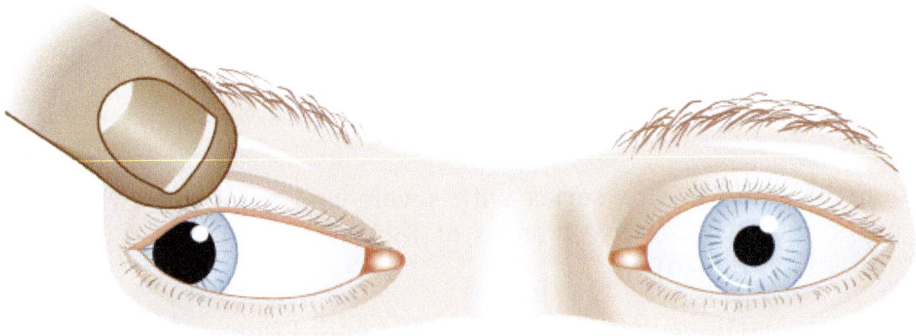

Figure 7.12. Clinical findings with oculomotor (III) nerve lesion. With the ptotic lid passively elevated, the affected (right) eye is abducted; it cannot adduct. On attempted downgaze, the unaffected superior oblique muscle, which is innervated by the trochlear (IV) nerve, causes the eye to turn inward.

Source: https://dl.mehrsys.ir/pdf-books/Clinical%20Neurology%209%20Edition%20(www.myuptodate.com).pdf.

b. **Trochlear (IV) Nerve Palsy:** When the superior oblique muscle is paralyzed by trochlear nerve lesions, the affected eye is elevated during primary (forward) gaze; the degree of elevation rises during adduction and falls during abduction. According to the Bielschowsky head-tilt test (Figure 7.13), elevation is greatest when the head is tilted toward the side of the affected eye and is eliminated by tilting in the opposite direction. When a patient looks down with the affected eye adducted or looks at the tip of their nose, the symptoms of diplopia are most noticeable. Of patients with unilateral palsies, about half have spontaneous head tilting, and a higher proportion have bilateral palsies. This behavior is meant to lessen or correct the diplopia.

c. **Abducens (VI) Nerve Palsy:** A lesion to the abducens nerve paralyzes the lateral rectus muscle, which leads to adduction of the affected eye during rest and unsuccessful abduction attempts (Figure 7.14). Diplopia manifests as a lateral gaze to the affected eye's side.

ii. **Gaze Palsy:** Caused by supranuclear lesions in the cerebral hemisphere or brainstem, gaze palsy is the reduced ability of a pair of yoked muscles (muscles that work together to move the two eyes in a specific direction) to move the eyes in voluntary gaze. In contrast to ocular palsies, gaze palsy typically affects both eyes and is treated with calorie stimulation. The pathophysiology and causes of binocular disorders of eye movement are covered in more detail in the section that follows. Mild impairment of upgaze in healthy elderly subjects is not unusual.

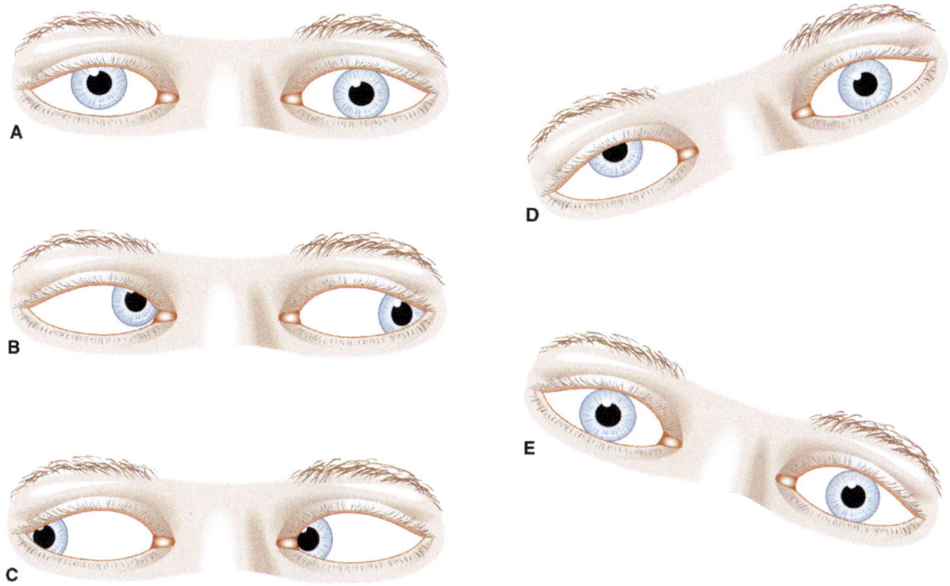

Figure 7.13. Clinical findings with trochlear (IV) nerve lesion. The affected (right) eye is elevated on forward gaze (A). The extent of elevation is increased with adduction (B) and decreased with abduction (C). Elevation increases with head tilting to the affected side (D) and decreases with head tilting in the opposite direction (E).

Source: https://dl.mehrsys.ir/pdf-books/Clinical%20Neurology%209%20Edition%20(www.myuptodate.com).pdf.

iii. **Internuclear Ophthalmoplegia:** A lesion of the medial longitudinal fasciculus, an ascending pathway in the brainstem that projects from the abducens (VI) to the contralateral oculomotor (III) nerve nucleus, causes internuclear ophthalmoplegia (INO) (Figure 7.6). The actions of the oculomotor (III) and abducens (VI) nerves during voluntary gaze or caloric-induced movement are uncoupled as a result of INO. The contralateral eye's adduction is impeded, but the excursion of the abducting eye is complete (Figure 7.15). The preserved adduction with convergence of INO sets it apart from oculomotor (III) nerve palsy, but it cannot be overcome by caloric stimulation. Usually, a brainstem stroke or multiple sclerosis is the cause.

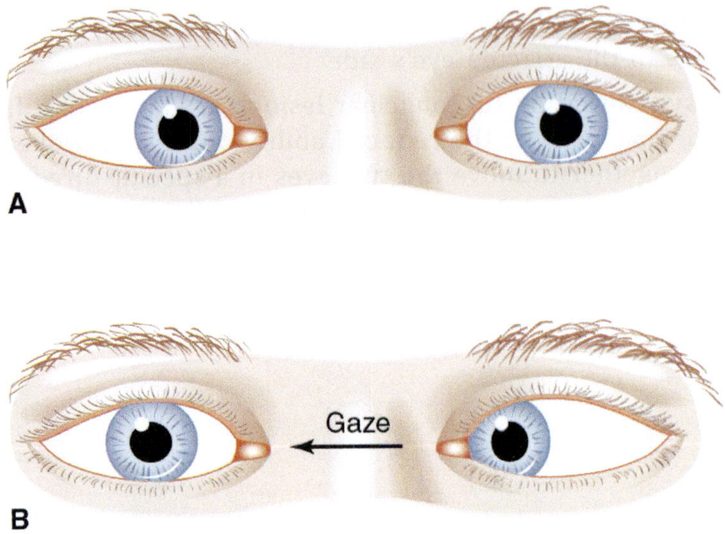

Figure 7.14. Clinical findings with abducens (VI) nerve lesion. The affected (right) eye is adducted at rest (A) and cannot be abducted (B).

Source: https://dl.mehrsys.ir/pdf-books/Clinical%20Neurology%209%20Edition%20(www.myuptodate.com).pdf.

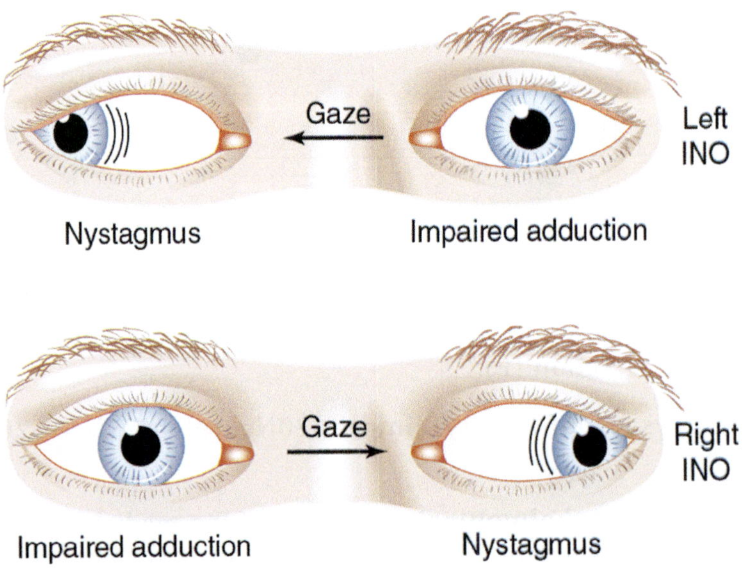

Figure 7.15. Eye movements in internuclear ophthalmoplegia (INO) resulting from a bilateral lesion of the medial longitudinal fasciculus.

Source: https://dl.mehrsys.ir/pdf-books/Clinical%20Neurology%209%20Edition%20(www.myuptodate.com).pdf.

iv. **One-and-a-Half Syndrome:** A syndrome that combines internuclear ophthalmoplegia with the incapacity to gaze sideways is caused by a pontine lesion that affects both the medial longitudinal fasciculus and the ipsilateral paramedian pontine reticular formation (lateral gaze center) (Figure 7.16). The contralateral eye can only move in abduction, which may be connected to nystagmus, while the ipsilateral eye remains motionless in the horizontal plane. Pontine hemorrhage, multiple sclerosis, and pontine infarct are among the causes.

2. **Diplopia Testing:** Examining the patient's eye movements should be done to ascertain the anatomical cause of double vision, or diplopia. In each of the six cardinal positions of gaze, the patient is instructed to fix their gaze on an object, like a flashlight (Figure 7.5). The flashlight's light falls at the same location on both corneas during normal conjugate gaze; a lack of this congruency indicates that the gaze is disconjugate. Each eye should be covered in turn when the patient reports diplopia in a particular direction of vision, and they should be asked to report which of the two images vanishes. Since it will never land on the fovea, the image that is displaced further in the direction of gaze is always referable to the weak eye. The red glass test is a variation on this process where one eye is covered with translucent red glass, plastic, or cellophane, making it possible to identify which eye produced each image.
3. **Nystagmus:** Nystagmus is a repetitive back-and-forth movement of the eyes. Pendular nystagmus, often starting in infancy, moves at the same speed in both directions. Jerk nystagmus involves a slow movement in one direction followed by a quick movement in the opposite direction, with the direction specified by the fast phase (such as leftward-beating nystagmus). Jerk nystagmus typically gets stronger when looking in the direction of the fast phase (known as Alexander's law).

Nystagmus is a normal component of the optokinetic response and the reflex eye movement response to caloric stimulation. It can also occur at the extremes of voluntary gaze in healthy subjects. Under other circumstances, on the other hand, it might be caused by sedative or anticonvulsant medications, or diseases of the cerebellum, central vestibular pathways, or peripheral vestibular apparatus.

The eyes should be examined in the primary position as well as in each of the cardinal positions of gaze in order to identify nystagmus (Figure 7.5). The position of gaze in which nystagmus occurs, its direction, and amplitude, as well as its precipitating factors (such as head position changes) and associated symptoms (like vertigo), are all described.

There are numerous types of nystagmus and associated ocular oscillations that have been identified, but the two most prevalent types are acquired pathologic jerk nystagmus syndromes.

i. **Gaze-Evoked Nystagmus:** When a patient tries to look away from the primary position in one or more directions, it can result in gaze-evoked nystagmus. The direction of gaze is where the fast phase of nystagmus occurs. When one looks in a single direction, nystagmus is frequently elicited, which indicates mild or early residual ocular palsy. Multidirectional gaze-evoked nystagmus can be caused by cerebellar or central vestibular dysfunction, but it is most commonly a side effect of anticonvulsant or sedative medications.

ii. **Vestibular Nystagmus:** A lesion of the peripheral vestibular apparatus can cause nystagmus, which is characterized by unidirectional, horizontal, or both horizontal and rotatory movements, and severe vertigo. Looking toward the fast phase causes its amplitude to increase. On the other hand, the accompanying vertigo in central vestibular nystagmus is usually mild and can be bidirectional, purely horizontal, vertical, or rotatory. Changes in head position can cause positional nystagmus, which can be caused by central or peripheral vestibular lesions. The presence of corticospinal tract abnormalities or additional cranial nerve abnormalities with central lesions, as well as hearing loss or tinnitus with peripheral lesions, are the most useful distinguishing characteristics.

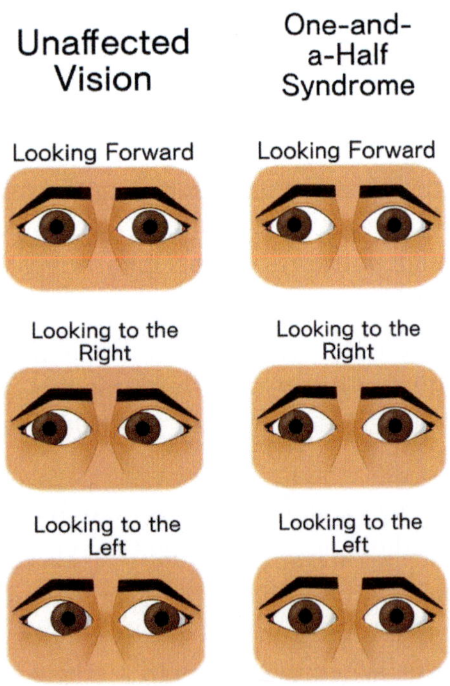

Figure 7.16. One-and-a-half syndrome. This results from a pontine lesion (shaded area) involving the paramedian pontine reticular formation (lateral gaze center) and medial longitudinal fasciculus, and sometimes also the abducens (VI) nucleus, and affecting the neuronal pathways indicated by dotted lines. Attempted gaze away from the lesion (A) activates the uninvolved right lateral gaze center and abducens (VI) nucleus; the right lateral rectus muscle contracts, and the right eye abducts normally. Involvement of the medial longitudinal fasciculus interrupts the pathway to the left oculomotor (III) nucleus, and the left eye fails to adduct. On attempted gaze toward the lesion (B), the left lateral gaze center cannot be activated, and the eyes do not move. There is a complete (bilateral) gaze palsy in one direction (toward the lesion) and one-half (unilateral) gaze palsy in the other direction (away from the lesion), accounting for the name of the syndrome.

7.2. Disorders of the Visual System

7.2.1. Monocular Disorders

Monocular visual loss is commonly associated with two reversible and two irreversible disorders. The sudden onset and quick resolution of transient monocular blindness are caused by optic nerve or retinal ischemia. Subacute, excruciating, unilateral visual loss with partial resolution is the result of optic neuritis. Giant cell (temporal) arteritis and idiopathic ischemic optic neuropathy both cause less reversible visual loss with an abrupt onset.

7.2.1.1. Transient Monocular Blindness

A usually painless, unilateral, transient diminution or loss of vision that occurs over seconds, reaches its maximum for one to five minutes, and resolves over ten to twenty minutes is known as transient monocular blindness (amaurosis fugax). While the etiology of both embolic and non-embolic episodes is known, the cause of these episodes is frequently still unknown. The majority of cases are caused by momentary ischemia of the retina or optic nerve. Emboli may be a common cause because of the appearance of embolic material in the retinal arteries during episodes. The frequency or duration of these episodes does not affect the increased risk of subsequent hemispheric stroke. Patients receiving medical treatment have a hemispheric transient ischemic attack (TIA) risk of only half that of patients not receiving medical treatment for transient monocular blindness.

Patients with transient monocular blindness are evaluated for diagnostic purposes and treated similarly to patients with hemispheric TIAs.

7.2.1.2. Autoimmune Optic Neuritis

The optic neuritis syndrome is caused by inflammation of the optic nerve. Acute demyelinating optic neuritis, or demyelination, is the most frequent cause. Inflammation of the parameningeal, meningeal, or intraocular spaces caused by viral infections or postviral syndromes are less frequent causes. Toxins (such as methanol and ethambutol), neurosyphilis, and vitamin B12 deficiency are uncommon causes. Unilateral visual acuity loss progresses over hours to days and reaches its peak in two weeks. In over 90% of cases, visual loss is accompanied by headache, globe tenderness, or eye pain, which is usually made worse by the movement of the eyes.

In visual field testing, a central scotoma, or blind spot, is linked to a reduction in visual acuity. When the nerve head is involved, examination of the fundus reveals unilateral disk swelling; however, when the inflammatory process is posterior to the optic disk (retrobulbar neuritis), as is most frequently seen in demyelinating disease, the fundus appears normal. Each pupil is the same size, but the affected eye's pupillary defect (also known as the Marcus Gunn pupil) causes less noticeable constriction in response to light. In a few weeks, vision recovery can start, and it might continue for a year. Most people's vision returns to normal.

In 25% of cases, optic neuritis is the initial sign of multiple sclerosis, and 70% of patients experience it at some point in their disease. Acute demyelinating optic neuritis is characterized by diffuse gadolinium enhancement of the optic nerve on MRI, and in 50–70% of these patients, T2-hyperintense lesions are also observed in the brain. 72% of optic neuritis patients in North America with a 15-year follow-up had one or more T2 lesions in their brains; by contrast, only about 25% of patients without T2 lesions went on to develop multiple sclerosis.

Methylprednisolone given intravenously at a rate of 1 g/d for three to five days, either in conjunction with or instead of an oral prednisone taper starting at 1 mg/kg/d for eleven days, can speed up recovery without changing the risk of multiple sclerosis or the ultimate visual outcome. If demyelinating lesions are observed on brain MRI, evolving data support immunomodulatory treatment for optic neuritis as presumed multiple sclerosis.

Devic disease was formerly known as neuromyelitis optica (NMO) spectrum disorder, which is characterized by bilateral spontaneous optic neuritis and transverse myelitis. Antibodies against aquaporin-4 are diagnostic.

7.2.1.3. Nonarteritic Anterior Ischemic Optic Neuropathy

One of the main causes of vision loss starting in middle age is ischemic infarction of the anterior portion of the optic nerve. The loss of vision always occurs suddenly, is monocular, usually painless, and does not have any prior ocular symptoms. The pattern of visual loss varies amongst patients; the visual deficit is typically maximal at onset and often subtotal. The course may occasionally be progressive or stuttering.

Upon examination, peripapillary hemorrhages and ipsilateral disk swelling are frequently observed. Even though ischemic optic neuropathy is frequently thought to have atherosclerotic origins, the occurrence of symptoms upon awakening is a common characteristic that points to nocturnal arterial hypotension, frequently caused by antihypertensive drugs. A structurally smaller disk than normal is present in patients with anterior ischemic optic neuropathy; within three to five years, 15 to 25% of these patients will experience problems in the other eye.

Improvement happens on its own over a six-month period. Optic atrophy is observed during ophthalmoscopic examination when disk swelling subsides. Corticosteroid therapy, consisting of 80 mg of prednisone per day for 14 days, tapered over a month, may improve recovery during the first two weeks of treatment. Aspirin doesn't work.

7.2.1.4. Giant Cell (Temporal) Arteritis

The most severe side effect of giant cell, or temporal, arteritis is arteritic infarction of the anterior portion of the optic nerve. Systemic symptoms like fever, malaise, sweats at night, headache, and weight loss are typical for this disorder. Polymyalgia rheumatica is also frequently present. Jaw claudication and tenderness in the scalp are possible. Temporary visual obscurations may occur before optic nerve infarction, but the loss of vision is typically abrupt and frequently complete. Examining the optic disk reveals that it is pale and enlarged. Usually, there is an increase in C-reactive protein and erythrocyte sedimentation rate. The final diagnosis is made through a temporal artery biopsy.

To preserve what vision remains, patients should receive corticosteroids right away (methylprednisolone 1,000 mg/d intravenously for at least three days, followed by prednisone 60–80 mg/d oral). It is possible to taper off prednisone gradually over several months while keeping an eye on the erythrocyte sedimentation rate.

It is crucial to differentiate giant cell arteritis from idiopathic or nonarteritic anterior ischemic optic neuropathy when considering treatment options for monocular visual loss. Giant cell arteritis patients may have premonitory symptoms and are typically older (70–80 years old). The most useful differential features are an elevated C-reactive protein and an erythrocyte sedimentation rate, which exceeds 50 mm/h (Westergren) in most, but not all, patients with giant cell arteritis.

7.2.2. Binocular Disorders

7.2.2.1. Papilledema

Papilledema is a passive, painless swelling of the disks that is usually bilateral and linked to elevated intracranial pressure. Before the disk swelling, there may be brief visual obscurations. Raised intracranial pressure is associated with nonspecific symptoms such as headache, nausea, vomiting, and diplopia, which is primarily caused by abducens (VI) nerve palsy.

Papilledema develops at varying rates depending on the underlying cause. Disk swelling may appear within hours of an abrupt increase in intracranial pressure, such as in subarachnoid or intracerebral hemorrhage, but it usually takes days to manifest. After the normal intracranial pressure is restored, the resolution of papilledema may take two to three months.

The funduscopic examination reveals the following in order of onset: hemorrhages in the nerve fiber layer, blurring of the disk surface with blurred margins, disk hyperemia, and blurring of the nerve fiber layer. Additionally, there are no venous pulsations, which indicates an intracranial pressure greater than about 200 mm Hg. Papilledema needs to be evaluated immediately in order to rule out meningeal carcinoma, sarcoidosis, or syphilis, which can all appear similar under the microscope, and to look for any intracranial masses. When the cerebrospinal fluid (CSF) pressure is elevated but the history, computed tomography (CT) scanning or MRI with contrast enhancement, meningeal inflammation, and other disorders associated with intracranial hypertension are excluded, the diagnosis of idiopathic intracranial hypertension (pseudotumor cerebri) is established by exclusion. The most prevalent kind, idiopathic, mostly affects obese women who are in their reproductive years. Prolonged elevation of intracranial pressure associated with papilledema can result in permanent visual loss, though it usually resolves on its own.

Less frequent causes of papilledema include congenital cyanotic heart disease and conditions linked to elevated levels of protein in the cerebrospinal fluid, like spinal cord tumors and idiopathic inflammatory polyneuropathy (Guillain-Barré syndrome).

7.2.2.2. Chiasmal Lesions

The most common symptom of a chiasmal lesion is visual impairment. Tumors are the main lesions, particularly those of pituitary origin (which can cause Cushing syndrome, amenorrhea, galactorrhea, headaches, and acromegaly). Berry aneurysms, multiple sclerosis, and trauma are additional causes. Bitemporal hemianopia is the classic pattern of chiasmal visual deficits (refer to Figure 7.7). Chiasmal visual loss develops gradually, with impairment in-depth perception occurring before lateral visual field loss, except for pituitary apoplexy caused by acute intrapituitary hemorrhage. Tumor expansion laterally into the cavernous sinus is suggested by associated involvement of the oculomotor (III), trochlear (IV), trigeminal (V), or abducens (VI) nerves.

Patients without tumors or elevated intracranial pressure who have an enlarged sella turcica may experience headache, endocrine abnormalities, and occasionally blurred or double vision. Women are more likely to experience this empty sella syndrome, which primarily affects them in their fourth and seventh decades of life. It is a symptomatic treatment.

7.2.2.3. Retrochiasmal Lesions

- **Optic Tract and Lateral Geniculate Body:** Infarction is typically the cause of lesions in the lateral geniculate body and optic tract. When this happens, the resultant abnormality of the visual field is usually a noncongruous homonymous hemianopia, meaning that the field defect differs between the two eyes. Thalamic lesions may be associated with hemisensory loss.
- **Optic Radiations:** A homonymous hemianopia that is congruent (bilaterally symmetric) is the result of optic radiation lesions. In the area of the field that is unaffected, visual acuity is normal. The field deficit is denser superiorly than inferiorly in the temporal lobe, where tumors

are the most common cause of lesions. This leads to a superior quadrantanopia, or "pie in the sky" deficit (see Figure 7.7).

A tumor or vascular disease may be the cause of lesions affecting the optic radiations in the parietal lobe, which are typically accompanied by contralateral weakness and sensory loss. In the acute stage, a gaze preference is typical, with the eyes conjugately shifted to the side of the parietal lesion. Figure 7.7 illustrates the two types of visual field abnormalities that can occur: inferior quadrantanopia and complete homonymous hemianopia. In contrast to pure temporal or occipital lobe lesions, the optokinetic response to a visual stimulus moved toward the lesion's side is compromised.

- **Occipital Cortex:** The contralateral visual field is typically affected by homonymous hemianopia, which is caused by lesions in the occipital cortex. The patient might not be aware of their vision impairment. Visual field abnormalities caused by vascular lesions in the occipital lobe may show sparing of macular vision (Figure 7.7). This is because the region of the occipital cortex in which the macula is represented is frequently supplied by branches of both the posterior and middle cerebral arteries (Figure 7.4). Bilateral cortical representation of the macular region of the visual field can also lead to macular sparing.

A posterior cerebral artery territory infarction is the most frequent cause of visual impairment in the occipital lobe. Less frequently occurring causes include watershed infarction following cardiac arrest, vertebral angiography, and occipital lobe arteriovenous malformations (AVMs). There may be more signs and symptoms of basilar artery ischemia. Unformed visual hallucinations, usually unilateral, stationary or moving, brief or flickering, and colored or not, are frequently linked to tumors and occipital lobe AVMs.

When both occipital lobes are affected, it can lead to cortical blindness. Despite this, pupillary reactions remain normal and partial preservation of central vision may occur due to sparing of the macula in both eyes. In cases of more severe lesions, a phenomenon known as Anton syndrome may manifest, where the individual denies their blindness.

7.3. Disorders of Eye Movement

7.3.1. Gaze Palsies

Gaze disorders can result from lesions in the brainstem or cortex that affect the conjugate (yoked) movement of the eyes. The eyes may move fully in milder gaze palsies, but they do so at a slower pace or with less amplitude when moving quickly.

- **Hemispheric Lesions:** Both eyes exhibit tonic deviation in the direction of the lesion and away from the side of the hemiparesis when there are acute hemispheric lesions (Figure 7.17A). For several days in awake patients (and possibly longer in comatose patients), this gaze deviation may occur. Gaze deviation can also result from seizures that involve the frontal gaze centers, as this drives the eyes away from the focal point of the seizure. The patient looks to the side of the seizure-induced motor activity when the ipsilateral motor cortex is also involved, resulting in focal motor seizures (Figure 7.17B).

- **Midbrain Lesions:** Upgaze paralysis may result from lesions to the dorsal midbrain, which affects the area responsible for voluntary upward gaze. Furthermore, all or some of the following characteristics of Parinaud syndrome may manifest: nystagmus (particularly on downward gaze and usually associated with retraction of the eyes), midsized pupils, preserved reflex vertical eye movements with the doll's head maneuver or Bell phenomenon (elevation of the eye upon eyelid closure), and light-near dissociation.
- **Pontine Lesions:** The paramedian pontine reticular formation is where the pontine gaze center is located (Figure 7.6). In contrast to hemispheric lesions, brainstem lesions at the level of the pontine gaze centers result in abnormalities of conjugate horizontal gaze but cause eye deviation toward the side of the hemiparesis rather than away from it (Figure 7.17C). This happens because the descending motor (pyramidal) pathways have not crossed at this level, but the corticobulbar pathways that control gaze have. Compared to hemispheric gaze pareses, brainstem gaze palsies are characterized by a significantly higher resistance to attempts to move the eyes (via the doll's head maneuver or caloric stimulation). Additionally, because the abducens (VI) nerve's nucleus is affected, gaze palsies resulting from brainstem lesions are frequently linked to abducens nerve palsies.

7.3.2. Internuclear Ophthalmoplegia

Lesions of the medial longitudinal fasciculus, which runs between the midpons and the oculomotor nerve nucleus, can cause internuclear ophthalmoplegia (INO) by severing the abducens (VI) nucleus from the contralateral oculomotor (III) nucleus (Figure 7.6). The side where oculomotor (III) nerve function is compromised determines the name of the INO site. INO causes the abducting eye's nystagmus and disconjugate gaze, which is characterized (Figure 7.15).

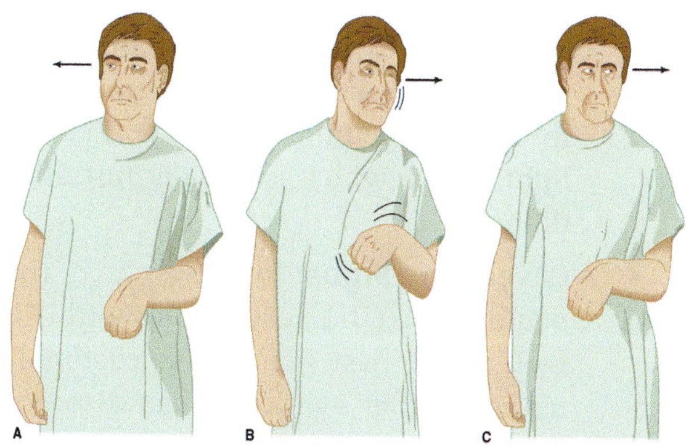

Figure 7.17. Disorders of gaze associated with hemispheric and brainstem lesions. (A) Destructive lesion in the frontal lobe of the right cerebral hemisphere. (B) Seizure arising from the frontal lobe of the right cerebral hemisphere. (C) Destructive lesion in the right pons. Arrows indicate the direction of gaze preference (away from the hemiparetic side in (A) and toward the convulsing or hemiparetic side in [B] and [C]).

Source: https://dl.mehrsys.ir/pdf-books/Clinical%20Neurology%209%20Edition%20(www.myuptodate.com).pdf.

An intrinsic brainstem disease is typically implied by an INO. Multiple sclerosis is the most common cause, particularly in young adults and patients with bilateral involvement. Stroke is most likely to occur in older patients and those with unilateral involvement. At least 80% of all cases have one of these two causes. Syringobulbia, Wernicke encephalopathy, brainstem encephalitis, intrinsic brainstem tumors, and sedative drug intoxication are among the less common causes. Myasthenia gravis needs to be ruled out in patients with isolated INO because it can mimic a lesion of the medial longitudinal fasciculus.

7.3.3. Ocular Nerve Palsies

7.3.3.1. Oculomotor (III) Nerve Lesions

Oculomotor (III) nerve lesions can happen at different levels. The most frequent causes are indicated in Table 7.3, and diabetes-related oculomotor problems are covered in more detail later.

- **Brainstem:** Other neurologic symptoms within the brainstem allow the lesion to be localized; the most common vascular syndromes are associated contralateral hemiplegia (Weber syndrome) and contralateral ataxia (Benedikt syndrome).
- Subarachnoid Space: The oculomotor (III) nerve is vulnerable to damage from trauma and posterior communicating artery aneurysms as it leaves the brainstem in the interpeduncular space. These compressive lesions usually affect the pupillary light reflex, which is usually not affected by ischemic lesions (like those caused by diabetes).
- **Cavernous Sinus:** In Figure 7.18, the cavernous sinus typically involves the oculomotor (III) nerve along with the trochlear (IV) and abducens (VI) nerves, as well as the first (V1) and occasionally the second (V2) division of the trigeminal nerve. Horner syndrome can also occur. Lesions of the oculomotor (III) nerve in the cavernous sinus often result in partial deficits that may or may not leave the pupil unaffected.
- **Orbit:** Optic (II) nerve involvement and exophthalmos are frequently linked to orbital lesions that affect the oculomotor (III) nerve, in contrast to cavernous sinus lesions. Nevertheless, disorders of the orbit and cavernous sinus may be clinically indistinguishable unless they are detected by CT scanning or MRI.

Table 7.3. Causes of Oculomotor (III), Trochlear (IV), and Abducens (VI) Nerve Lesions

Cause	Nerve III	Nerve IV	Nerve VI	Multiple
	Percent of cases			
Unknown	24	32	26	12
Vasculopathy[3]	20	18	12	4
Aneurysm	16	1	4	8
Trauma	15	29	5	18
Neoplasm	13	5	22	36
Other[4]	12	15	21	22

[1] Data from Richards BW, Jones FR Jr, Younge BR. Causes and prognosis in 4,278 cases of paralysis of the oculomotor, trochlear, and abducens cranial nerves. Am J Ophthalmol. 1992;113:489–496.

[2] Percent of all cases by nerve: III, 25%; IV, 12%; VI, 43%; multiple, 13%.

[3] Includes diabetes.

[4] Includes (in order of frequency) congenital, neurosurgical, multiple sclerosis, stroke, meningitis or encephalitis, carotid cavernous fistula, myasthenia, ophthalmoplegic migraine, hydrocephalus, subarachnoid hemorrhage, arteriovenous malformation, spinocerebellar atrophy, sinus disease, radiation, chemotherapy, and herpes zoster.

7.3.3.2. Trochlear (IV) Nerve Lesions

An isolated trochlear (IV) nerve palsy is frequently caused by head trauma, which is frequently mild (Table 7.3). Trochlear palsies frequently occur for no apparent reason in middle-aged and elderly patients, though they are frequently linked to vascular disease or diabetes. The best course of treatment for individuals with isolated nontraumatic trochlear (IV) nerve palsies in whom diabetes, myasthenia, thyroid dysfunction, and orbital mass lesions have been ruled out is observation.

7.3.3.3. Abducens (VI) Nerve Lesions

Patients who have lesions on the abducens (VI) nerve report weakness in the lateral rectus muscle, which results in horizontal diplopia. Disorders of the abducens (VI) nerve or the muscle itself can cause lateral rectus palsies; both of these possibilities need to be looked into. Table 7.3 provides an overview of the causes of lesions to the abducens (VI) nerve. The most common causes of abducens (VI) nerve involvement in elderly patients are vascular disease, diabetes, or idiopathic conditions; however, erythrocyte sedimentation rate testing should be performed to rule out the uncommon manifestation of giant cell arteritis. Imaging of the base of the skull is recommended to rule out tumors other than nasopharyngeal carcinoma. Patients with painless abducens palsy can be treated conservatively if the aforementioned studies show no abnormalities, there are no additional systemic or neurological symptoms, and there is no rise in intracranial pressure. Prednisone (60 mg/d orally for 5 days) may provide a significant improvement in painful abducens (VI) nerve palsy, supporting a preliminary diagnosis of idiopathic inflammation of the cavernous sinus (Tolosa-Hunt syndrome) or superior orbital fissure (superior orbital fissure syndrome). When corticosteroid treatment is not working to relieve the pain, a CT scan or MRI of the cavernous sinus should be performed, and in certain situations, an angiography. The underlying lesion is localized to the cavernous sinus when there is a concurrent Horner syndrome.

7.3.3.4. Diabetic Ophthalmoplegias

Patients with diabetes mellitus may develop an isolated lesion of the oculomotor (III), trochlear (IV), or abducens (VI) nerve; noninvasive imaging tests (MRI or CT scanning) show no abnormalities. Pupilar sparing is a feature of diabetic oculomotor (III) nerve lesions, which is typically explained by infarction of the central part of the nerve with sparing of the more peripherally located fibers that mediate pupillary constriction. In addition to compressive, infiltrative, or inflammatory lesions of the oculomotor (III) nerve, pupil-sparing oculomotor palsies can also be observed in cases of infarcts, hemorrhages, or tumors affecting the oculomotor (III) nucleus or fascicle within the midbrain. When pain is experienced, it may be severe enough to indicate that aneurysmal expansion is most likely the cause.

In individuals with established diabetes, exophthalmos and painful ophthalmoplegia necessitate immediate medical attention to rule out the possibility of a fungal infection in the orbit, cavernous sinus, or paranasal sinus caused by mucormycosis. Typically, a nasal mucosa biopsy is used to make the diagnosis. Amphotericin B therapy must be started right away, and necrotic tissue must be surgically debrided.

7.3.3.5. Painful Ophthalmoplegias

Lesions anywhere from the posterior fossa to the orbit can cause one or more of the ocular motor nerves to malfunction and cause pain (Table 7.4). A thorough record of the clinical course, a globe examination and palpation for proptosis (which localizes the process to the orbit or anterior cavernous sinus), auscultation over the globe to find a bruit (which supports a diagnosis of carotid artery–cavernous sinus fistula or another vascular anomaly), and a diabetes evaluation should all be included in the evaluation. Blood glucose, orbital CT or MRI, carotid arteriography, and orbital venography are useful laboratory tests.

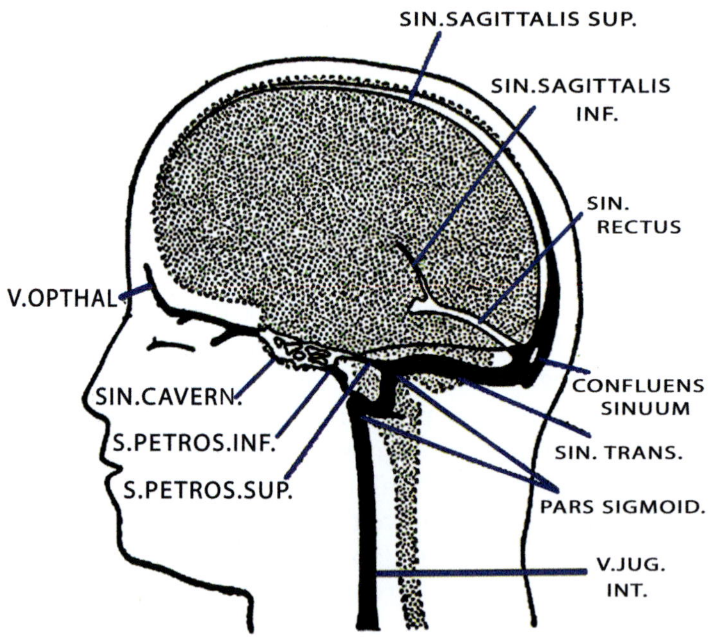

Figure 7.18. Position of cranial nerves in the cavernous sinus and adjacent structures. Note that a lesion in the cavernous sinus spares the optic (II) and mandibular (V3) nerves, a lesion in the superior orbital fissure additionally spares the maxillary (V2) nerve, and a lesion in the orbital apex spares both V2 and V3 but may involve II.

Source: By User: Wikid77 (clarifying Gray's image) – Derivative of Wikimedia Image:Gray488. png., Public Domain, https://commons.wikimedia.org/w/index.php?curid=2945470.

The particular diagnosis for these disorders determines the course of therapy. When corticosteroids (prednisone 60–100 mg/d orally) are administered, the idiopathic inflammation of the orbit (orbital pseudotumor) or cavernous sinus (Tolosa-Hunt syndrome) significantly improves. However, during corticosteroid therapy, the pain and ocular symptoms linked to some neoplasms may also temporarily improve, so a biopsy may be necessary to determine the precise etiologic diagnosis.

7.3.4. Myasthenia Gravis

Approximately 90% of patients with myasthenia eventually experience ocular muscle involvement; over 60% of patients exhibit this condition at initial presentation. Pupilary responses are consistently normal, the syndrome is painless, and there are no abnormal sensory experiences. An intravenous edrophonium (Tensilon) positive response validates the diagnosis.

Table 7.4. Diagnosis of Painful Ophthalmoplegia

Tolosa-Hunt Syndrome	Recurrent Painful Ophthalmoplegic Neuropathy	
DESCRIPTION	Unilateral orbital or periorbital pain associated with paresis of one or more between the 3rd, 4th and/or 6th cranial nerves caused by a granulomatous inflammation in the cavernous sinus, superior orbital fissure or orbit	Repeated attacks of paresis of one or more ocular cranial nerves (commonly the 3rd), with ipsilateral headache
DIAGNOSTIC CRITERIA	A. Unilateral orbital or periorbital headache fulfilling criterion C	A. At least two attacks fulfilling criterion B
		B. Both of the following:
	B. Both of the following:	
	1. granulomatous inflammation of the cavernous sinus, superior orbital fissure or orbit, demonstrated by MRI or biopsy	1. unilateral headache
		2. ipsilateral paresis of one, two or all three ocular motor nerves
	2. paresis of one or more of the ipsilateral the 3rd, 4th and/or 6th cranial nerves	C. Orbital, parasellar or posterior fossa lesion has been excluded by appropriate investigation

	C. Evidence of causation demonstrated by both of the following:	D. Not better accounted for by another ICHD-3 diagnosis
	1. headache is ipsilateral to the granulomatous inflammation	
	2. headache has preceded paresis of the the 3rd, 4th and/or 6th nerves by ≤ 2 weeks, or developed with it	
	D. Not better accounted for by another ICHD-3 diagnosis	
COMMENTS	Some reported cases of Tolosa-Hunt syndrome had additional involvement of the 5th nerve (commonly the first division) or optic, 7th or 8th nerves. Sympathetic innervation of the pupil is occasionally affected	Some data suggest that headache can develop up to 14 days prior to ocular motor paresis
	Careful follow-up is required to exclude other causes of painful ophthalmoplegia such as tumors, vasculitis, basal meningitis, sarcoid or diabetes mellitus	Gadolinium enhancement or nerve thickening can be demonstrated using MRI
	Pain and paresis of Tolosa-Hunt syndrome resolve when adequately treated with corticosteroids	

Source: Frattini, D., Iodice, A., Spagnoli, C. et al. Tolosa-Hunt syndrome and recurrent painful ophthalmoplegic neuropathy, case reports: what to do and when?. Ital J Pediatr., 49, 157 (2023). https://doi.org/10.1186/s13052-023-01541-5.

7.3.5. Ocular Myopathies

Ocular myopathies are usually bilateral, painless syndromes that preserve pupillary function. The most prevalent is hyperthyroidism myopathy, which can cause double vision starting in midlife or later in life. At the time of diagnosis, many patients are otherwise clinically euthyroid. The most frequent symptom is double vision when elevating the globe, but in less severe cases, there may also be lid retraction when staring or lid lag when rapidly moving the eye up and down. Exophthalmos is a typical finding, particularly in more advanced cases (Figure 7.11). The forced duction test, which identifies mechanical resistance to forced movement of the anesthetized globe in the orbit, can be used to confirm the diagnosis. Usually, this restrictive ocular myopathy resolves on its own. When necessary, the patient should receive treatment for hyperthyroidism and be referred for thyroid function testing.

A class of syndromes known as progressive external ophthalmoplegias is defined by a symmetric, slowly progressing impairment of ocular movement that is unresponsive to caloric stimulation. There is no pain and no loss of puffery function, though ptosis may be noticeable. Ocular or oculopharyngeal muscular dystrophy can cause this clinical picture. Myotonic dystrophy is suggested as a diagnosis when progressive external ophthalmoplegia is accompanied by myotonic contraction upon percussion of muscle groups, most commonly the thenar group in the palm. Progressive external ophthalmoplegia in Kearns-Sayre-Daroff syndrome is accompanied by pigmentary degeneration of the retina, cardiac conduction defects, cerebellar ataxia, and elevated CSF protein levels. This syndrome has been linked to deletions in muscle mitochondrial DNA. Rough red fibers in the muscle biopsy indicate the presence of aberrant mitochondria. Parkinson's disease and progressive supranuclear palsy are disorders that mimic progressive external ophthalmoplegia; however, in these cases, oculocephalic or caloric stimulation can compensate for the impairment of eye movements, which are typically vertical.

A Closer Look

Ophthalmoplegia

Ophthalmoplegia is the paralysis of the muscles outside the eye that regulate its movements. The third (oculomotor), fourth (trochlear), or sixth (abducens) cranial nerves are typically affected by ophthalmoplegia. The defining symptom in all three cases is double vision. Oculomotor paralysis affects the muscles that control the eye, causing it to drift outward and slightly downward and making it difficult for it to turn inward and upward. Additionally, the pupil may enlarge and the affected eye's upper lid typically droops, a condition known as ptosis. An abnormally large pupil raises the risk of a cerebral aneurysm. This may be connected to discomfort. The eye that is affected by trochanterial paralysis exhibits a vertical deviation due to the involvement of the superior oblique muscle. Another ocular muscle, the lateral rectus, is also affected by paralysis of the abducens nerve, which causes the affected eye to turn inward toward the nose rather than fully outward.

Ophthalmoplegia can result from a variety of conditions that affect the nervous system, such as multiple sclerosis, cerebral tumors, migraines, vascular (blood vessel) disease, such as diabetes, trauma, complications from viral infections, and congenital abnormalities. Even though it is typically accompanied by other muscle symptoms, ophthalmoplegia can also develop as a side effect of muscular disorders like myasthenia gravis. If possible, ophthalmoplegia treatment aims to address any underlying conditions. Isolated nerve palsies often go away on their own with time, and the only treatment for them is to patch the affected eye to stop any temporary double vision. For those who have had ophthalmoplegia for a long time, prism-equipped glasses or surgery may be beneficial.

Summary

- The term "neuro-ophthalmologic disease" refers to a broad range of visual issues that are associated with the optic nerve, eye movements, and the visual-related brain regions.
- Ocular muscles have differential innervation, which makes it possible to differentiate between disorders of the ocular muscles and disorders affecting cranial nerves based on the pattern of their involvement in pathologic conditions.
- The abducens (VI) nerve nucleus is situated in the pons in a similarly dorsal and periventricular position to that of the oculomotor (III) and trochlear (IV) nerve nuclei, which are situated in the dorsal midbrain, ventral to the cerebral aqueduct (of Sylvius).
- The optic disk is typically easily identified as a slightly oval, yellowish structure located nasally at the posterior pole of the eye.
- Eye movements caused by a patient's sequential fixation on a series of targets that are passing in front of their eyes, like telephone poles seen from a moving train, are known as optokinetic nystagmus.
- A lesion of the medial longitudinal fasciculus, an ascending pathway in the brainstem that projects from the abducens (VI) to the contralateral oculomotor (III) nerve nucleus, causes internuclear ophthalmoplegia (INO)
- The sudden onset and quick resolution of transient monocular blindness are caused by optic nerve or retinal ischemia.
- Devic disease was formerly known as neuromyelitis Optica (NMO) spectrum disorder, which is characterized by bilateral spontaneous optic neuritis and transverse myelitis.

References

1. Biousse, V., & Newman, N. J. (2009). *Neuro-Ophthalmology Illustrated.* Stuttgart: Thieme.
2. Foroozan, R. (2018). Neuro-Ophthalmology in Clinical Practice: An Approach to Diplopia. *Asia-Pacific Journal of Ophthalmology, 7*(3), 186–193.
3. Fraser, J. A., & Plant, G. T. (2019). Neuro-Ophthalmology in the Emergency Department. *Emergency Medicine Clinics, 37*(4), 777–794.
4. Galetta, K. M., & Galetta, S. L. (2018). Neuro-Ophthalmology: What the Neurologist Should Know. *Continuum: Lifelong Learning in Neurology, 24*(4), 1223–1254.
5. Hayreh, S. S. (2013). Ischemic optic neuropathies. *Graefes Arch Clin Exp Ophthalmol., 251*, 1873–1884.
6. Kennard, C., & Leigh, R. J. (Eds.). (2011). *Neuro-Ophthalmology.* Handbook of Clinical Neurology, Vol 102. Amsterdam: Elsevier.
7. Lee, A. G., Brazis, P. W., & Galetta, S. L. (2010). *Neuro-Ophthalmology Review Manual.* Lippincott Williams & Wilkins.
8. Liu, G. T., Volpe, N. J., & Galetta, S. L. (2010). *Liu, Volpe, and Galetta's Neuro-Ophthalmology: Diagnosis and Management.* Saunders.

9. Miller, N. R., & Newman, N. J. (Eds.). (2005). *Walsh & Hoyt's Clinical Neuro-Ophthalmology* (6th ed.). Philadelphia, PA: Lippincott Williams & Wilkins.

10. Miller, N. R., Newman, N. J., & Biousse, V. (2018). *Walsh & Hoyt's Clinical Neuro-Ophthalmology: The Essentials*. Lippincott Williams & Wilkins.

11. Peragallo, J. H., & Newman, N. J. (2019). Ischemic Optic Neuropathies. *Handbook of Clinical Neurology, 157*, 485–503.

12. Petzold, A., Islam, N., Hu, H. H., & Plant, G. T. (2013). Embolic and nonembolic transient monocular visual field loss: A clinicopathologic review. *Surv. Ophthalmol., 58*, 42–62.

13. Prasad, S., & Volpe, N. J. (2010). Paralytic strabismus: Third, fourth and sixth nerve palsy. *Neurol. Clin., 28*, 803–833.

14. Rizzo, J. F., & Lessell, S. (2012). *Neuro-Ophthalmology Illustrated*. Thieme.

15. Toosy, A. T., Mason, D. F., & Miller, D. H. (2014). Optic neuritis. *Lancet Neurol., 13*, 83–99.

Chapter

SEIZURES AND SYNCOPE

8

Contents

Introduction

Two different medical conditions that are distinguished by a brief loss of consciousness are seizures and syncope. Abnormal electrical activity in the brain causes seizures, which change a person's awareness, movement, or behavior. These may result from epilepsy, brain trauma, or other neurological disorders and present as convulsions, staring spells, or loss of consciousness. Medical history, neurological examination, and imaging and EEG tests are commonly used in the diagnosis process. Surgical procedures or antiepileptic drugs are frequently used in treatment.

Syncope, also referred to as fainting, is characterized by an abrupt drop in consciousness caused by insufficient blood supply to the brain. It could be caused by orthostatic hypotension, cardiac problems, or vasovagal reactions. Prodromal symptoms, such as nausea or vertigo, frequently occur before syncope. A physical examination, an ECG, a medical history, and other tests are used in the diagnosis process. The goal of management is to address the underlying causes, which may include medication or lifestyle changes.

Although both conditions involve a loss of consciousness, they stem from different causes and require unique diagnostic and treatment strategies. It is important to recognize these distinctions to provide precise diagnosis and personalized care.

Orientation and Directional Terms

Term	Definition	Illustration
Orthostatic hypotension	Orthostatic hypotension, also known as postural hypotension, is a medical condition that causes a sudden drop in blood pressure when standing up from a seated or Lying position.	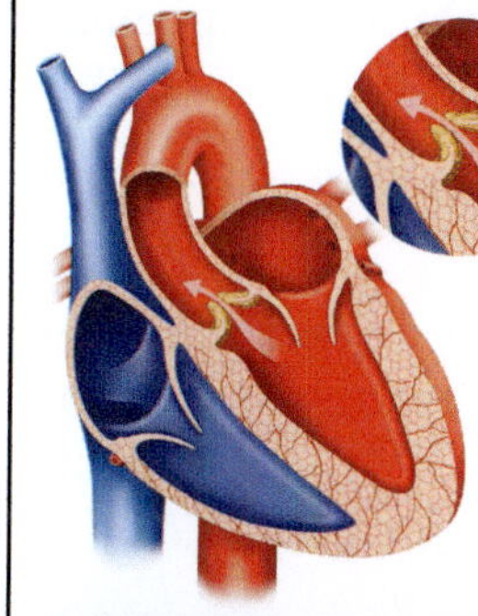
Encephalopathy	Encephalopathy means any disorder or disease of the brain, especially chronic degenerative conditions.	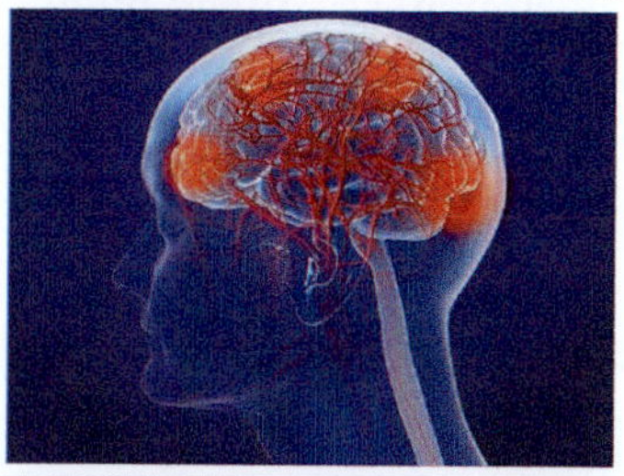
Embolic infarction	An embolic infarction, also known as an ischemic stroke, occurs when a blood clot (embolus) travels from another part of the body to the brain and blocks blood flow.	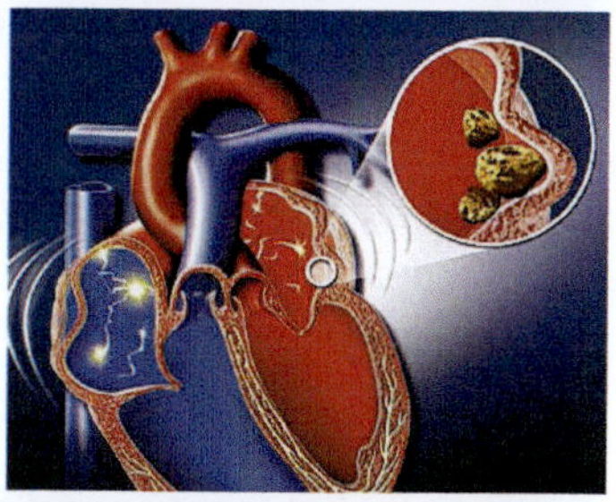
Proteinuria	Proteinuria is high levels of protein in your urine. Causes may include relatively harmless conditions, including dehydration or intense exercise, or more serious, including kidney disease or immune disorders.	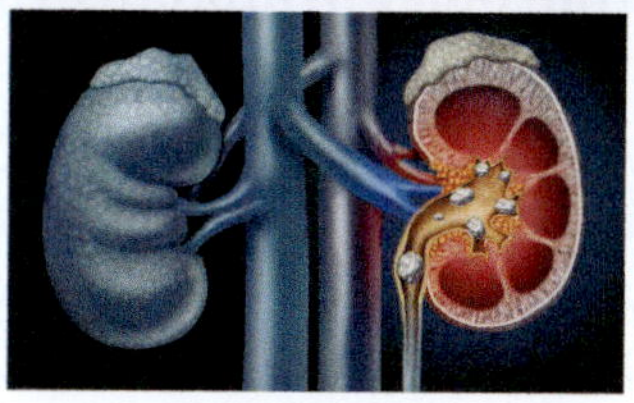
Pupillary dilatation	Pupillary dilation, also known as mydriasis, is when the black center of the eye is larger than normal.	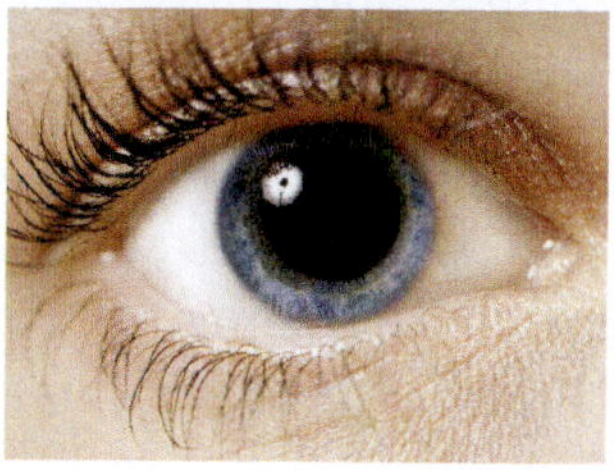

8.1. Episodic LOSS of Consciousness

When the brainstem reticular activating system or both cerebral hemispheres are not functioning properly, consciousness is lost. Anatomical regions that experience periodic dysfunction give rise to brief, frequently recurring episodes of unconsciousness. Episodic loss of consciousness has two main causes.

8.1.1. Seizures

Disorders known as seizures are typified by transient neurologic symptoms or signs that arise from abnormal, hypersynchronous, paroxysmal electrical neuronal activity in the cerebral cortex.

8.1.2. Syncope

Loss of consciousness caused by decreased blood flow to the brainstem or both cerebral hemispheres is known as syncope. It may be brought on by orthostatic hypotension, reduced cardiac output, pancerebral hypoperfusion from vasovagal reflexes, or selective brainstem hypoperfusion from vertebrobasilar ischemia.

8.1.3. Approach to Diagnosis

The causes, methods of diagnosis, and courses of treatment for seizures and syncope vary. Assess whether the circumstances surrounding the incident, or any accompanying symptoms or indicators, point to a medical condition that needs to be treated right away, such as hypoglycemia, meningitis, head trauma, cardiac arrhythmia, or acute pulmonary embolism. Evaluate the quantity and degree of similarity or dissimilarity among the spells. One pathophysiologic process can be assumed if all spells are the same. The key differentiating characteristics should be determined as explained below.

8.1.3.1. Events at Onset of Spell

- **Prodromal Symptoms (Aura):** Ask about early symptoms and prodromal symptoms. A witness might be important. Some seizures have brief, recognizable premonitory symptoms (aura) that may help identify the specific central nervous system (CNS) abnormality causing the seizures. Be aware that a patient may experience multiple types of auras. Epilepsy with temporal lobe origin is frequently accompanied by visceral or déjà vu sensations, olfactory or gustatory hallucinations, and a fearful sensation. Diminished cerebral blood flow is indicated by progressive lightheadedness, dizziness, and fainting (e.g., simple faints, cardiac arrhythmias, orthostatic hypotension).
- **Posture When Loss of Consciousness Occurs:** While standing or sitting, orthostatic hypotension and simple faints can happen. Seizures or cardiac arrhythmias are suspected of being the cause of episodes that also or exclusively occur in the recumbent position, though syncope caused by powerful emotional stimuli (such as phlebotomy) can also happen in this position.
- **Relationship to Physical Exertion:** Exertion-induced syncope is typically caused by cardiac arrhythmias or blockages in the outflow, such as atrial myxoma, obstructive

hypertrophic cardiomyopathy, and aortic stenosis.

- **Focal Symptoms:** The contralateral frontoparietal cortex may be the source of focal motor or sensory phenomena, such as forced head turning, hemifacial paresthesias, or involuntary jerking of one hand. Epilepsy with temporal lobe origin is frequently accompanied by visceral or déjà vu sensations, olfactory or gustatory hallucinations, and a fearful sensation.

8.1.3.2. Events during the Spell

- **Tonic Stiffening and Clonic Movement:** Loss of consciousness is the hallmark of generalized tonic-clonic seizures, also known as grand mal or major motor seizures. Clonic (jerking) movements of the extremities follow tonic stiffening.
- **Flaccidity:** Typically, cerebral hypoperfusion results in flaccid inresponsiveness.
- **Brief Stiffening or Jerking:** Hypoperfusion-induced loss of consciousness rarely lasts longer than 10 to 20 seconds, and postictal confusion does not usually follow unless there has been a severe and prolonged brain ischemia. Additionally, jerking or stiffening movements may be a result of cerebral hypoperfusion, particularly if the hypoperfusion lasts longer than expected due to the patient's inability to fall or adopt a recumbent position. Sometimes called convulsive syncope, this condition resolves on its own and doesn't need to be treated with anticonvulsants.

8.1.3.3. Events after the Spell

- **Prompt Recovery of Consciousness:** A simple faint can be recovered from in 20 to 30 seconds, with full lucidity returning shortly thereafter.
- **Brief Confusion:** A generalized tonic-clonic seizure is followed by a postictal state, which is a period of confusion, disorientation, or agitation. Usually, the period of confusion lasts only a few minutes. Even though this kind of behavior is frequently very obvious to onlookers, the patient might not remember it.
- **Prolonged Confusion:** Status epilepticus may be followed by a prolonged postictal state or altered state of consciousness. Patients with persistent nonconvulsive seizures, metabolic encephalopathy, or diffuse structural cerebral disease (such as dementia, other cognitive impairment, or encephalitis) may also experience it following a single seizure.
- **Tongue Biting:** The patient may notice biting of the lateral aspect of the tongue after a generalized tonic-clonic seizure, which is highly specific for this type of seizure.
- **Urinary Incontinence:** Urine incontinence can happen during a syncope or a seizure. Incontinence of the feces is rare.

8.2. Seizure

A seizure is a brief disruption of brain activity caused by an aberrant neuronal discharge. A common cause of sudden unconsciousness is epilepsy, a collection of disorders marked by recurrent seizures. About 1% of the general population has epilepsy, and 10% of people will experience a seizure in their lifetime.

A patient who is convulsing violently or a known epileptic who has had a seizure reported usually present no diagnostic challenges. However, the diagnosis must frequently be made after the fact because the majority of seizures happen outside of hospitals without the attention of medical professionals. The aura linked to focal onset seizures and the postictal confusional state that ensues after generalized tonic-clonic seizures are the two historical features most suggestive of a seizure.

8.2.1. Etiology

Primary central nervous system dysfunction, underlying metabolic disorders, and systemic diseases can all cause seizures. This distinction is important because therapy needs to focus on both seizure control and the underlying disorder. Table 8.1 provides a list of common neurologic and systemic disorders that cause seizures. The patient's age may be useful in determining the origin of the seizures (Figure 8.1).

Table 8.1. Common Causes of New-Onset Seizures

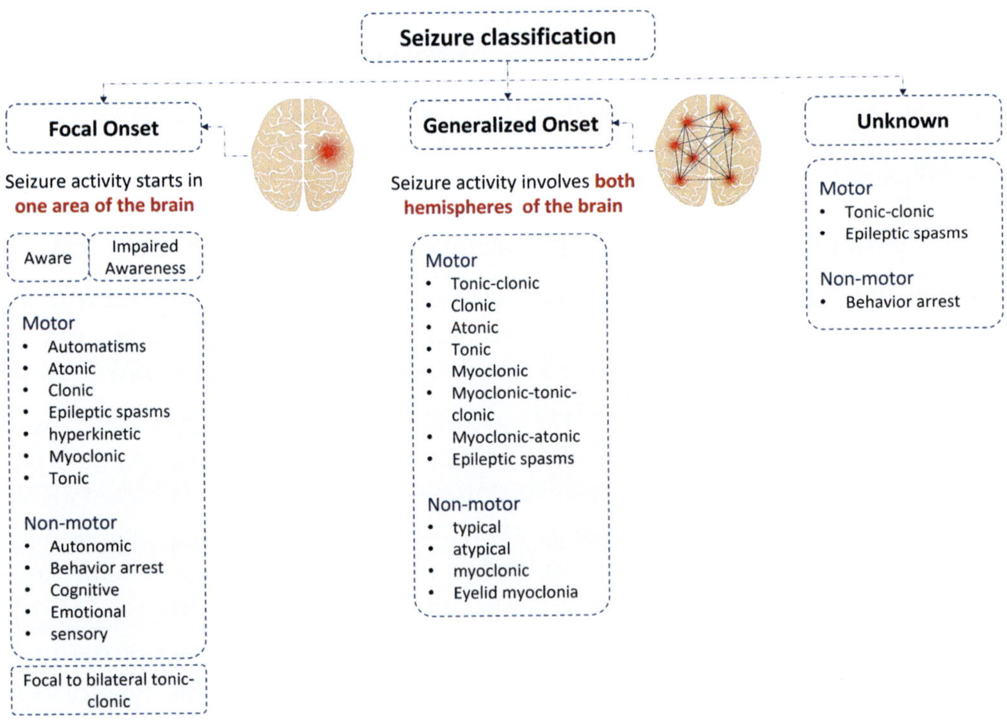

Source: Djemal A, Bouchaala D, Fakhfakh A, Kanoun O. Wearable Electromyography Classification of Epileptic Seizures: A Feasibility Study. *Bioengineering*. 2023; 10(6):703. https://doi.org/10.3390/bioengineering10060703.

Complexity exists in both the genetic component of epilepsy and how it responds to therapy. Mutations in one gene (e.g., SCN1A sodium channel subunit) can cause multiple epileptic phenotypes, and mutations in multiple genes can result in a single epileptic syndrome (e.g., juvenile myoclonic epilepsy). Genes encoding for GABA, nicotinic cholinergic, sodium, calcium, potassium, and chloride channels, as well as enzymes, have all been linked to an increased risk of epilepsy.

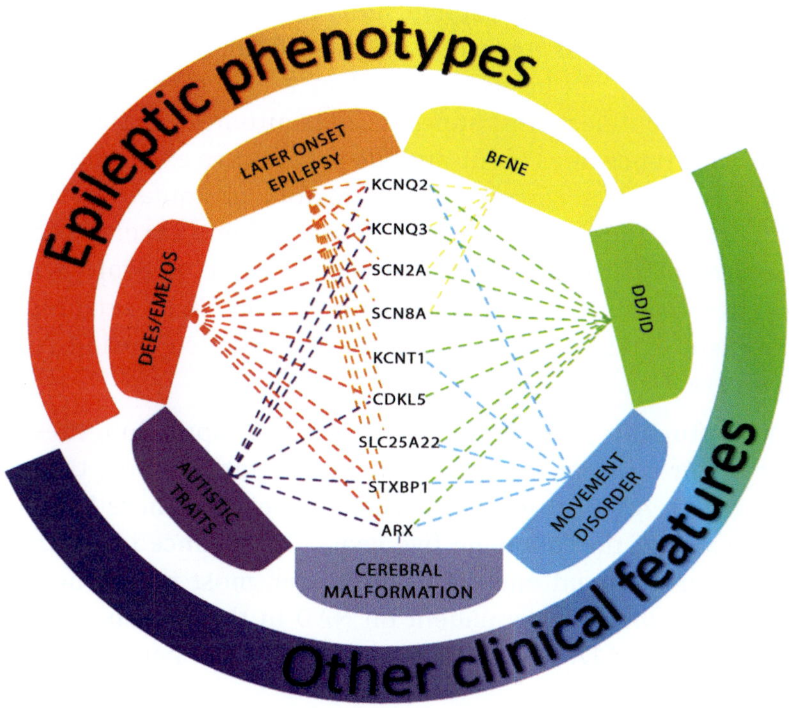

Figure 8.1. Causes of seizures.

Source: Spoto G, Saia MC, Amore G, Gitto E, Loddo G, Mainieri G, Nicotera AG, Di Rosa G. Neonatal Seizures: An Overview of Genetic Causes and Treatment Options. *Brain Sciences*. 2021; 11(10):1295. https://doi.org/10.3390/brainsci11101295.

8.2.1.1. Primary Neurologic Disorders

- **Benign Febrile Convulsions:** Between two and five percent of children between the ages of 6 months and 5 years experience benign febrile convulsions. These typically happen on the first day of a febrile illness (temperature > 100 °F or 38 °C), and they do not result from a central nervous system infection (meningitis or encephalitis). A family history of benign febrile convulsions or other seizure disorders could exist. Frequent convulsions have been associated with mutations in multiple genes, such as the G protein-coupled receptor MASS1, the inositol monophosphatase IMPA2, the sodium channel subunits SCN1A, SCN1B, and SCN2A, the potassium channel subunits KCNQ2, KCNQ3, and KCNA1, and the GABA receptor subunits GABRG2 and GABRD.

  Benign febrile convulsions are characterized by focal features absent and a duration of less than 10 to 15 minutes. Less than 10% of patients have more than three seizures, while about two-thirds only have one. 90% of recurrences happen within two years of the original episode. Children younger than eighteen months old or those with a family history of febrile seizures are more likely to experience seizures during the first hour of fever.

Treatment for benign febrile convulsions is usually not necessary because they usually go away on their own. However, for prolonged convulsions (lasting more than 15 minutes), diazepam (0.03 mg/kg orally, intramuscularly, or intravenously) or 0.00 mg/kg rectally, or buccal midazolam (0.05 mg/kg; maximum, 10 mg), can be used. The chance of a recurrence may be reduced with such treatment. When a febrile illness first appears, intermittent oral diazepam may help prevent further recurrences if a recurrence does occur and the parents are especially worried. Patients who have prolonged, focal, or multiple seizures; a family history of nonfebrile seizures; or persistent neurologic abnormalities have the highest chance of developing a chronic seizure disorder, which affects two to six percent of patients. Since phenobarbital or valproic acid use is associated with significant morbidity and does not alter the risk of nonfebrile seizures, it is generally not recommended to administer these medications over an extended period to reduce the risk of subsequent afebrile seizures.

- **Idiopathic (Cryptogenic) Seizures:** In the general population, these cause two-thirds of new-onset seizures. From the second to the seventh decade, there is a wide range of ages (Figure 8.1). After an initial unprovoked seizure, there is about a 35% chance of a recurrence within the following five years. The chance of another seizure rises to about 75% after a second one. In the first year, most recurrences take place. The malic enzyme ME2, which is dependent on NAD in the mitochondria, and the calcium channel subunits CACNA1A and CACNB4 are among the genes linked to idiopathic generalized epilepsy.
- **Head Trauma:** Head trauma is frequently linked to epilepsy, especially in cases where it happens during pregnancy, is associated with a depressed skull fracture, or results in an intracerebral or subdural hematoma. However, seizures that happen within the first week following non-incisive head trauma are not indicative of a long-term seizure disorder. Although prophylactic anticonvulsant medication treatment is frequently administered to patients with severe head injuries, this practice has come under scrutiny because a consistent decrease in the incidence of posttraumatic seizures has not been shown.
- **Stroke:** 5 to 15% of patients experience seizures following a stroke that affects the cerebral cortex. These seizures can be caused by intracerebral hemorrhage, thrombotic or embolic infarction, or both. Similar to head trauma, prolonged anticonvulsant therapy may not be necessary, and early seizures are not always a sign of chronic epilepsy. Vascular malformations can cause seizures even when they do not rupture, most likely because they irritate nearby brain tissue.
- **Mass Lesions:** Seizures may occur in conjunction with mass lesions such as brain tumors or abscesses. The most frequent tumors linked to seizures are meningiomas, glioblastomas, and astrocytomas, which is consistent with their high frequency among tumors affecting the cerebral hemispheres.
- **Meningitis or Encephalitis:** Seizures can also result from fungal, bacterial, viral, or parasitic infections, such as tuberculous or Haemophilus influenzae, herpes simplex,

or cysticercosis. In individuals suffering from AIDS, seizures are typically linked to dementia associated with HIV; however, they can also be caused by toxoplasmosis or cryptococcal meningitis.

- **Developmental Anomalies:** Cortical dysgenesis and neuronal migration disorders can predispose to epilepsy.

8.2.1.2. Systemic Disorder

Seizures linked to metabolic and other systemic disorders, such as drug overdose and withdrawal syndromes, may subside when the underlying abnormality is corrected. Under these circumstances, the patient is not diagnosed with epilepsy.

1. Hypoglycemia can produce seizures, especially with serum glucose levels of 20 to 30 mg/dL, but neurologic manifestations of hypoglycemia are also related to the rate at which serum glucose levels fall.
2. Hyponatremia may be associated with seizures at serum sodium levels less than 120 mEq/L or at higher levels after a rapid decline.
3. Hyperosmolar states, including both hyperosmolar nonketotic hyperglycemia and hypernatremia, may lead to seizures when serum osmolality rises above approximately 330 mOsm/L.
4. Hypocalcemia with serum calcium levels in the range of 4.3 to 9.2 mg/dL can produce seizures with or without tetany.
5. Uremia can cause seizures, especially when it develops rapidly, but this tendency correlates poorly with absolute serum urea nitrogen levels.
6. Hepatic encephalopathy is sometimes accompanied by generalized or multifocal seizures.
7. Porphyria is a disorder of heme biosynthesis that produces both neuropathy and seizures. The latter may be difficult to treat because most anticonvulsants can exacerbate metabolic abnormalities. Case reports attest to the safety and efficacy of gabapentin, pregabalin, and levetiracetam in porphyria.
8. Drug overdose can exacerbate epilepsy or cause seizures in nonepileptic patients. Generalized tonic– clonic seizures are most common, but focal or multifocal partial seizures can also occur. The drugs most frequently associated with seizures are antidepressants, antipsychotics, cocaine, insulin, isoniazid, lidocaine, and methylxanthines (Table 8.2).
9. Drug withdrawal, especially withdrawal from ethanol or sedative drugs, may be accompanied by one or more generalized tonic–clonic seizures that usually resolve spontaneously. Alcohol withdrawal seizures occur within 48 hours after cessation or reduction of ethanol intake in 90% of cases and are characterized by brief flurries of one to six attacks that resolve within 12 hours. Acute abstinence from sedative drugs can also produce seizures in patients habituated to more than 600 to 800 mg/d of secobarbital or equivalent doses of other short-acting sedatives. Seizures from sedative

drug withdrawal typically occur 2 to 4 days after abstinence but may be delayed for up to 1 week. Focal seizures are rarely due to alcohol or sedative drug withdrawal alone; they suggest an additional focal cerebral lesion that requires evaluation.

10. Global cerebral ischemia from cardiac arrest, cardiac arrhythmias, or hypotension may produce, at onset, a few tonic or tonic–clonic movements that resemble seizures, but they probably reflect abnormal brainstem activity instead.

Table 8.2. Major Categories of Drugs Reported to Cause Seizures

Antibiotics (quinolones, penicillins, isoniazid)
Anticholinesterases (organophosphates, physostigmine)
Antidepressants (tricyclic, monocyclic, heterocyclic; selective serotonin reuptake inhibitors)
Antihistamines
Antipsychotics (phenothiazines, butyrophenones, atypicals)
Chemotherapeutics (etoposide, ifosfamide, cisplatin)
Cyclosporine, FK 506 (tacrolimus)
Hypoglycemic agents (including insulin)
Hypo-osmolar parenteral solutions
Lithium
Local anesthetics (bupivacaine, lidocaine, procaine, etidocaine)
Methylxanthines (theophylline, aminophylline)
Narcotic analgesics (fentanyl, meperidine, pentazocine, propoxyphene)
Phencyclidine
Sympathomimetics (amphetamines, cocaine, ecstasy[1], ephedrine, phenylpropanolamine, terbutaline)

[1] Methylenedioxymethamphetamine (MDMA).

Source: https://dl.mehrsys.ir/pdf-books/Clinical%20Neurology%209%20Edition%20(www.myuptodate.com).pdf.

Global ischemia can also be linked to myoclonus that occurs spontaneously or myoclonus that is triggered by movement (action myoclonus) once consciousness returns. There are also instances of partial or generalized tonic-clonic seizures, which need to be identified and treated because they may only show minor facial or ocular movements. However, a poor prognosis is not always indicated by isolated seizures following global cerebral ischemia.

11. Hypertensive encephalopathy may be accompanied by generalized tonic– clonic or partial seizures.
12. Eclampsia refers to the occurrence of seizures or coma in a pregnant woman with hypertension, proteinuria, and edema (preeclampsia). As in hypertensive encephalopathy in nonpregnant patients, cerebral edema, ischemia, and hemorrhage may contribute to neurologic complications. Magnesium sulfate has been widely used to treat eclamptic seizures and may be superior for this purpose to anticonvulsants such as phenytoin.
13. Hyperthermia can result from infection, exposure (heat stroke), hypothalamic lesions, or drugs such as phencyclidine, as well as anticholinergics or neuroleptics and inhalational anesthetics or neuromuscular blocking agents (malignant hyperthermia). Clinical features of severe hyperthermia (42°C, or 107°F) include seizures, confusional states or coma, shock, and renal failure. Treatment is with antipyretics and artificial cooling to reduce body temperature immediately to 39°C (102°F) and anticonvulsants and more specific therapy (e.g., antibiotics for infection, dantrolene for malignant hyperthermia) where indicated. Patients who survive may be left with ataxia as a result of the special vulnerability of cerebellar neurons to hyperthermia.

8.2.1.3. Nonepileptic Seizures

Seizures or seizures resembling seizures (nonepileptic or psychogenic seizures) could be signs of a mental illness like somatization disorder, conversion disorder, factitious disorder with physical symptoms, or deception.

Seizures that are not epileptic can typically be differentiated based on clinical features and electroencephalogram (EEG) results. There may be warning and preparation before the attack in patients with nonepileptic seizures that resemble tonic-clonic attacks; typically, there is no tonic phase, and the clonic phase consists of violent thrashing movements during which the patient is rarely hurt or incontinent. Ocular ictal closure is frequent. There may be abnormal movements of all limbs without loss of consciousness in certain cases; during an apparent loss of consciousness, there may be goal-directed behavior, screaming, or the uttering of obscenities in other cases. After the attack, there are no unusual clinical symptoms or postictal confusion. If the EEG is taken during an episode, postictal slowing does not happen and there is no organized seizure activity visible. Frontal lobe seizures should be considered in the differential diagnosis. These seizures can be distinguished by very brief postictal states and unusual midline movements, such as pelvic thrusting or cycling. Abnormalities in ictal EEG may also go undetected.

Recognizing that many patients with non-epileptic seizures also experience real epileptic attacks necessitates the prescription of anticonvulsant drugs at a dosage based on empirical evidence. Referrals to psychiatry could be beneficial.

8.2.2. Classification and Clinical Findings

8.2.2.1. Classification

Seizures are classified as follows:

- **Generalized Seizures**

- o Tonic–clonic (grand mal)
- o Absence (petit mal)
- o Other types (tonic, clonic, myoclonic, atonic)

- **Partial (Focal) Seizures**
  - o Simple partial (with preservation of consciousness)
  - o Complex partial (temporal lobe, psychomotor, or focal seizures with dyscognitive features)
  - o Partial seizures with secondary generalization

8.2.2.2. Generalized Seizures

- **Generalized Tonic–Clonic Seizures:** Attacks known as generalized tonic-clonic seizures cause loss of consciousness, typically with no aura or other warning signs. When a warning does materialize, it typically takes the form of vague symptoms.
  - o **Tonic Phase:** Initially, there are two signs: limb muscles contract tonically for 10 to 30 seconds, causing flexion and then extension, especially in the back and neck (Figure 8.2). The symptoms start off unconscious. Tone trauma can result from the tonic contraction of the masticatory muscles and the expiration-induced vocalization (cry or moan) and cyanosis of the respiratory muscles. The patient may sustain injuries when they fall to the ground.
  - o **Clonic Phase:** The clonic phase of symmetric limb jerking, which lasts for an extra 30 to 60 seconds or more, comes after the tonic phase and involves alternating muscle contraction and relaxation. As soon as the tonic phase ends, ventilation attempts resume, and the cyanosis goes away. Saliva may foam in the mouth. Gradually, the jerking lessens until at last the muscles become flaccid and all movements stop. Urinary incontinence may result from detrusor muscle contraction or sphincteric relaxation.
  - o **Recovery:** After losing consciousness, the patient frequently experiences postictal confusion and headaches. Complete orientation typically takes ten to thirty minutes, or longer in patients who have preexisting metabolic or structural brain disorders, status epilepticus (see next section), or both. In cases of idiopathic epilepsy or seizures with a metabolic cause, physical examination during the postictal state is typically normal with the exception of the possibility of temporary extensor plantar responses (Babinski sign). Even in cases where the patient is unconscious, the pupils always respond to light.
  - o **Status Epilepticus:** Seizures that last five to thirty minutes without ending on their own or that occur so frequently that complete consciousness is not regained between episodes are arbitrary criteria for defining status epilepticus. Status epilepticus is a medical emergency because, if left untreated, it can result in excitotoxic neuronal damage, circulatory collapse, or permanent brain damage from hyperpyrexia.

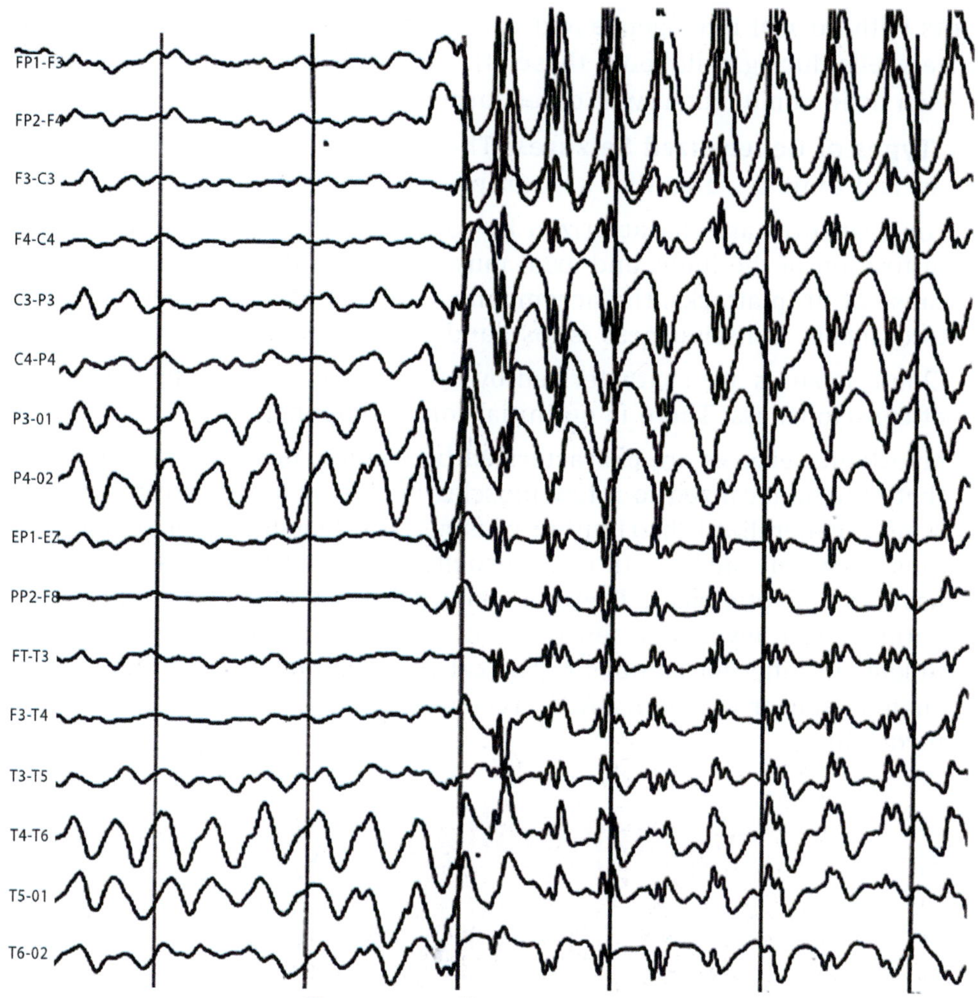

Figure 8.2. Generalized tonic–clonic seizure.

Source: CC BY-SA 2.0, https://commons.wikimedia.org/w/index.php?curid=845554.

- **Absence (Petit Mal) Seizures:** These are hereditary seizures that usually start in childhood and very seldom last into adolescence. The voltage-gated calcium channel and GABAA receptor subunits, malic enzyme 2, and inhibin alpha precursor are among the genes associated with childhood absence epilepsy. The spells are characterized by a brief (5–10 seconds) loss of consciousness combined with normal posture. It's common to see subtle motor manifestations like a slight head turn or blinking of the eyes. More intricate automatic motions, or automatisms, are not common. Complete orientation occurs right away following the end of a seizure.

  A child may experience up to several hundred spells every day, which could impair their social and academic performance and lead to misconceptions about their mental retardation. Hyperventilation is a characteristic that induces the spells. During a seizure, the EEG pattern displays 3-Hz spike-wave activity (Figure 8.3). The majority of patients with normal intelligence and background activity on the EEG only experience absence spells during childhood; these attacks rarely persist into adulthood, either on their own or in conjunction with other forms of seizures.

- **Other Types of Generalized Seizures:** These consist of myoclonic seizures, clonic seizures, and tonic seizures that are not preceded by a clonic phase.
    - o Tonic seizures are characterized by continuous muscle contraction that can lead to fixation of the limbs and axial musculature in flexion or extension and are a cause of drop attacks; the accompanying arrest of ventilatory movements leads to cyanosis. Consciousness is lost, and there is no clonic phase to these seizures.
    - o Clonic seizures are characterized by repetitive clonic jerking accompanied by loss of consciousness. There is no initial tonic component.
    - o Myoclonic seizures are characterized by sudden, brief, shock-like contractions that may be localized to a few muscles or one or more extremities or may have a more generalized distribution causing falls. Juvenile myoclonic epilepsy is the most common cause, with onset usually in adolescence. Not all myoclonic jerks have an epileptic basis. There is a family history of seizures in one-third of patients with myoclonic seizures. The disorder is genetically heterogeneous, with linkage in different families to the calcium channel beta4 subunit, CASR calcium channel sensor receptor, $GABA_A$ receptor alpha one and delta subunits, and myoclonin1.

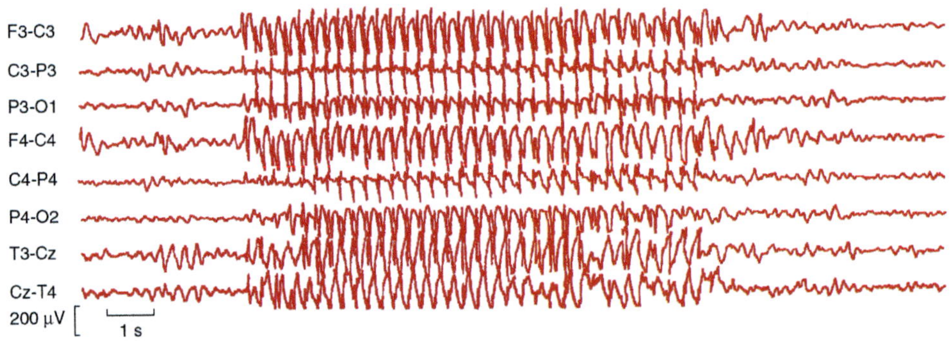

Figure 8.3. EEG of a patient with typical absence (petit mal) seizures, showing a burst of generalized 3-Hz spike-wave activity (center of record) that is bilaterally symmetric and bisynchronous. Odd-numbered leads indicate electrode placements over the left side of the head; even numbers, over the right side.

Source: https://dl.mehrsys.ir/pdf-books/Clinical%20Neurology%209%20Edition%20(www.myuptodate.com).pdf.

Rare hereditary neurodegenerative disorders such as Unverricht-Lundborg disease, Lafora body disease, neuronal ceroid lipofuscinosis, and mitochondrial encephalomyopathy can also be linked to myoclonic seizures, characterized by mutations in cystatin B, laforin, and other genes. Myoclonus epilepsy can be detected through ragged red fibers in a skeletal muscle biopsy.

- o Atonic seizures result from loss of postural tone, sometimes after a myoclonic jerk, leading to a fall or drop attack. They are most common in developmental disorders such as the Lennox-Gastaut syndrome.

8.2.2.3. Partial (Focal) Seizures

- **Simple Partial Seizures:** Depending on the cortical region involved, motor, sensory, or autonomic phenomena may precede simple partial seizures. For instance, there may be self-limited clonic movements of a single muscle group in the face, limb, or pharynx. These movements may also be recurrent, continuous, or extend to encompass adjacent areas of the motor cortex (Jacksonian march).

Autonomic symptoms such as pallor, flushing, sweating, piloerection, pupillary dilatation, vomiting, borborygmi, and hypersalivation may occur during a seizure. Psychic symptoms can include memory distortions like déjà vu, forced thinking, cognitive deficits, affective disturbances like fear or depression, hallucinations, or illusions. Simple partial seizures typically do not affect consciousness unless they spread to other areas of the brain, leading to tonic-clonic seizures. The aura precedes loss of consciousness during a seizure and can sometimes be the only symptom of the epileptic discharge.

A focal neurologic deficit, such as Todd paralysis or hemiparesis, can be present for 30 to 36 hours in the postictal state and is indicative of an underlying focal brain lesion.

- **Complex Partial Seizures:** Partial seizures in which consciousness, responsiveness, or memory are compromised are known as complex partial seizures. Previously known as temporal lobe or psychomotor seizures, they are also occasionally referred to as focal seizures with dyscognitive features. The temporal lobe or medial frontal lobe are typically where the seizure discharge originates, though it can come from another location. Though they can take many different forms, the symptoms are typically generalized to each patient. Auras can trigger the start of an episode. The most frequent symptoms are epigastric, but there are also affective (fear), psychic (déjà vu), and sensory (olfactory hallucinations) symptoms. Then, consciousness is compromised. Typically, seizures last one to three minutes. The motor manifestations of complex partial seizures are typified by coordinated involuntary motor activity, also known as automatism. About 75% of patients experience orobuccolingual movements, while the remaining 50% exhibit other facial, neck, or hand movements. Bilateral limb movements, fumbling with objects, and sitting up or standing are less common. There could be a secondary generalization of the seizure.

8.2.3. Diagnosis

Based on the clinical identification of one of the previously described seizure types, a seizure diagnosis is made. When separating seizures from other causes of loss of consciousness, the EEG can be a useful confirmatory test (Figure 8.4). A normal or mildly abnormal EEG, however, never rules out the diagnosis of epilepsy. Spike-wave complexes, polyspike discharges, and aberrant spikes are specific EEG characteristics that are suggestive of epilepsy.

Table 8.3 presents a standard diagnostic evaluation for patients who have recently started having seizures. Since they don't require anticonvulsants, metabolic and toxic disorders that can cause seizures (Table 8.1) should be ruled out.

It's important to get a seizure evaluated right away to rule out a structural brain lesion if it's clearly focal or starts after age 25. Computed tomography (CT) scans are insufficient for this purpose; magnetic resonance imaging (MRI) is necessary. The likelihood of recurrence should be taken into consideration when deciding whether to start long-term anticonvulsant therapy if no cause is identified. In 30 to 70% of untreated adult patients, recurrence of one or more seizures can be anticipated within 3 to 4 years following a single generalized tonic-clonic seizure.

8.2.4. Treatment

8.2.4.1. Principles of Treatment

If the cause of the seizures is known, therapy should focus on that. Anticonvulsants typically have little effect on seizures linked to metabolic and systemic disorders, but they stop when the underlying abnormality is corrected. Self-limited seizures resulting from acute withdrawal from alcohol and other sedative drugs typically do not require anticonvulsant medication therapy. Anticonvulsant medication therapy must be used to control convulsions caused by acute head trauma and other structural brain lesions as soon as possible. Anticonvulsants are used to treat idiopathic epilepsy.

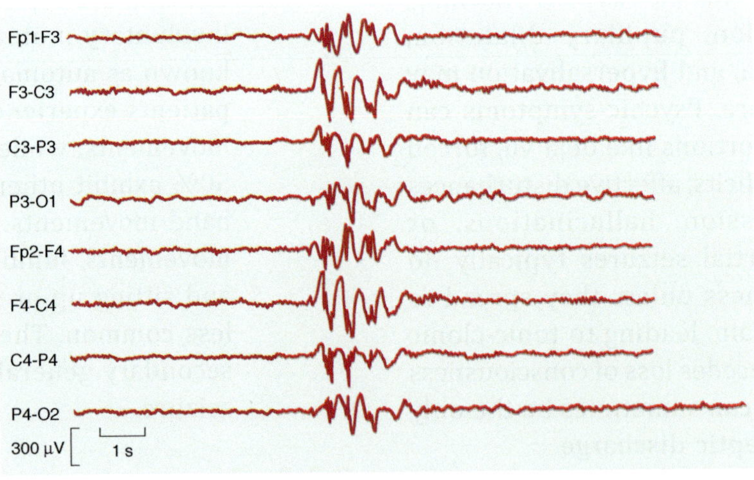

Figure 8.4. EEG of a patient with idiopathic (primary generalized) epilepsy. A burst of generalized epileptiform activity (center) is seen on a relatively normal background. These findings, obtained at a time when the patient was not experiencing seizures, support the clinical diagnosis of epilepsy. Odd-numbered leads indicate electrode placements over the left side of the head; even numbers, over the right side.

Source: https://dl.mehrsys.ir/pdf-books/Clinical%20Neurology%209%20Edition%20(www.myuptodate.com).pdf.

Table 8.3. Evaluation of a New Seizure Disorder in a Stable Patient

History (including medications and drug exposure)
General physical examination
Complete neurologic examination
Blood studies
Fasting glucose
Serum electrolytes
Serum calcium
Renal function studies
Hepatic function studies
Complete blood count
Serum FTA-ABS
EEG (abnormal in 20%-60% of first EEGs; 60%-90% with repeated EEGs)
Brain MRI (especially with abnormal neurologic examination, progressive disorder, or onset of seizures after age 25 years)

Source: https://dl.mehrsys.ir/pdf-books/Clinical%20Neurology%209%20Edition%20(www.myuptodate.com).pdf.

There are four key principles of management:

- **Establish the Diagnosis of Epilepsy Before Starting Drug Therapy**: Therapeutic trials of anticonvulsant drugs intended to establish or reject a diagnosis of epilepsy may yield incorrect diagnoses.
- **Choose the Right Drug for the Seizure Type**: Absence seizures, for example, do not respond to most drugs used for complex partial or generalized tonic–clonic seizures.
- **Treat the Seizures, Rather Than the Serum Drug Levels:** Control of seizures is achieved at different drug levels in different patients.
- **Evaluate One Drug at a Time:** In most cases, seizures can be controlled with a single drug. Therefore, beginning therapy with multiple drugs may expose patients to increased drug toxicity without added therapeutic benefit.

8.2.4.2. Anticonvulsant Drug

The majority of anticonvulsants work in the brain by either blocking excitatory (glutamatergic) or potentiating inhibitory (GABAergic) synaptic transmission. Figure 8.5 shows drugs that act at GABAergic synapses and their molecular targets; Figure 8.6 shows drugs that act at glutamatergic synapses and their molecular targets. Table 8.4 lists common anticonvulsant medications along with their dosages and modes of administration.

8.2.4.3. Treatment Strategies

Most patients with epilepsy fall into one of the following treatment categories.

- **New Seizures:** After a single seizure, the majority of epileptologists do not advise long-term anticonvulsant medication therapy unless an underlying cause is identified, such as a brain tumor, that is likely to result in recurrent seizures and cannot be treated. Nonetheless, anticonvulsant medication is necessary for recurrent seizures, and oral loading schedules, as shown in Table 8.4, can be employed if this kind of therapy is to be given. It should be noted that starting a medication at its daily maintenance dose results in stable drug levels in the serum only after about five half-lives have passed. For this reason, loading doses should be administered to patients who have seizures frequently in order to quickly reach therapeutic drug levels.
    - **Partial (Including Complex Partial) or Secondarily Generalized Tonic–Clonic Seizures**: Phenytoin, carbamazepine, oxcarbazepine, levetiraceatam, topiramate, zonisamide, sodium valproate and lamotrigine are appropriate drugs of first choice for treating these seizure types. Aside from ethosuximide (and perhaps rufinamide), all currently available seizure medications have demonstrated efficacy in treating partial seizures. As none of the newest medications (including lacosamide, perampanel, ezogabine, and eslicarbazepine) have demonstrated superior efficacy or side-effect profiles, they should not be used for initial therapy. Gabapentin is usually not used for initial seizure treatment as its short half-life is a significant limitation. Tiagabine, felbamate, vigabatrin, barbiturates, and benzodiazepines are not used for initial treatment due to their side-effect profiles.
    - **Generalized Seizures:** Valproic acid is effective for all types of primary generalized seizures, but is not recommended as the initial treatment in women of childbearing age because of its potential teratogenicity. Similarly, levetiracetam, topiramate, lamotrigine, and zonisamide can be used successfully in generalized epilepsies.
    - **Absence Seizures:** Absence attacks of the petit mal variety are treated with sodium valproate or ethosuximide. The former has the advantage of also protecting tonic–clonic seizures but has caused fatalities from hepatic damage in children younger than 10 (usually < 2) years of age. Levetiracetam, topiramate, zonisamide and lamotrigine may also be used for absence seizures. As with valproate, they protect tonic– clonic seizures, as well.
    - **Myoclonic Seizures:** These are treated with sodium valproate, levetiracetam, zonisamide, or clonazepam.
- **Recurrent Seizures on Drug Therapy**
    - **Determining Serum Levels of Drugs:** Blood levels of anticonvulsant drugs the patient has been taking should be measured in samples taken just before a scheduled dose. For a single breakthrough seizure, no acute change in medication is mandated, even if there has been no interruption of drug therapy and anticonvulsant drug levels are in the therapeutic range, but a slight increase in

prescribed dose may be considered. If the history or serum drug levels suggest that treatment has been interrupted, the prescribed drug should be started again as for new seizures.

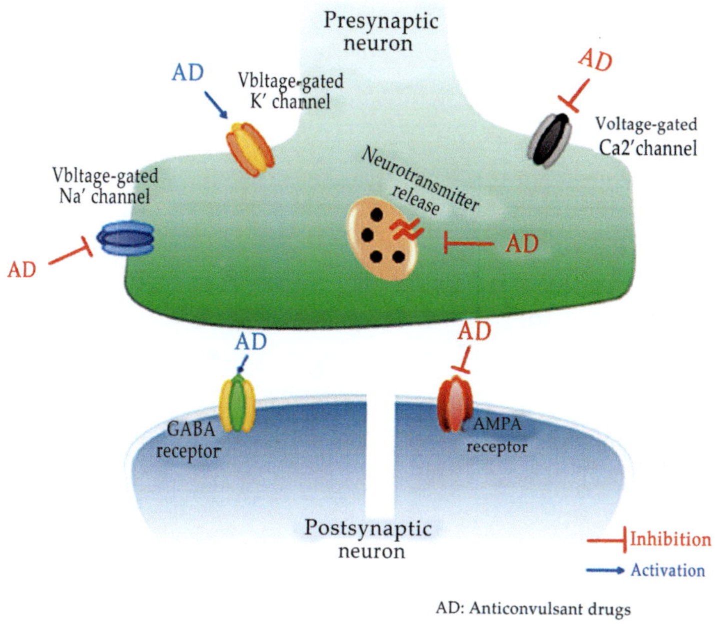

Figure 8.5. Known and potential sites of action of anticonvulsant drugs at inhibitory GABAergic synapses: (1) GABA transporters (tiagabine); (2) GABA transaminase (vigabatrin); (3) GABAA receptors (benzodiazepines, barbiturates); and (4) GABAB receptors. Abbreviations: GABA-T, GABA transaminase; GAT, GABA transporter; VG, voltage-gated ion channel; (N) and (T), calcium channel subtypes. Small circles in the intercellular space represent GABA molecules.

Source: da Fonsêca DV, da Silva Maia Bezerra Filho C, Lima TC, de Almeida RN, de Sousa DP. Anticonvulsant Essential Oils and Their Relationship with Oxidative Stress in Epilepsy. *Biomolecules*. 2019; 9(12):835. https://doi.org/10.3390/biom9120835.

- o **Changing to a Different Drug:** A different anticonvulsant should be introduced only if seizures continue to occur after maximum therapeutic benefit has been achieved with the initial drug. This means that blood levels of the drug are in the therapeutic range and that drug toxicity precludes further dosage increments. An anticonvulsant that has failed to alter seizure frequency should be discontinued gradually once therapeutic levels of the new drug have been achieved. Transition to monotherapy with a different drug is recommended before trials of two-drug combination therapy.

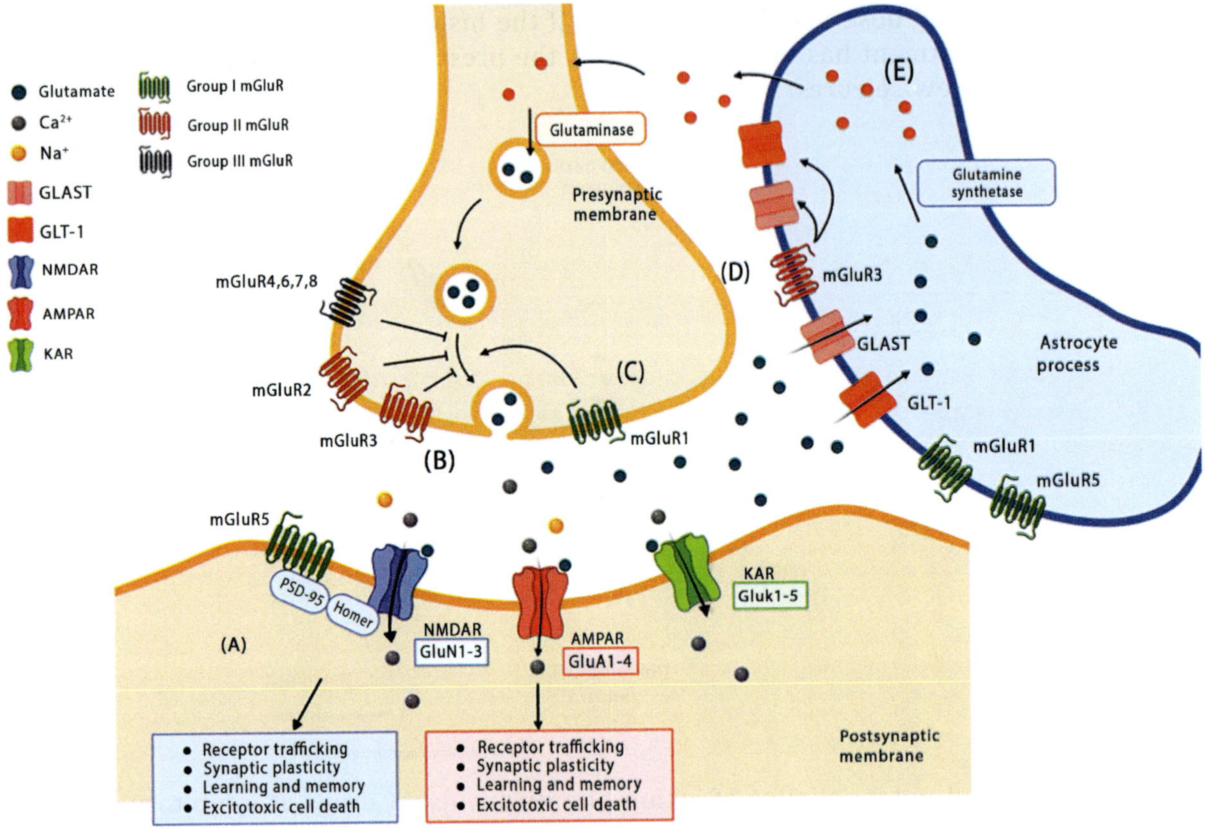

Figure 8.6. Known and potential sites of action of anticonvulsant drugs at excitatory glutamatergic synapses: (1) voltage-gated sodium channels (phenytoin, carbamazepine, lamotrigine); (2) voltage-gated calcium channels (ethosuximide, lamotrigine, gabapentin, pregabalin); (3) voltage-gated potassium channels; (4) synaptic vesicle glycoprotein 2A (levetiracetam); (5) collapsin-related mediator protein-2; (6) AMPA-preferring glutamate receptors (phenobarbital, topiramate, lamotrigine); (7) NMDA-preferring glutamate receptors (felbamate). Abbreviations: EAAT, excitatory amino acid transporter; mGluR, metabotropic glutamate receptor; (N), (P/Q) and (T), calcium channel subtypes; NTFs, neurotrophic factors. Small circles in the intercellular space represent glutamate molecules.

Source: Chen T-S, Huang T-H, Lai M-C, Huang C-W. The Role of Glutamate Receptors in Epilepsy. *Biomedicines*. 2023; 11(3):783. https://doi.org/10.3390/biomedicines11030783.

- **Treating refractory seizures:** In some patients, disabling seizures persist despite trials of major anticonvulsants, alone and in combination, and at the highest doses the patient can tolerate. When no treatable cause can be found, seizures are not due to a progressive neurodegenerative disease, and medical treatment has been unsuccessful for at least 2 years, evaluation for possible surgical therapy should be considered.

Table 8.4. Summary of Anticonvulsant Drug Therapy

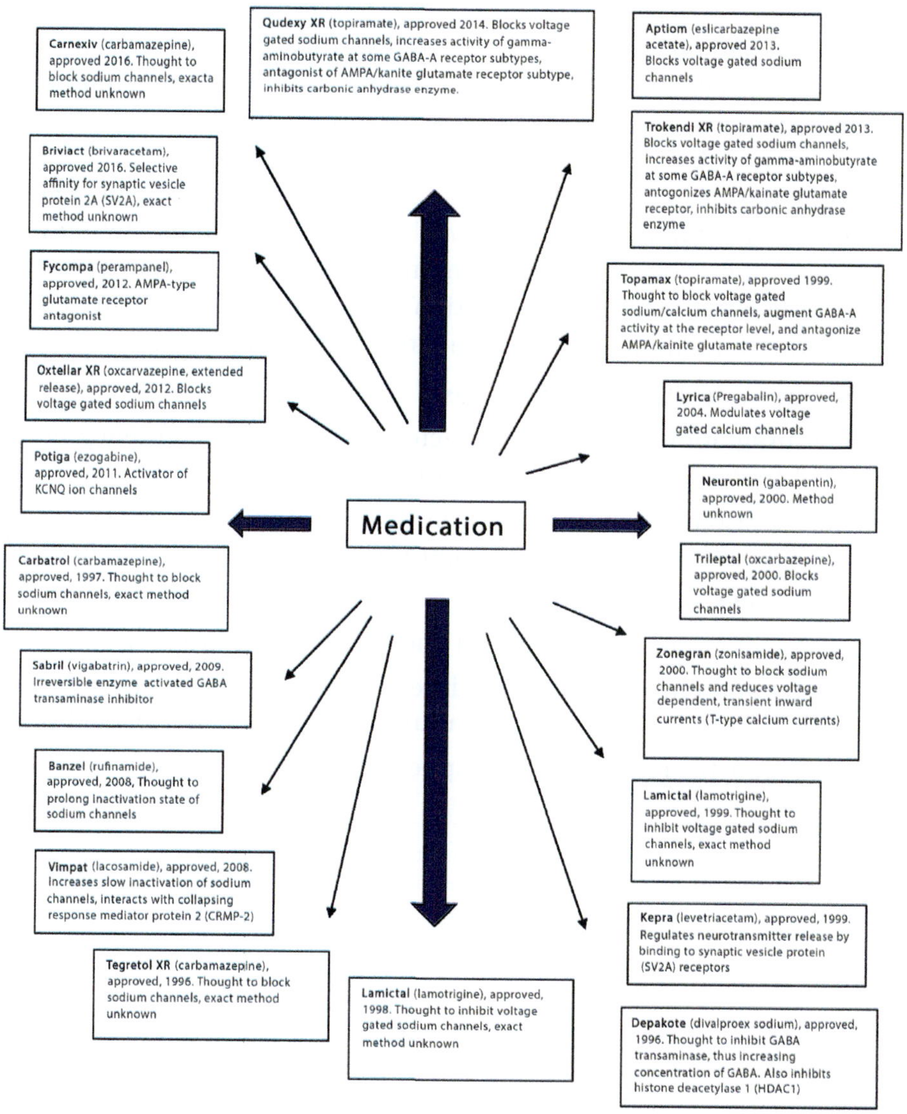

Source: Smolarz B, Makowska M, Romanowicz H. Pharmacogenetics of Drug-Resistant Epilepsy (Review of Literature). *International Journal of Molecular Sciences.* 2021; 22(21):11696. https://doi.org/10.3390/ijms222111696.

A thorough history and neurologic examination are the first steps in the presurgical evaluation process. These are used to determine the origin of seizures, where they occur in the brain, and whether previous medical treatments were effective. The epileptogenic zone of the brain is located through electrophysiologic and magnetic resonance imaging (MRI) investigations. Numerous electrophysiologic techniques are available for use: intracranial or invasive EEG, which records activity from electrodes placed over the surface of the brain (subdural electrodes) or inserted into the brain (depth electrodes); electrocorticography, which records activity from the surface of the brain intraoperatively; and EEG, which records cerebral electrical activity from the scalp noninvasively. Surgical excision may be necessary when an epileptogenic zone can be identified in this way and its removal is not anticipated to cause undue neurologic impairment.

Approximately 50% of patients with complex partial seizures originating from a single temporal lobe are candidates for surgery; a unilateral anterior temporal lobectomy eliminates seizures and auras in 25% of these patients and significantly lowers their frequency in the remaining 25%. For the treatment of intractable epilepsy, hemispherectomy and corpus callosum section are occasionally employed. It has been demonstrated that stimulating the left vagal (X) nerve can reduce the frequency of seizures in adults and children with refractory epilepsy by up to 50%. Afferent responses from the vagus nerve are received in the nucleus tractus solitarius in the medulla and project widely, though the exact mechanism of action is unknown. Two cutting-edge experimental therapies are deep brain stimulation and transcranial magnetic stimulation.

- **Multiple Seizures or Status Epilepticus**
    - **Early Management**: Status epilepticus is a medical emergency because of its potential to cause irreversible brain injury and death.
        - Immediate attention should be given to ensure that the airway is patent and the patient is positioned to prevent aspiration of stomach contents.
        - The laboratory studies listed in Table 8.5 should be ordered without delay.
        - Dextrose (50 mL of 50% solution) should be given intravenously.
        - Meningitis and encephalitis should be considered, especially if fever and meningeal signs are present, and a lumbar puncture performed if indicated.

Table 8.5. Advanced Diagnostic Techniques for Epilepsy

Name of Imaging Technique	Study Population/ Disease Model	Indication	Location/ Tissue Examined	Effect in Epilepsy	AUC	Ref.
T1 and T2 weighted MRI	4-AP-induced seizures in rats	Diagnostic biomarker of epilepsy	Brain	In the cerebral cortex, hippocampus, amygdala, and medial thalamus, T2 relaxation time changes (recovered completely after 3 days)	-------	[3]
TSPO-PET	Kainic acid-induced SE in rats	Predictive biomarker of SE and SRS	Brain	Unregulated TSPO expression 14 days post-SE predicts SRS frequency and comorbidities associated with chronic SE	-------	[52]

iECEEG scalp EEG	Epileptic foci vs. other brain areas in humans assessed during epilepsy surgery	Diagnostic biomarker to identify epileptic foci	Brain	Existence of HFOs Conventional HFOs with waveform similarity Spikes	--------	**[89]**
fMRI	Patients with IGE vs. healthy controls	Diagnostic and predictive biomarker of IGE	Brain	Reduced DNM functional connectivity between anterior and posterior cortical seeds, seizure duration is positively associated with RSFC between Para hippocampal gyri and the PCC and negatively associated with connectivity between PCC and frontal lobe	---------	**[90]**
TARC/sICAM5 ratio assisted with video-EEG monitoring	Patients with focal epilepsy	Diagnostic biomarker for drug-resistant focal epilepsy	Blood/plasma	Increased TARC/sICAM5 ratio of these two proteins serves a vital role in epileptogenesis, as one is inducer of inflammation and the other inhibits it.	1.000	**[91]**
PET	Kainic acid-induced SE in rats	Diagnostic biomarker of SE	Brain	Decreased GABA receptor density and affinity in the hippocampus	---------	**[92]**

MRI	Hyperthermia-induced SE rats, with or without epilepsy	Diagnostic biomarker of epilepsy or prognostic biomarker of epilepsy development in hyperthermia-induced SE rats	Brain tissue regions–amygdala, thalamus	T2 relaxation time decreased in basolateral and medial amygdala	0.910 (Basolateral amygdala) 0.820 (Medial amygdala)	[93]
FDG-PET	Pilocarpine-induced SE	Diagnostic biomarker of SE	Brain	Decreased glucose metabolism, along with decreased brain connectivity	---------	[94]
PET	Pilocarpine-induced SE in rats	Diagnostic biomarker of SE	Brain	Decrease in global mGluR5 metabotropic glutamate receptor. Decreased focal in amygdala and hippocampus during chronic SE	--------	[95]
MRI	PTZ-induced seizures test in seizure susceptible or non-susceptible rats after TBI induction	Diagnostic biomarker of augmented seizure susceptibility after TBI	Brain tissue–cortex, hippocampus, thalamus	Decreased T2 relaxation time in medial thalamus	0.780	[96]
				Appearance of T1σ in S1 cortex, S1 HC, and Prh cortex	0.881 (S1 cortex) 0.857 (S1 HC) 0.929 (Prh cortex)	
				Appearance of T2 in the thalamus	0.893	
DTI-MRI	Patients with h benign vs. refractory mTLE (age and sex-harmonized)	Diagnostic biomarker for drug-resistant mTLE	Brain tissue–temporal lobe gray and white matter	Increased ipsilateral MD	0.670	[97]
				Decreased ipsilateral FA	0.770	
				Decreased ipsilateral HC volume	0.670	

FDG-PET	Pilocarpine-induced TLE	Prognostic biomarker of TLE	Brain	Decreased glucose metabolism in the hippocampus at the latent phase of the disease and neuronal loss	-------	[98]
DTI/DWI-MRI	Right and left TLE patients vs. healthy individuals	Diagnostic biomarker for TLE	Brain tissue–anterior corpus callosum	Reduced local diffusion homogeneity	RmTLE 0.935 LmTLE 0.919	[99]
MRS	Kainic acid-induced SE and amygdala kindling in rats	Biomarker of epilepsy	Brain	Sodium selenate prevents changes in mIns, NAA levels, volumetric changes, and FA	---------	[100]
T1 and T2 weighted MRI	Lithium–pilocarpine-induced SE in rats	Diagnostic biomarker of SE	Brain	T2 in the amygdala after 30 days of SE induction, strongly correlated with hyperactivity in the novel open field	--------	[101]
T1 and T2 weighted MRI	Kainic acid-induced MTLE in mouse	Diagnostic biomarker of MTLE	Brain	Hippocampal paroxysmal discharges (number and duration) are associated with T2 relaxation time	--------	[102]
Gadolinium-MRI	Patients with epilepsy vs. without epilepsy after TBI	Diagnostic biomarker for PTE in patients with TBI	Cerebral cortex	Area of gadolinium leakage around cortical lesion after TBI	0.850	[103]
Intracortical EEG	Rats having epilepsy vs. rats deprived of epilepsy after lateral fluid-percussion-induced TBI	Diagnostic biomarker for PTE in rats after lateral fluid-percussion induced TBI	Brain	Incidence of perilesional pHFOs and rHFOSs throughout the first 2 post-TBI weeks only in rats that will grow PTE	---------	[104]

MRS	Pilocarpine-induced SE -P21 rats which develop epilepsy vs. P21 rats which does not develop epilepsy	Diagnostic and prognostic biomarker for epilepsy and SE	Septal pole of the hippocampus	Augmented hippocampal mIns/tCr after 72 days of SE induction	0.830	**[105]**
MRS	Pilocarpine-induced SE in rats	Biomarker of SE	Brain	Increased expression of mIns post SE induction	-------	**[105]**
Combination of EEG and fMRI	Kainic acid-induced SE in Rhesus Monkey	Diagnostic biomarker of SE	Brain	Functional brain network disruption in chronic SE	------	**[106]**
MRI	Rats with or deprived of epilepsy after paraoxan-induced SE	Diagnostic and prognostic biomarker for epilepsy and SE	BBB pathology in the piriform network	Amplified T2-weighted signal	0.720	**[107]**
HMGB1-acetylated	65 patients with drug-resistant epilepsy and electrically induced rat SE model	Diagnostic biomarker for drug refractoriness	plasma	Acts on RAGE and TLR and increased expression in epilepsy	1	**[108]**
HMGB1- total	65 patients with drug-resistant epilepsy and electrically induced rat SE model	Diagnostic biomarker for epileptogenesis	plasma	Acts on RAGE and TLR and increased expression in epilepsy	1	**[108]**
HMGB1- bisulfide	65 patients with drug-resistant epilepsy and electrically induced rat SE model	Prognostic biomarker for SE	plasma	Acts on RAGE and TLR and increased expression in epilepsy	1	**[108]**
Diffusion MRI	Kainic acid and pilocarpine-induced SE in rats	Diagnostic biomarker of SE	Brain	Longitudinal changes in hippocampal diffusion due to astrocyte processes	-------	**[109]**

Diffusion MRI	Spontaneous recurrent seizures in cats	Diagnostic biomarker of epilepsy	Brain	Microstructural changes and hypoperfusion in the hippocampus and parietal cortex during ictal periods in cats	-------	**[110]**
Sleep EEG	Rats having epilepsy vs. rats deprived of epilepsy after lateral fluid-percussion-induced TBI	Diagnostic biomarker for PTE in rats after lateral fluid-percussion-induced TBI	Brain	Decrease of the extend of sleep occurrence of spindles at conversion from N3 to REM	0.907	**[111]**
Electrophysiology Interictal VEP-visual hyper excitability assessed using contrast response function	Patients having idiopathic generalized epilepsy vs. healthy individuals	Diagnostic biomarker for idiopathic generalized epilepsy	Brain	Relative lack of gain control at high contrasts	0.870	**[112]**
fMRI	17 patients with drug-resistant TLE with good post-operative seizure control vs. healthy controls	Diagnostic biomarker of TLE	Brain	fALFF reduction in ipsilateral amygdala	-------	**[113]**
Diffusion MRI	Spontaneous recurrent seizures in cats	Diagnostic biomarker of epilepsy	Brain	Decreased postictal hippocampal perfusion compared to ictal state	-------	**[114]**
TSPO-PET	Electrically induced SE in rats	Prognostic biomarker of SE	Brain	Unregulated TSPO expression up to 10 weeks after SE induction	-------	**[115]**

Theta dynamics in EEG	Rats with or without epilepsy after photo thrombotic stroke, Rats with or without epilepsy after bilateral hippocampal electrical stimulation-induced SE	Diagnostic biomarker of epilepsy or prognostic biomarker of epilepsy development in rodents having a brain injury	Brain	Absolute slope value of dynamic change in theta band	0.910	**[116]**
PET	Pilocarpine-induced SE in rats	Prognostic and diagnostic biomarker of SE	Brain	48 h after SE induction, the permeability of BBB gets increased in the hippocampus, piriform cortex, thalamus, and amygdala	------	**[117]**
EEG	Patients having acute anterior circulation ischemic stroke, which developed into epilepsy vs. not developed into epilepsy	Diagnostic biomarker of epilepsy or prognostic biomarker of acute anterior circulation ischemic stroke developing into epilepsy	Brain	Background asymmetry, Interictal epileptiform activity	0.810	**[118]**
EEG	Two cohort studies with-Patients having idiopathic generalized epilepsy and generalized spike-wave discharges on EEG, who are drug-resistant vs. drug-responsive	Diagnostic biomarker of drug resistance in idiopathic generalized epilepsy	Brain	Appearance of generalized polyspikes (burst of generalized rhythmic spikes lasting less than 1 s) in EEG during sleep	------	**[119]**
MEG coupled with behavioral evaluation	Human and animal models TLE	Early diagnostic biomarker of TLE	Brain	Coherence and alteration of theta and gamma rhythms	--------	**[120]**

EEG	Three different rodent models of epilepsy	Diagnostic and prognostic biomarker of epilepsy	Brain	Decrease in the non-linear dynamics dimension in EEG	≥0.886 in different models	**[121]**
EEG	A child with type 1 RCDP	Diagnostic biomarker of impending epilepsy	Brain	Transition from normal background to the appearance of focal epileptiform abnormality	-------	**[122]**
Interictal scalp EEG	22 children having CSWS	Predictive biomarker of seizures and cognitive outcome in CSWS	Brain	Presence of interictal HFOs around 80–250 Hz range (ripple band) and they are negatively associated with average IQ	-------	**[123]**
intracranial and scalp EEG	11 patients (6 M, 5 F; age range 21–41 years)	Diagnostic biomarker of postictal generalized EEG suppression	Brain	Delta- gamma phase-amplitude coupling (gradual decrease of phase-frequency in the coupling between delta, 0.5–4 Hz and gamma, 30+ Hz, followed by an increased coupling between the phase of 0.5–1.5 Hz signal and amplitude of 30–50 Hz signal)	-------	**[124]**
Scalp EEG	30 patients, suspected to have infantile spasms	Objective biomarker for active epileptic spasm	Brain	Increased HFO rates and coupling were identified between HFOs and SWA.	0.80–0.98	**[125]**

iEEG	11 patients having TLE (6 M, 5 F)	Diagnostic biomarker of SOZ	Brain	High amplitude of HFOs was observed in SOZs, and measuring the amplitude of HFOs serves a greater advantage over measuring the rate of HFOs, in the case of SOZ identification	0.948–0.960	**[126]**
MRS	35 patients with IGE (avg. age-32) vs. 35 healthy individuals (avg. age-31)	Diagnostic biomarker of IGE	Brain	Upregulated Cr expression in left thalamus (no difference in right thalamus). Downregulated NAA expression in right and left thalamus. Downregulated NAA/Cr ration in right and left thalamus.	-------	**[127]**
^{18}F-FDG-PET/rs-fMRI	Patients with mTLE-HS vs. healthy individuals	Biomarker of epilepsy surgery in patients having mTLE-HS	Bain	Positive correlation between SUVR and rs-fMRI metrics, spatial correlation between SUVR and fMRI across the gray matter, and Higher fALFF/SUVR couplings, suggested altered bioenergetic coupling across gray matter and it was also found to be associated with seizure outcome.	------	**[128]**

[11 C] UCB-J PET	12 patients having TLE vs. 12 healthy controls	Diagnostic and predictive biomarker of TLE		Reduced [11 C] UCB-J binding in the seizure onset zone of patients having TLE		**[129]**
MRS	Kainic acid-induced MTLE in mouse (KA-MTLE model)	Biomarker of epileptic zone in MTLE	Brain	Upregulated GABA expression in the epileptic zone of mouse	------	**[130]**
iEEG	27 patients with SOZ in different parts of the hemisphere	Predictive biomarker of seizures	Brain	Temporal trends in HFO rates can predict preictal state and can differentiate between preictal and interictal periods for a few patients.	0.80	**[131]**

AUC: area under the curve; RCDP: rhizomelic chondrodysplasia punctata; HFO: high-frequency oscillations; SWA: slow-wave activity; iEEG: intracranial electroencephalogram; SOZ: seizure onset zone; CSWS: continuous spike-and-wave during sleep; fALFF: fractional amplitude of low-frequency fluctuations; IGE: idiopathic generalized epilepsy; DNM: default mode network; RSFC: resting-state functional connectivity; PCC: posterior cingulate cortex; 4-AP: 4-aminopyridine; SRS: spontaneous recurrent seizures; Cr: creatine; NAA: N-acetyl aspartate; mTLE-HS: medial temporal lobe epilepsy patients with hippocampal sclerosis; rs-fMRI: resting-state functional MRI; SUVR: 18 F-FDG standardized uptake value ratio; fALFF: fractional amplitude of low-frequency fluctuations.

Source: Bandopadhyay R, Singh T, Ghoneim MM, Alshehri S, Angelopoulou E, Paudel YN, Piperi C, Ahmad J, Alhakamy NA, Alfaleh MA, et al. Recent Developments in Diagnosis of Epilepsy: Scope of MicroRNA and Technological Advancements. *Biology*. 2021; 10(11):1097. https://doi.org/10.3390/biology10111097.

If the cause of the seizures is unknown, patients should also have lumbar punctures unless there are indications of focal brain dysfunction or elevated intracranial pressure. In the absence of infection, postictal pleocytosis is seen in the cerebrospinal fluid (CSF) of about 2% of patients who have a single generalized tonic-clonic seizure (and 15% of those who have status epilepticus). Up to 80/μL of white blood cells may be present, with a polymorphonuclear or mononuclear predominance. While glucose concentration is normal and Gram stain is negative, there may be a slight increase in serum protein content. Within two to five days, the postictal pleocytosis goes away.

- **Drug Therapy to Control Seizures:** Every effort must be made to establish a precise etiologic diagnosis so that treatment of the underlying disorder can be started. Because generalized seizure activity per se damages the brain if it persists for more than 30 minutes, drug therapy to terminate seizures should be instituted immediately. An outline for rapid pharmacologic control of multiple seizures is presented in Table 8.6.

Table 8.6. Prehospital Management of Status Epilepticus. Regardless of the choice of Benzodiazepine, no Increased Frequency of Adverse Outcomes Was Appreciated, as Per the Prehospital Treatment of Status Epilepticus (PHTSE) Trial [2, 17, 22–24, 26, 27].

Benzodiazepines			
Drug and Route	Clinical Application	Dose	Maximum Dose
Lorazepam—IV/IM	Limited use in prehospital setting due to difficulty to stock in emergency vehicles and required refrigeration.	2 mg–4 mg	8 mg
Diazepam—IV/IM/PR	Rectal mucosa allows rapid effectiveness within 5–10 min	5 mg–10 mg	20 mg
Midazolam—IM/SL	All modes of administration can be used safely in prehospital setting.	10 mg (5 mg if <50 kg)	10 mg

* PO = per os (mouth), IV = Intravenous, IM = Intramuscular, PR = per rectum, SL = sublingual.

Source: Billington M, Kandalaft OR, Aisiku IP. Adult Status Epilepticus: A Review of the Prehospital and Emergency Department Management. *Journal of Clinical Medicine*. 2016; 5(9):74. https://doi.org/10.3390/jcm5090074.

- **Management of Hyperthermia**: The systemic physiologic consequences of status epilepticus are related to increased motor activity and high levels of circulating catecholamines; they include hyperthermia (temperature elevation to 42–43°C [108–109°F] in the absence of infection), lactic acidosis (pH < 7.00), and peripheral blood leukocytosis (elevation to 30,000 cells/µL). These derangements resolve after cessation of the seizures. Only hyperthermia, which is known to increase the risk of brain damage from status epilepticus, requires specific attention. Severe hyperthermia must be treated with a cooling blanket and, if necessary, the induction of motor paralysis with a neuromuscular blocking agent. Mild or moderate hyperthermia (101–102°F), not requiring specific intervention, may persist for 24 to 48 hours after seizure cessation. Lactic acidosis resolves spontaneously over 1 hour and should not be treated. Infection should, of course, be excluded.

8.2.4.4. Discontinuing Anticonvulsants

Patients with epilepsy (usually children) who have been seizure-free for two to five years while taking medication may want to stop taking anticonvulsants. The chance of a seizure recurrence in patients with normal intelligence and neurologic examination may be as low as 25%. Recurrence risk factors include EEG slowing or spikes (maximum risk when both are present). When anticonvulsants are to be stopped, one medication at a time is weaned off gradually for about six weeks. After stopping medication, recurrence of seizures has been observed in about 20% of children and 40% of adults; in these cases, previous medication should be resumed at the previously efficacious dosages.

8.2.4.5. Complications of Epilepsy and Anticonvulsant Therapy

- **Complications of Epilepsy:** Following an epilepsy diagnosis, the patient should be informed of the dangers of swimming alone and cautioned against working near moving machinery or at heights. There is also the matter of driving. Notifying the state government of an epilepsy diagnosis is required in many states.
- **Side Effects of Anticonvulsant Drugs:** Anticonvulsant medications almost universally carry the risk of hepatic toxicity and blood dyscrasias. Because of this, tests for liver function and a complete blood count should be performed both before starting these medications and periodically while the patient is receiving treatment. The tests should be run twice during the first few weeks to months and then every six to twelve months after that, according to the authors. In the first eight weeks of treatment, lamotrigine has a 1:1000 incidence of Stevens-Johnson syndrome. Even at therapeutic dosages, the majority of anticonvulsant medications, particularly barbiturates, have some effect on cognitive function.

Table 8.7. Examples of Barriers to Epilepsy Diagnosis and Treatment

Epilepsy diagnostic status	Barriers
Pre-diagnosis	• Distance to healthcare facility • Local customs or beliefs • Lack of seizure unknowledge • Superstitions • Discrimination and stigma • Lack of family/social support • Denial or minimization of symptoms • Lack of diagnostic services (e.g., EEG) • Poor healthcare worker education
Post-diagnosis	• Cost and availability of medications • Side effects of medications • Inefficacy of medications • Cost of medications • Medication non-compliance • Drug resistance • Distance to healthcare facility • Cost of medical care • Lack of specialists • Lack of seizure/epilepsy education • Lack of caregiver support • Discrimination and stigma • Medical comorbidities

Source: Pellinen J (2022) Treatment gaps in epilepsy. Front. Epidemiol. 2:976039. doi: 10.3389/fepid.2022.976039.

- **Drug Interactions:** The metabolism and absorption of anticonvulsants can be affected by several medications when taken concurrently. Table 8.8 provides a summary of the anticonvulsant level changes. Oral contraceptives may become less effective as a result of the cytochrome P450 system being induced by several anticonvulsants, including carbamazepine, primidone, phenytoin, phenobarbital, topiramate, felbamate, and oxcarbazepine.

Table 8.8. Some Major Anticonvulsant Drug Interactions

Drug combinations	References	Efficacy	Potential drug-drug interaction and side effects	Seizure types and/or epileptic syndromes
VPA + LTG	(51)	VPA + LTG > CBZ or PHT+ LTG	VPA-LTG combination shows supra-additive or additive effects. VPA acts as an enzymatic metabolic inhibitor, thus the addition of LTG to VPA led to a reduction in lamotrigine clearance, resulting in an increase of its plasma concentration. This combination augments the probability of lamotrigine-induced hypersensitivity and the development of both postural and action tremor. Lamotrigine should be slowly titrated with small initial dose.	Focal refractory seizures; no-specified DRE; possible combination therapy for absence seizures (67).
VPA + ETX	(52)	VPA + ETX> VPA or ETX as monotherapy	The interaction between VPA and ETX in terms of pharmacokinetic effects is not clear. It may lead to elevated serum ETX levels, even if neurotoxic effects are less than additive antiseizure effects.	Absence seizures
LTG + LEV	(53)	LTG + LEV > LEV as monotherapy	Supra-additive effect. Levetiracetam has not been reported to cause relevant pharmacokinetic drug interactions. It is not an enzyme-inducer, thus an interaction with LCM seems unlikely.	Idiopathic generalized epilepsy and post-traumatic focal epilepsy

LCM + LEV	(54, 55)	LCM + LEV > LCM + other ASMs (e.g., VPA, TPM, PB)	Supra-additive effect (may be due to different mechanism of actions). A clinically relevant interaction between LEV with LCM seems unlikely. Attention must be paid to using LCM in patients with arrhythmias or long QT syndrome and LEV in patients with neuropsychiatric disorders.	Focal onset seizures in adults.
VPA + CLB + STP	(58–60)	VPA + CLB + STP >>> VPA + CLB in duotherapy	The supra-additive effect of the STP-CLB combination may be due to pharmacokinetic drug interactions, as STP is known to act by inhibiting the metabolism of norclobazam, thus increasing its serum levels and possibly leading to more side effects (neurotoxicity effect). Common side effects are drowsiness and loss of appetite.	Dravet Syndrome

Source: Fattorusso A, Matricardi S, Mencaroni E, Dell'Isola GB, Di Cara G, Striano P and Verrotti A (2021) The Pharmacoresistant Epilepsy: An Overview on Existant and New Emerging Therapies. Front. Neurol. 12:674483. doi: 10.3389/fneur.2021.674483.

- **Epilepsy and Anticonvulsant Therapy in Pregnancy**
  - **Teratogenic Effects of Epilepsy:** The incidence of stillbirth, microcephaly, mental retardation, and seizure disorders is increased in children born to epileptic mothers.
  - **Teratogenic Effects of Anticonvulsant Treatment:** Anticonvulsant therapy during pregnancy is also associated with a greater than normal frequency of congenital malformations—especially cleft palate, cleft lip, and cardiac anomalies. Such malformations are about twice as common in the offspring of medicated than of unmedicated epileptic mothers, but because patients with more severe epilepsy are more likely to be treated, it is difficult to know whether epilepsy or its treatment is the more important risk factor.
  - **Differences in Teratogenesis Among Anticonvulsants:** Among commonly used anticonvulsants, valproic acid and to some degree carbamazepine are associated with an increased incidence of neural tube defects (2% and 0.5%, respectively). Teratogenic effects have been reported with most established anticonvulsants and some (e.g., phenytoin) have been implicated in causing a specific pattern of defects. Based on current data, the safest anticonvulsant in pregnancy is lamotrigine. Levetiracetam also appears safe.

- **Folate Deficiency:** Several anticonvulsants can lower serum folate levels. As dietary deficiency of folic acid is associated with neural tube defects, folate supplementation (1 mg/d) should be provided for all women of childbearing age who take antiepileptic drugs.
- **Withdrawing Anticonvulsants Before Pregnancy:** When an epileptic patient who has been seizure free for several years is contemplating pregnancy, an attempt should be made to assess whether anticonvulsant drugs can be safely withdrawn before conception. In contrast to generalized tonic–clonic seizures, partial and absence seizures present little risk to the fetus, and it may be possible to tolerate imperfect control of these seizures during pregnancy to avoid fetal drug exposure. If anticonvulsant therapy is continued during pregnancy, it is best to maintain treatment with a single drug that has been shown effective for the patient's seizures, using a dose that avoids clinical toxicity. Status epilepticus is treated as described previously for nonpregnant patients.
- **Anticonvulsant Levels in Pregnancy:** Plasma levels of anticonvulsant drugs may decrease during pregnancy because of the patient's enhanced drug metabolism, and higher doses may be required to maintain control of seizures. It is therefore important to monitor drug levels closely in this setting. This is particularly important with lamotrigine as the dose often needs to be doubled or tripled during pregnancy to maintain adequate blood levels.

8.2.5. Prognosis

Just about one-third of patients will experience another unprovoked seizure within three to five years, meaning they will not develop epilepsy. However, the chance of a subsequent seizure approaching 75% means that anticonvulsants should be initiated if a second seizure happens. Most patients can have their seizures well controlled, if not completely eliminated, with the right anticonvulsant medication treatment. Patients should see a doctor a few months after starting treatment in order to monitor seizure frequency and adjust dosage.

8.3. Syncope

An intermittent loss of consciousness accompanied by a change in postural tone is known as syncope. The pathophysiology is different from that of seizures, involving global hypoperfusion of the brain or brainstem. Table 8.9 to the most common causes of syncope.

8.3.1. Vasovagal Syncope (Simple Faints)

Vasovagal syncope affects people of all ages. Genetic influences might be important. Emotional stimulation, pain, seeing blood, exhaustion, medical equipment, blood loss, and extended periods of immobility are examples of precipitating factors. Syncope and CNS hypoperfusion are caused by vagally mediated reductions in arterial blood pressure and heart rate. There is a chance that cerebral ischemia will cause transient tonic-clonic movements.

Vasovagal episodes rarely start in a horizontal position (such as during phlebotomy or the insertion of an intrauterine device); instead, they usually start when the patient is standing or sitting. Syncope is typically preceded by a 30- to 60-second prodrome that can include tachycardia, lassitude, yawning, nausea, pallor, diaphoresis, salivation, and blurred vision.

Table 8.9. Common Causes of Syncope (TLOC: Temporay Loss of Consciousness)

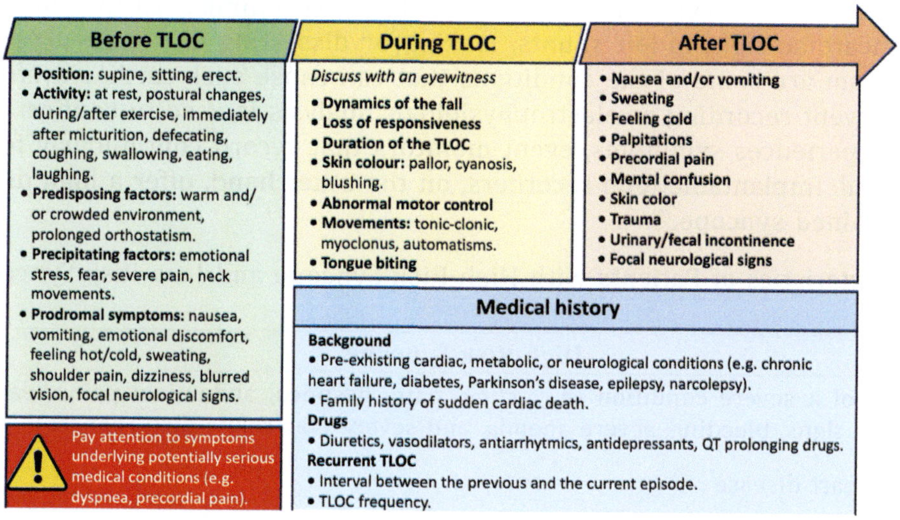

Source: Martone AM, Parrini I, Ciciarello F, Galluzzo V, Cacciatore S, Massaro C, Giordano R, Giani T, Landi G, Gulizia MM, et al. Recent Advances and Future Directions in Syncope Management: A Comprehensive Narrative Review. *Journal of Clinical Medicine.* 2024; 13(3):727. https://doi.org/10.3390/jcm13030727.

The patient is often pale, diaphoretic, and has dilated pupils before losing consciousness and collapsing to the floor. Breathing keeps going. The globes are turning upward while the eyes stay open. As consciousness wanes, tachycardia gives way to bradycardia. Abnormal movements may occur during unconsciousness, especially if the patient is largely vertical. These movements are primarily tonic or opisthotonic, but seizure-like tonic-clonic activity can occasionally be observed, which can result in an incorrect epilepsy diagnosis. Incontinence of the urine may also happen.

After assuming the horizontal position, the patient regains consciousness very quickly (20–30 seconds), though there may be some lingering anxiety, headache, nausea, dizziness, pallor, diaphoresis, and the urge to urinate. Either there is no postictal confusional state with agitation and disorientation, or it lasts for less than 30 seconds. Recurrence of syncope is possible, particularly if the patient stands for the next half hour.

Usually, the only interventions required are reassurance and advice to steer clear of triggers. By causing syncope during a head-up tilt test, recurrent vasovagal syncope—also known as neurally mediated or neurocardiogenic syncope—can be identified. The selective serotonin reuptake inhibitor paroxetine (10–40 mg/d) or the alpha-agonist midodrine (5 mg three times daily) can both relieve the bradycardia and hypotension associated with syncope. Tilt training might be advantageous. Artificial pacing doesn't work.

8.3.2. Cardiovascular Syncope

When syncope happens in a recumbent position, during or after physical exertion, or in a patient who has a known heart condition, a cardiovascular cause is suggested. The most common cause of cardiac disease-related loss of consciousness is an abrupt drop in cardiac output, which leads to cerebral hypoperfusion. Cardiac arrest, brady- or tachyarrhythmias, cardiac inflow or outflow obstruction, intracardiac right-to-left shunts, leaking or dissecting aortic aneurysms, and acute pulmonary embolism are some of the conditions that can cause such cardiac dysfunction (Table 8.10). Long-term event recording or electrophysiologic analysis is used to confirm the diagnosis. When a patient experiences symptoms, event monitors that record continuously for up to three years may be useful. Implantable loop recorders, on the other hand, offer a high diagnostic yield in cases of unexplained syncope.

Table 8.10. Characteristics of Patients with High-Risk Syncope and Low-Risk Syncope

	High-Risk Syncope
•	"Red flags" of a severe condition (e.g., chest pain, dyspnea, abdominal pain, headache, focal neurological signs, bleeding, severe anemia, and severe electrolyte disturbances)
•	Structural heart disease
•	Syncope in the supine position or during exercise
•	Sudden onset of palpitations followed by syncope
•	Family history of sudden death at a young age
•	Absence of prodromes or short prodromes and structural heart disease/abnormal ECG
•	Syncope in the sitting position and structural heart disease/abnormal ECG
•	Unexplained BP < 90 mmHg
•	Unknown systolic murmur
•	Major ECG criteria for cardiac syncope:
o	Signs of acute ischemia;
o	Second-degree AV block Mobitz II or third-degree AV block;
o	Low ventricular response atrial fibrillation (<40 bpm), sinus bradycardia (<40 bpm), or repetitive sinoatrial block or pauses > 3 s and weakness at the rest state;
o	Bundle-branch block;
o	Intraventricular conduction disturbance;
o	Ventricular hypertrophy or Q waves (ischemic heart disease or cardiomyopathy);
o	Sustained/not sustained VT;
o	PM or ICD malfunction;

o Brugada pattern;
o QTc interval > 460 ms in repeated 12-lead ECG (long QT syndrome).
• Minor ECG criteria (suggesting syncope of cardiac origin only if the history is consistent with arrhythmic syncope):
o Second-degree AV block Mobitz I and first-degree AV block with a long PR interval;
o Bifascicular block;
o Mild sinus bradycardia (40–50 bpm);
o Unexplained or low ventricular rate response AF (40–50 bpm) without negative chronotropic drugs;
o Signs of early repolarization;
o Ventricular hypertrophy signs consistent with hypertrophic cardiomyopathy;
o Paroxysmal VT and AF;
o Short QT interval;
o Atypical Brugada patterns;
o Negative T-waves in right precordial leads;
o Epsilon waves (right ventricular arrhythmogenic cardiomyopathy).
Low-Risk Syncope
• Definite criteria for classic vasovagal syncope (e.g., emotional triggers or prolonged orthostatism associated with typical prodromal symptoms);
• Definite criteria for situational syncope (e.g., during/immediately after urination, coughing, defecation, swallowing, or laughing);
• Definite criteria for orthostatic syncope (e.g., documented OH after prolonged standing, temporal link with the beginning or changes in vasodilator therapy, TLOC preceded by pain radiating from the neck to the shoulders and trunk).
o Definite criteria for reflex syncope (e.g., absence of cardiac disease, long history of syncope, syncope after typical triggers even without prodromes, after exercise, after neck compression/rotation, syncope without triggering factors but preceded/followed by nausea and/or vomiting, TLOC in the supine position but preceded by nausea, abdominal pain, or urgency to defecate.

Abbreviations: AF: atrial fibrillation; AV: atrioventricular; BP: blood pressure; ECG: electrocardiogram; ICD: implantable cardiac defibrillator; OH: orthostatic hypotension; PM: pacemaker; QTc: corrected QT interval; TLOC: temporary loss of consciousness; VT: ventricular tachycardia.

Source: Martone AM, Parrini I, Ciciarello F, Galluzzo V, Cacciatore S, Massaro C, Giordano R, Giani T, Landi G, Gulizia MM, et al. Recent Advances and Future Directions in Syncope Management: A Comprehensive Narrative Review. *Journal of Clinical Medicine*. 2024; 13(3):727. https://doi.org/10.3390/jcm13030727.

8.3.2.1. Cardiac Arrest

Any cause of cardiac arrest (ventricular fibrillation or asystole) will cause the patient to lose consciousness in 3–5 seconds if they are standing or in 15 seconds if they are lying down. As cerebral hypoperfusion lasts longer, seizures and fecal and urine incontinence may occur.

8.3.2.2. Tachyarrhythmias

- **Supraventricular Tachyarrhythmias:** Atrial flutter, atrial fibrillation, and other supraventricular tachyarrhythmias can be either paroxysmal or persistent. Palpitations that occur suddenly and briefly may precede syncope.

A heart rate of over 160–200 beats per minute decreases cardiac output through myocardial ischemia or a reduction in the ventricular filling time. Half of normal people in an upright posture will experience syncope from prolonged tachycardia of 180 to 200 beats per minute; in patients with underlying cardiac disease, a heart rate of 135 beats per minute may reduce cardiac output to the point of unconsciousness. When their tachyarrhythmias stop, patients with sinus node dysfunction may experience severe bradycardia or even asystole. When arrhythmias are shown during a symptomatic episode, the diagnosis is made.

Postural tachycardia syndrome (POTS) is a condition that primarily affects young women. It is characterized by an increase in heart rate of 30 beats per minute or more upon standing from a supine position. Other symptoms, such as presyncopal symptoms, are also present. Usually, there is no significant change in blood pressure.

- **Ventricular Tachyarrhythmias:** Prolonged electrocardiogram monitoring of certain syncope patients reveals the presence of ventricular tachyarrhythmias, which include ventricular tachycardia and multiform, frequent, or paired premature ventricular contractions. Ventricular tachycardia-related syncope is distinguished by a very short prodrome (less than 5 seconds). There is a close relationship between the duration of the arrhythmia and syncope. Premature ventricular contractions that occur frequently or repeatedly are indicative of sudden death even though they do not always correspond with syncopal symptoms. Young adults without structural heart disease (Brugada syndrome) who have elevated ST segments in the right precordium are at risk for ventricular arrhythmias and sudden death. Numerous genes have been linked to this, especially those that deal with sodium channels.
- **Mitral Valve Prolapse:** Mitral valve prolapse, also known as click-murmur syndrome, is a common condition that can cause ventricular and supraventricular arrhythmias as well as syncope in a small number of cases. Dyspnea, exhaustion, and nonexertional chest pain are additional symptoms. Bradycardia and severe ventricular arrhythmias could happen. The ECG may exhibit regular premature ventricular contractions, nonspecific ST-T wave changes, or be normal. Echocardiography is used for diagnosis.
- **Prolonged QT Syndrome:** Congenital prolonged QT-interval syndrome is inherited as an autosomal dominant form without

deafness or as an autosomal recessive form with paroxysmal ventricular arrhythmias (usually torsades de pointes), syncope, and sudden death. Potassium channels (KCNE1, KCNE2, KCNH2, KCNJ2, KCNJ5, KCNQ1), sodium channels (SCN4B, SCN5A), calcium channels (CACNA13), A kinase anchor protein 9 (AKAP9), ankyrin 2 (ANK2), caveolin 3 (CAV3), and α-1 syntrophin (SNTA1) are among the genes linked to prolonged QT syndrome. There are also sporadic cases. QT prolongation can also be brought on by antiarrhythmic medications and electrolyte imbalances (hypomagnesemia, hypocalcemia, and hypokalemia). In hereditary cases, β-blockers may be helpful.

8.3.2.3. Bradyarrhythmias

- **Sinoatrial Node Disease:** Diseases of the sinoatrial node (such as sick sinus syndrome) can result in sinus arrest with a slow atrial, junctional, or idioventricular escape rhythm, prolonged sinus pauses, or syncope with profound sinus bradycardia. Mutations in the type V voltage-gated sodium channel alpha subunit (SCN5A) and hyperpolarization-activated cyclic nucleotide-gated potassium channel 4 (HCN4) genes, respectively, are the cause of this disorder, which can be inherited as an autosomal recessive or dominant condition. Patients should see a cardiologist right away because many times they will require a permanent pacemaker. Both kinds of arrhythmias can be found in tachycardia-bradycardia syndrome, a kind of sick sinus syndrome.
- **Complete Heart Block:** Third-degree atrioventricular block, or complete heart block, is frequently the cause of bradyarrhythmia-induced syncope. An irregular tracing may not show intermittent conduction abnormalities, but a routine ECG can readily identify permanent atrioventricular conduction abnormalities. An ECG taken after the episode with a normal PR interval does not rule out the diagnosis of transient complete heart block. Patients should be admitted to the hospital right away if they have syncope and a confirmed or suspected complete heart block. An atrioventricular block is highly likely in patients who have experienced an acute inferior myocardial infarction.

8.3.2.4. Cardiac Inflow Obstruction

While embolic episodes are the typical presentation of atrial or ventricular myxomas and atrial thrombi, they can also cause a blockage of the left ventricle's inflow or outflow, which causes a sharp drop in cardiac output and syncope. A classic, though rare, history of syncope is one in which there is a change in position. An echocardiogram can validate the diagnosis. The myxoma should be surgically removed. Any procedure or medication that lowers heart rate or venous return can cause syncope and abruptly insufficient cardiac output in patients with constrictive pericarditis or pericardial tamponade.

8.2.2.5. Cardiac Outflow Obstruction

- **Aortic Stenosis:** Severe aortic stenosis, whether congenital or acquired, usually results in loss of consciousness following exercise and is frequently accompanied by dyspnea, angina, and diaphoresis. Acute left ventricular failure that causes coronary hypoperfusion and ventricular fibrillation, or sudden increases in left ventricular pressure that activate baroreceptors and cause peripheral vasodilation, could be the pathophysiology. The diagnosis can be verified with echocardiography.

Symptomatic aortic stenosis necessitates valve replacement; in the absence of therapy, the prognosis following aortic syncope ranges from 18 months to 3 years.

- **Pulmonary Stenosis:** Syncope can result from severe pulmonary stenosis, particularly after physical activity. The cause is a hemodynamic process resembling that of aortic stenosis.

8.3.2.6. Hypertrophic Cardiomyopathy

A class of congenital cardiomyopathies known as hypertrophic cardiomyopathy are inherited as autosomal dominant disorders with varying degrees of severity. Numerous genes have been connected to this. Usually, between the second and fourth decades, symptoms start to appear. While syncope occurs in 30% of patients and is the presenting complaint in 10% of patients, dyspnea is the most common presenting complaint. Exercise is usually when syncope first appears, but post-tussive and orthostatic episodes can also happen. Transient arrhythmias, blockages in the left ventricle's outflow or inflow, or both can cause syncope. Echocardiography can verify the diagnosis. An implanted cardioverter defibrillator can stop potentially fatal ventricular arrhythmias, while propranolol may manage symptoms.

8.3.2.7. Dissecting Aortic Aneurysm

Acute aortic dissection patients typically exhibit isolated syncope in 5–10% of cases; additional neurologic abnormalities may or may not be present. 15% of patients report no pain during the dissection.

8.3.2.8. Pulmonary Hypertension and Pulmonary Embolus

Pulmonary hypertension may manifest as syncope, which is frequently exertional. It is typical to have a history of exertional dyspnea, and a blood gas analysis reveals hypoxemia even during rest. About 20% of patients with massive pulmonary embolism present with syncope as their primary symptom. After they recover, these patients frequently report feeling anxious, dyspneic, and experiencing pleuritic chest pain. These large emboli are frequently accompanied by arterial hypoxemia, tachycardia, tachypnea, and hypotension.

8.3.3. Cerebrovascular Syncope

Although it is rare, cerebral vascular disease is a frequently suspected cause of episodes of unconsciousness.

- **Basilar Artery Insufficiency:** Transient ischemic attacks in the basilar artery typically happen after the sixth decade. Diffuse brainstem ischemia may be indicated by the combination of symptoms that include drop attacks, occipital headaches, dysphagia, dysarthria, vertigo, and other sensory or motor symptoms. Attacks usually begin suddenly and last for a short while (seconds to minutes), but recovery from unconsciousness usually takes much longer (30–60 minutes or more). Basilar artery insufficiency is rarely the cause of isolated unconsciousness without additional signs of brainstem ischemia. Strokes occur in about one-fifth of cases, and two-thirds of patients experience recurrent attacks.

- **Subclavian Steal Syndrome:** Subclavian or innominate artery stenosis causes retrograde blood flow in the vertebral artery, diverting flow from the brainstem and resulting in hypoperfusion. This condition is known as subclavian steal syndrome. There is variation in the degree of symptomatic subclavian artery stenosis, but stenosis as minor as ~40% can occasionally cause symptoms. There is almost always a difference in the blood pressure readings taken in the two arms, with the average difference being a systolic pressure decrease of 45 mm Hg in the arm that receives blood flow from the stenotic vessel. There may be signs of vertebrobasilar ischemia or distal limb ischemia. Although stroke is uncommon, cerebrovascular risk factors should be changed. Procedures like revascularization and angiography might be taken into account.
- **Migraine:** About 10% of migraine patients experience syncope during the headache, frequently upon abruptly standing up, indicating that orthostatic hypotension is the cause of their loss of consciousness; autonomic neuropathy may also be present. Compared to syncope alone, syncopal migraine causes both longer periods of unconsciousness and longer periods of recovery. Some people experience symptoms from basilar migraine that are comparable to those from transient ischemic attacks in the basilar artery. Prophylactic antimigraine medications frequently work well to stop attacks.
- **Takayasu Disease:** Young Asian women are most commonly affected by Takayasu disease, also known as pulseless arteritis, which is a panarteritis of the aorta and its major branches. Cerebral hypoperfusion frequently manifests as syncope, confusion, and impaired vision. There are myalgias, arthralgias, and fever with widespread symptoms. Activities like exercising, standing, or head movement can cause precipitation. Examining both arms reveals low blood pressure and either absent or reduced brachial pulses. There may be an increase in C reactive protein and erythrocyte sedimentation rate. Treatment with corticosteroids is recommended.
- **Carotid Sinus Syncope:** Rarely occurs carotid sinus syncope. Males are impacted twice as frequently as females, and the majority of those impacted are older than 60. Certain medications, such as methyldopa, digitalis, and propranolol, have been linked to carotid sinus syncope. When bradycardia/hypotension (carotid sinus hypersensitivity) is produced and spontaneous syncope is replicated after a 10-second carotid sinus massage, carotid sinus syncope is diagnosed. Older men frequently experience carotid sinus

hypersensitivity without syncope. Pacing is the method used to treat symptomatic patients.

When symptoms arise from compression of a normal carotid artery contralateral to an occluded internal carotid artery, carotid sinus syncope may be misdiagnosed. Patients who have had a recent transient ischemic attack (TIA), stroke, or carotid bruit should not receive carotid sinus massage.

8.3.4. Orthostatic Hypotension

Men experience orthostatic hypotension more frequently than women, and it is most prevalent in the sixth and seventh decades of life. Still, it can manifest in teenagers as well. When someone loses consciousness, it usually happens when they stand up quickly, stand still for a long time (especially after exercising), or stand up after lying down for a long time (especially in older people).

Orthostatic hypotension (Table 8.11) can be caused by a variety of conditions, but it usually stems from either hypovolemia or autonomic dysfunction. Drugs, autonomic neuropathy, or central nervous system disorders affecting sympathetic pathways in the hypothalamus, brainstem, or spinal cord could be the cause of the latter.

Table 8.11. Causes of Orthostatic Hypotension: Orthostatic Challenge Tests

Test	Method	Results
Active standing test	Measure the BP in clinostatism and after rapid orthostatism at minute 0, minute 1, and minute 3	• A symptomatic SBP fall of >20 mmHg or a DBP fall of > 10 mmHg, or absolute an BP value of ≤90 mmHg indicates OH; • In reflex OH, the HR increases slightly (<10 bpm); • In hypovolemia, the HR increases significantly.
Tilt test	• Place the patient in the supine position for at least 5 min (without IVC) or at least 20 min (with IVC); • Tilt the table to an angle of 60–70° for 20–45 min (passive phase); • If nothing happens during the passive phase, repeat the test after the administration of 300–400 µg of sublingual nitroglycerin (pharmacological phase); • Lower the table in less than 15 s; • Record a video for additional information if necessary.	• Positive if syncope occurs • Low specificity and sensitivity in patients with syncope of uncertain cause

Valsalva maneuver	Indicated in patients with suspected reflex syncope or to confirm the tendency of hypotension induced by situational syncope	Results can help diagnose neurogenic syncope or confirm hypotension tendency induced with situational syncope
Deep breathing test	Indicated in patients with OH of suspected neurogenic origin	Results can provide information about reflex syncope
ABPM	Identifies any drops in BP occurring in the 24 h.	Can identify different patterns: dipping (BP falls > 10% at night compared with daytime) or non-dipping (BP falls < 10% at night), or reverse dipping (BP rises at night)

Source: Martone AM, Parrini I, Ciciarello F, Galluzzo V, Cacciatore S, Massaro C, Giordano R, Giani T, Landi G, Gulizia MM, et al. Recent Advances and Future Directions in Syncope Management: A Comprehensive Narrative Review. *Journal of Clinical Medicine*. 2024; 13(3):727. https://doi.org/10.3390/jcm13030727.

Abbreviations: ABPM: 24-h ambulatory blood pressure monitoring; BP: blood pressure; DBP: diastolic blood pressure; HR: heart rate; IVC: venous cannulation; SBP: systolic blood pressure; TLOC: temporary loss of consciousness.

Neurodegenerative diseases may also exhibit orthostatic hypotension. Isolated postganglionic sympathetic neuron degeneration is linked to idiopathic orthostatic hypotension. Preganglionic sympathetic neuron degeneration coexists with parkinsonian, pyramidal, cerebellar, or lower motor neuron symptoms in multisystem atrophy (Shy-Drager syndrome).

When a patient stands from a laying position and their blood pressure drops by at least 20 mm Hg systolic or 10 mm Hg diastolic in 3 minutes, it is considered classic orthostatic hypotension. Postural orthostatic tachycardia syndrome (POTS), which is most common in young women, is defined as severe orthostatic intolerance accompanied by heart rate increases (>120/min) without significant hypotension or syncope.

To determine the cause of the disorder, a comprehensive general physical and neurologic examination, as well as laboratory tests (hematocrit, stool occult blood, serum glucose and electrolytes, FTA-ABS, nerve conduction studies), should be performed. Stopping any medication that could be causing orthostatic hypotension is advised, especially diuretics, venodilators like nitrates, and vasodilators like α-agonists. The patient should be advised to use waist-high elasticized support stockings, raise the head of the bed on blocks, and stand up gradually. When you wake up and drink 500 mL of water before getting out of bed, your blood pressure goes up for an hour. The precise cause of hypotension determines the other course of treatment.

Fludrocortisone, a strong mineralocorticoid, is beneficial in diabetic neuropathy and idiopathic cases when taken orally in doses starting at 0.1 mg/d and progressively increased to 0.5 mg/d as needed. Although its exact mechanism of action is unknown, its advantages could include heightened plasma volume and responsiveness to norepinephrine in circulation. One of the adverse effects is recumbent hypertension. An alternative is to use midodrine, an α-adrenergic receptor agonist, starting at 2.5 mg two or three times per day.

8.3.5. Miscellaneous Causes of Syncope

- **Cough Syncope:** Although it has also been documented in children, middle-aged men with chronic obstructive pulmonary disease are the main population affected by cough (tussive) syncope. It doesn't take long to start coughing, and it happens right before unconsciousness. In a supine position, the patient may experience cough syncope. Prodromal symptoms are absent, and unconsciousness lasts for a short while—often just a few seconds. Consciousness returns to normal quickly. It is common to have a history of similar episodes, and the patient can be made to cough on request to elicit symptoms. The reason could be a drop in cerebral blood flow due to elevated intracranial pressure, which is caused by a cough that raises intrathoracic pressure and transfers that pressure to the intracranial compartment through venous or spinal connections. Additional information is consistent with a cough-induced decrease in total peripheral resistance mediated by baroreflex.

  Antitussive medications like dextromethorphan are the only treatment options; otherwise, the condition is usually benign.
- **Micturition Syncope:** Micturition syncope is a cerebral hypoperfusion event that primarily affects men, most likely as a result of standing while urinating. It is caused by peripheral blood pooling in addition to vagally induced bradycardia. Episodes may happen right before, during, or following micturition. They tend to happen more frequently at night following extended periods of recumbency sleep. Sitting down to urinate usually gets rid of the symptoms.
- **Glossopharyngeal Neuralgia:** A rare syndrome called glossopharyngeal neuralgia is characterized by excruciating, paroxysmal pain that is localized to the tonsillar pillar and sometimes the external auditory meatus. Contact with or movement of the tonsillar pillars causes pain, particularly when swallowing or speaking. A glossopharyngeal-vagal reflex arc is triggered during syncope, resulting in a brief bradyarrhythmia that causes cerebral hypoperfusion. For the majority of patients, an oral dose of 400–1000 mg/d of carbamazepine will prevent bradycardia and pain.
- **Psychogenic Syncope:** The diagnosis of psychogenic syncope is one of exclusion and is frequently made incorrectly. Absence of any prodrome, potential secondary gain, strange stances and motions, lack of pallor, recurrent spells, and an extended period of apparent in responsiveness are suggestive characteristics. During an episode, the eyes are closed. Psychogenic spells are rarely accompanied by incontinence or injury, and they rarely happen when the patient is by themselves. The majority of patients are either young or have a well-established conversion disorder

history. A diagnosis made after the third decade is dubious without such a history.

Without the slowing that usually follows unconsciousness from a seizure and happens with cerebral hypoperfusion, the EEG is normal during psychogenic unconsciousness. Caloric testing can differentiate between psychogenic unresponsiveness and coma due to a metabolic or structural lesion. It causes nystagmus in conscious patients and tonic eye deviation in unconscious patients.

A Closer Look

Guillain-Barré syndrome

The immune system of the body targets a portion of the peripheral nervous system in Guillain-Barré syndrome. The nerves that transmit pain, temperature, and touch sensations can all be impacted by the syndrome, in addition to the ones that govern muscle movement. Muscle weakness, numbness in the arms and/or legs, and difficulties breathing or swallowing can arise from this.

People of all ages can be affected by this uncommon condition, though adults and men are more likely to have it. Most people recover without serious, long-term neurological consequences after a few weeks of symptoms.

Weakness or tingling sensations are among the initial signs of Guillain-Barré syndrome. Usually beginning in the legs, they can also spread to the face and arms. Some individuals may develop paralysis in their arms, legs, or facial muscles as a result of these symptoms. Breathing becomes difficult in about one-third of cases due to damage to the chest muscles.

Speaking and swallowing abilities may be impacted in severe Guillain-Barré syndrome cases. People who are affected by these cases should receive treatment in intensive care units as they are thought to be life-threatening. Even in the most severe cases of Guillain-Barré syndrome, the majority of patients fully recover, though some still feel weak.

Even in the best of circumstances, complications from Guillain-Barré syndrome can cause death in a small percentage of cases. These complications can include heart arrest, blood infections, lung clots, or paralysis of the breathing muscles.

GBS, or Guillain-Barré syndrome, is uncommon. Although the exact cause is unknown, most cases are related to bacterial or viral infections. The body itself is attacked by the immune system as a result. One of the most frequent causes of gastroenteritis (including symptoms of nausea, vomiting, and diarrhea) is an infection with the bacteria *Campylobacter jejuni*. Infections with the cytomegalovirus, Epstein-Barr virus, Zika virus, or the flu can also cause people to contract GBS.

There is a very slim possibility that receiving vaccinations will raise a person's risk of contracting GBS. Studies reveal that vaccinations meant to prevent infections—in this case, the flu vaccine—have a significantly lower risk of causing GBS in humans than do infections like the flu. GBS can occasionally be caused by surgery.

Deep tendon reflex loss or diminution is one of the neurological examination findings that go toward making the diagnosis. Although they shouldn't postpone treatment, lumbar punctures and electromyography (EMG) may be performed for supportive information. Tests to determine the underlying trigger, like blood tests, are not necessary to diagnose GBS and shouldn't postpone treatment. Respiratory difficulties should be closely monitored in anyone suspected of having GBS.

Summary

- Disorders known as seizures are typified by transient neurologic symptoms or signs that arise from abnormal, hypersynchronous, paroxysmal electrical neuronal activity in the cerebral cortex.
- Loss of consciousness caused by decreased blood flow to the brainstem or both cerebral hemispheres is known as syncope.
- Hypoperfusion-induced loss of consciousness rarely lasts longer than 10 to 20 seconds, and postictal confusion does not usually follow unless there has been severe and prolonged brain ischemia.
- A seizure is a brief disruption of brain activity caused by an aberrant neuronal discharge.
- Head trauma is frequently linked to epilepsy, especially in cases where it happens during pregnancy, is associated with a depressed skull fracture, or results in an intracerebral or subdural hematoma.
- Eclampsia refers to the occurrence of seizures or coma in a pregnant woman with hypertension, proteinuria, and edema (preeclampsia).
- Attacks known as generalized tonic-clonic seizures cause loss of consciousness, typically with no aura or other warning signs.
- Patients with epilepsy (usually children) who have been seizure-free for two to five years while taking medication may want to stop taking anticonvulsants.
- Vasovagal syncope affects people of all ages. Genetic influences might be important. Emotional stimulation, pain, seeing blood, exhaustion, medical equipment, blood loss, and extended periods of immobility are examples of precipitating factors.
- Prolonged electrocardiogram monitoring of certain syncope patients reveals the presence of ventricular tachyarrhythmias, which include ventricular tachycardia and multiform, frequent, or paired premature ventricular contractions.
- A class of congenital cardiomyopathies known as hypertrophic cardiomyopathy are inherited as autosomal dominant disorders with varying degrees of severity.

References

1. Angus-leppan, h. (2014). First seizures in adults. *Bmj, 348*, g2470.
2. Aydin, m. A., Salukhe, t. V., Wilke, i., & Willems, s. (2010). Management and therapy of vasovagal syncope: a review. *World j cardiol., 26*, 308–315.
3. Betensky, b. P., Jaeger, j. R., & Woo, e. Y. (2011). Unequal blood pressures: a manifestation of subclavian steal. *Am. J. Med., 124*, E1–e2.
4. Brignole, m., & Menozzi, c. (2011). The natural history of carotid sinus syncope and the effect of cardiac pacing. *Europace, 13*, 462–464.
5. Curfman, d., Chilungu, m., Daroff, r. B., Et al. (2012). Syncopal migraine. *Clin. Auton. Res., 22*, 17–23.

6. Delgado-escueta, a. V., Koeleman, b. P. C., Bailey, j. N., Medina, m. T., & Duron, r. M. (2013). The quest for juvenile myoclonic epilepsy genes. *Epilepsy behav., 28*(Suppl 1), s52–s57.

7. Edvardsson, n., Frykman, v., Van mechelen, r., Et al., On behalf of the picture study investigators. (2011). Use of an implantable loop recorder to increase the diagnostic yield in unexplained syncope: results from the picture registry. *Europace, 13*, 262–269.

8. Engel, j., & Pedley, t. A. (Eds.). (2007). *Epilepsy: a comprehensive textbook* (2nd ed.). Philadelphia, pa: lippincott williams & wilkins.

9. Hatoum, t., & Sheldon, r. (2014). A practical approach to investigation of syncope. *Can. J. Cardiol., 30*, 671–674.

10. Hilz, m. J., Marthol, h., & Neundörfer, b. (2002). Syncope – a systematic overview of classification, pathogenesis, diagnosis and management. *Fortschr. Neurol. Psychiatr., 70*, 95–107.

11. Jetter, g. M., & Cavazos, j. E. (2008). Epilepsy in the elderly. *Semin. Neurol., 28*, 336–341.

12. Moya, a., Sutton, r., Ammirati, f., Et al. (2009). Guidelines for the diagnosis and management of syncope (version 2009). Task force for the diagnosis and management of syncope; european society of cardiology (esc); european heart rhythm association (ehra); heart failure association (hfa); heart rhythm society (hrs). *Eur. Heart j., 30*, 2631–2671.

13. Olde nordkamp, l. R. A. (2013). Syncope. In: de jong, j. S. S. G., & Van der waals, f. (Eds.), *Textbook of cardiology*. The netherlands: cardionetworks foundation and the health[e] foundation. Retrieved from http://www.Textbookofcardiology.Org

14. Raj, s. R., & Coffin, s. (2013). Medical therapy and physical maneuvers in the treatment of vasovagal syncope and orthostatic hypotension. *Prog. Cardiovasc. Dis., 55*, 425–433.

15. Soteriades, e. S., Evans, j. C., Larson, m. G., Et al. (2002). Incidence and prognosis of syncope. *N. Engl. J. Med., 347*, 878–885.

16. Stefan, h., & Theodore, w. H. (2012). Epilepsy. In handbook of clinical neurology, vols 107 and 108. Amsterdam: elsevier.

17. Van dijk, j. G., Thijs, r. D., Benditt, d. G., & Wieling, w. (2009). A guide to disorders causing transient loss of consciousness: focus on syncope. *Nat. Rev. Neurol., 5*, 438–448.

18. Yalçin, ö. (2012). Genes and molecular mechanisms involved in the epileptogenesis of idiopathic absence epilepsies. *Seizure, 21*, 79–86.

Chapter

SENSORY DISORDERS

9

Contents

Introduction

A vast spectrum of illnesses that impact one or more of the sensory systems—vision, hearing, taste, smell, and touch—are referred to as sensory disorders. These conditions can significantly lower a person's quality of life because they frequently cause abnormalities or impairments in sensory perception, which make it harder for the affected person to understand and react to their surroundings.

The ability to see clearly or at all is impacted by conditions like cataracts, glaucoma, and macular degeneration, which can result in blurred vision, loss of peripheral vision, or even blindness. Similar to this, hearing impairments such as mixed, sensorineural, and conductive hearing loss can make it difficult to hear sounds or comprehend speech.

Anosmia and dysgeusia, two disorders that impair taste and smell, can make it difficult for a person to appreciate food and drink or to recognize possible dangers like spoiled food. Touch-related sensory disorders, such as sensory processing disorder or neuropathic pain, can produce pain, discomfort, or changed sensitivity to tactile stimuli.

All things considered, sensory disorders can have a substantial impact on a person's capacity to navigate and interact with their environment, underscoring the significance of early detection, intervention, and support services to maximize sensory function and improve general well-being.

Orientation and Directional Terms

Term	Definition	Illustration
Dysgeusia	Dysgeusia, also known as parageusia, is a taste disorder that causes a person to experience a distorted sense of taste, such as a foul, salty, rancid, or metallic taste in the mouth.	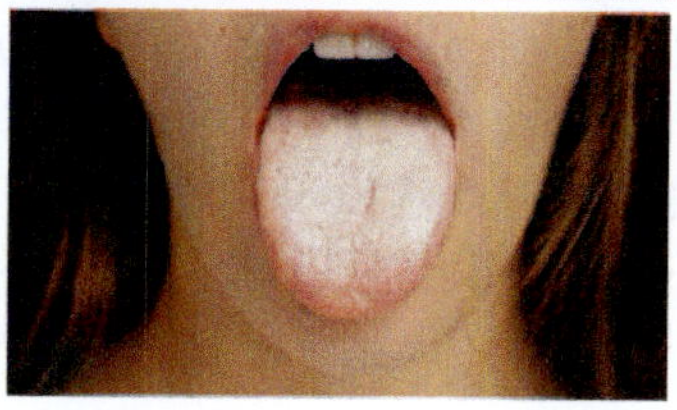
Somatic sensation	Somatic sensation is the physiological process that converts physical stimuli into neural signals.	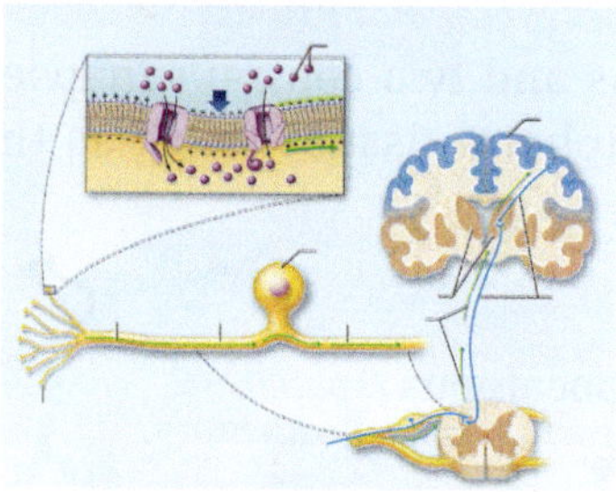
Sensory cortex	The sensory cortex is the part of the brain that processes and interprets sensory information, and is located on the brain's outer surface.	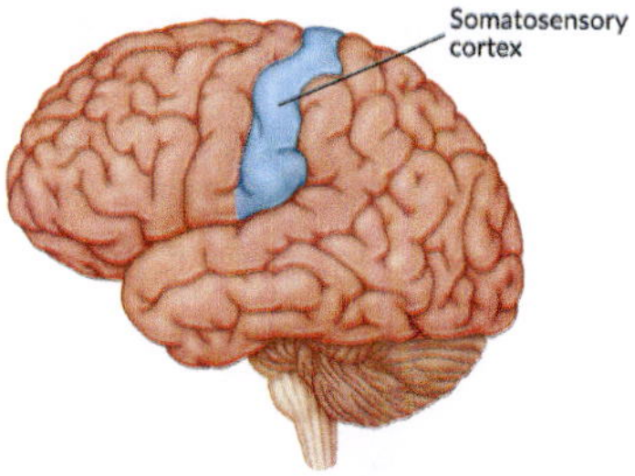
Cutaneous sensation	Cutaneous sensation is a sensation caused by stimulation of the skin's end organs, such as warmth, cold, contact, or pain.	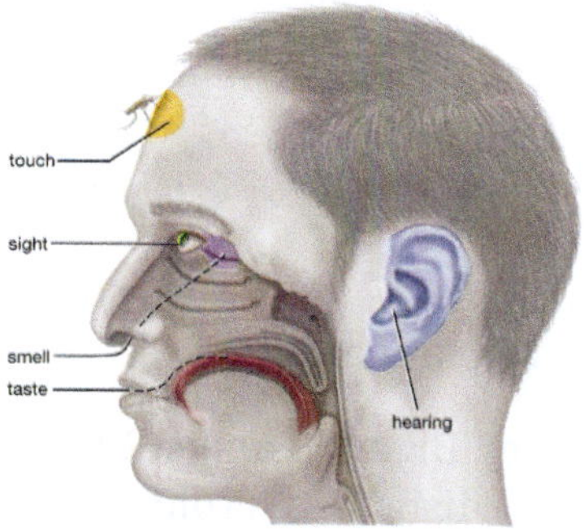
Spinothalamic tract	The spinothalamic tract (STT) is a sensory pathway in the nervous system that carries information about pain, temperature, pressure, and touch from the skin to the thalamus.	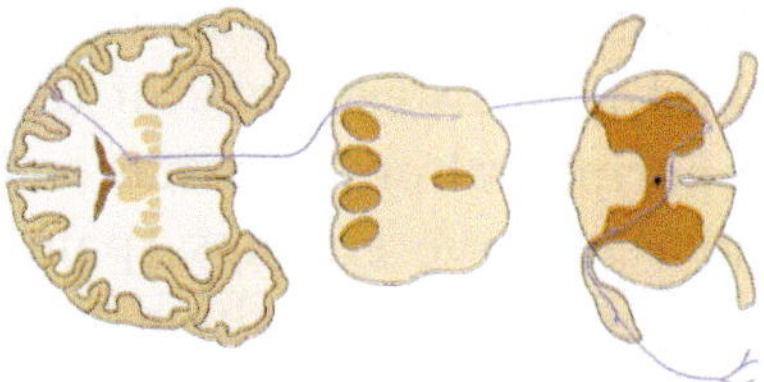

9.1. Diagnosis Approach of Sensory Disorders

Understanding the functional anatomy of the sensory components of the nervous system is necessary to interpret the clinical signs and history of patients with disorders of somatic sensation. In this context, "somatic sensation" refers to the following: touch or pressure, vibration, joint position, pain, and temperature; it also includes more sophisticated functions (like two-point discrimination, stereognosis, and graphesthesia) that depend on these primary sensory modalities. Special senses (like smell, vision, taste, and hearing) are not included in this definition.

9.1.1. Functional Anatomy of the Somatic Sensory Pathways

Three neurons and two central synapses make up the sensory pathway that connects the cerebral cortex to peripheral tissues (such as the skin or joints) (Figure 9.1).

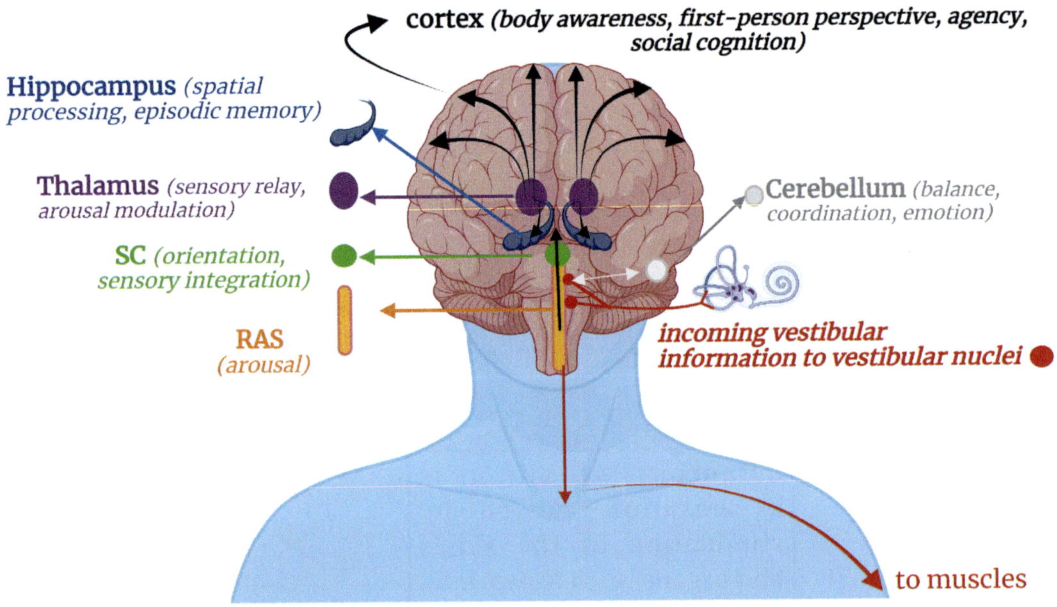

Figure 9.1. Sensory pathways conveying touch, pressure, vibration, joint position, pain, and temperature sensation.

Source: Kearney BE and Lanius RA (2022) The brain-body disconnect: A somatic sensory basis for trauma-related disorders. Front. Neurosci. 16:1015749. doi: 10.3389/fnins.2022.1015749.

Dorsal root ganglia are home to the cell bodies of first-order sensory neurons originating from the limbs and trunk. Every one of these neurons sends a central process that enters the spinal cord and a peripheral process that ends in a free nerve ending or encapsulated sensory receptor. Apart from free nerve endings (pain, itching), sensory receptors are relatively specialized for specific sensations. These include Meissner corpuscles, Merkel corpuscles, and hair cells (touch); Krause end-bulbs (cold); and Ruffini corpuscles (heat). Depending on the kind of sensation, first-order sensory neurons synapse centrally at a different location. The medulla is where the gracile and cuneate nuclei of the spinal cord synapse when fibers mediating touch, pressure, or postural sensation in the limbs and trunk ascend in the posterior columns of the spinal cord. Additional fibers in the limbs and trunk that facilitate touch as well as those that serve pain, temperature, and itch perception synapse on neurons in the posterior horns of the spinal cord, specifically in the substantia gelatinosa. The trigeminal (V) nerve carries first-order sensory neurons from the face into the pons. These neurons have cell bodies in the trigeminal (gasserian) ganglion. Facial touch and pressure-related fibers synapse in the main sensory nucleus of the trigeminal (V) nerve, while facial pain- and temperature-related fibers synapse in the spinal trigeminal (V) nerve nucleus.

Second-order sensory neurons ascend in the medial lemniscus and cross the midline, with their cell bodies located in the cuneate and gracile nuclei. Although fibers mediating touch pass upward in the anterior spinothalamic tract, fibers mediating pain, itch, and temperature typically travel in the lateral spinothalamic tract. Second-order sensory neurons that originate in the posterior horns of the spinal cord cross the midline and ascend in the anterolateral part of the cord.

Fibers from the face connect the second-order sensory neurons from the limbs and trunk in the brainstem. The facial fibers transmit pain, itch, and temperature information from the spinal trigeminal (V) nerve nucleus to the ipsilateral thalamus via the trigeminothalamic tract, and they mediate facial touch and pressure sensation from the main trigeminal (V) nerve sensory nucleus via the trigeminal lemniscus. The ventral posterolateral (VPL) nucleus in the thalamus is where medial lemniscal and spinothalamic fibers synapse. Additionally, spinothalamic fibers synapse in the intralaminar (ILa) and ventral posteroinferior (VPI) nuclei. Finally, fibers in the trigeminal lemniscus and trigeminothalamic tract synapse in the ventral posteromedial (VPM) nucleus. Furthermore, some spinothalamic sensory neurons of second order send collaterals to the reticular formation.

From the thalamus, third-order sensory neurons project to the ipsilateral cerebral cortex. Fibers from ILa also project to the striatum, cingulate gyrus, and prefrontal cortex. Fibers from VPL, VPI, and VPM mainly go to the primary somatosensory cortex in the postcentral gyrus.

9.1.2. History

Pain, unusual sensations, or loss of feeling are examples of sensory disturbances. While dysesthesia refers to any unpleasant sensation caused by a normally painless stimulus, paresthesia refers to abnormal spontaneous sensations like burning, tingling, or pins and needles. Patients often use the term "numbness" to refer to a feeling of weakness, heaviness, or deadness in a particular part of their body. It can also refer to any kind of sensory impairment; therefore, it is important to always clarify the meaning of this word when it is used.

The location of sensory symptoms, their mode of onset and progression, their episodic or constant nature, the specific factors that cause, exacerbate, or relieve them, and the presence of comorbid symptoms should all be determined.

The origin of the symptoms may be reflected in their location. For instance, sensory abnormalities affecting every limb may indicate a brainstem or cervical cord lesion, peripheral neuropathy, or a metabolic disorder like hyperventilation syndrome. One side of the body or one entire limb affected indicates a central lesion (brain or spinal cord). In addition to the face, hemisphere or brainstem lesions can also cause lateralized sensory symptoms. Other symptoms and indicators include dysarthria, weakness, vertigo, diplopia, disequilibrium, and ataxia with brainstem disorders, or aphasia, apraxia, and visual field defects with hemispheric disease. Depending on the exact distribution, the involvement of a portion of a limb or a distinct area of the trunk increases the risk of a nerve or root lesion. When there is a root lesion, the symptoms can be related to movements of the neck or back, and the pain is frequently noticeable.

The progression of sensory complaints offers insight into their underlying cause. Periodic or recurrent short-term symptoms could be signs of ischemic events, sensory seizures, or metabolic problems like those that come with hyperventilation. Periodic, localized symptoms that happen regularly could point to the diagnosis or an external trigger. For instance, the patient is usually awakened from sleep at night by the pain and paresthesias associated with carpal tunnel syndrome (median nerve compression at the wrist).

9.1.3. Sensory Examination

After testing each sensory modality in turn, the distribution of any abnormality is plotted, paying special attention to the normal peripheral and root nerve territories. Anesthesia is the total loss of appreciation for touch; hypesthesia is the partial loss; and hyperesthesia is the increased sensitivity. Analgesia, hypalgesia, hyperalgesia, and hyperpathia are the corresponding terms for appreciating pain; allodynia is the term for misinterpreting a minor tactile sensation as pain.

9.1.3.1. Primary Sensory Modalities

- **Light Touch:** A cotton wool swab that is gently applied to a small area of skin is used to assess the appreciation of light touch. With their eyes closed, the patient indicates whenever they feel a stimulus. The ability to perceive light touch is dependent upon fibers that pass through the gracile (leg) and cuneate (arm) fasciculi in the posterior column of the spinal cord ipsilaterally (Figures 9.1 and 9.2), on fibers in the contralateral anterior spinothalamic tract, and on the medial lemniscus of the brainstem (Figure 9.3).
- **Pinprick and Temperature:** Asking the patient to describe whether a pin (as opposed to a hypodermic needle, which could pierce the skin and draw blood) feels blunt or sharp is how pinprick appreciation is measured.

It's important to distinguish between the appreciation of touch or pressure and that of sharpness. The pin should be handled carefully and disposed of after use as it may be an infection source. The assessment of temperature appreciation involves putting hot or cold water containers on the skin. Applying the side of a metal tuning fork to various body parts can be a convenient way to test for cold; heat testing is typically not included in the standard examination. The functions of the lateral spinothalamic tract determines the perception of temperature and pinprick (Figures 9.1 and 9.2). After ascending for two or three segments from their level of entry into the cord, the afferent fibers cross in front of the central canal.

- **Deep Pressure:** Applying pressure to tendons, like the Achilles tendon at the ankle, is one way to measure deep pressure sensibility.
- **Vibration:** After placing a tuning fork (128 Hz) over a bony prominence and vibrating it, the patient is asked to report whether they feel a vibration or just pressure. The ability to appreciate vibration below the knees is often compromised in many elderly, healthy patients.

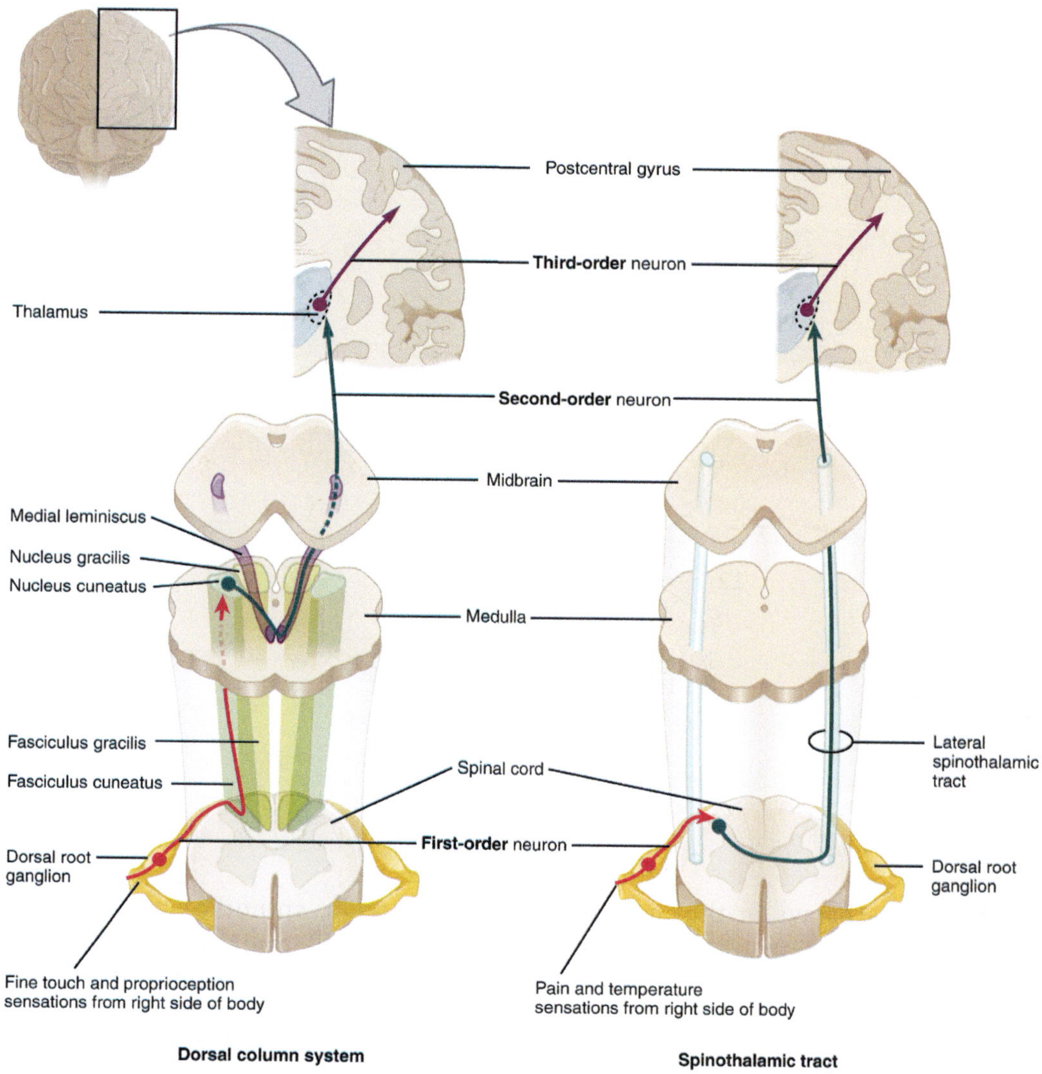

Figure 9.2. Location and lamination of sensory pathways in the spinal cord.

Source: https://open.oregonstate.education/aandp/chapter/14-5-sensory-and-motor-pathways/#:~:text=1%20%E2%80%93%20Ascending%20Sensory%20Pathways%20of,%2C%20mouth%2C%20and%20nasal%20cavity.

- **Joint Position:** When the patient's fingers and toes move passively in small directions, the terminal interphalangeal joints are asked to be pointed out. When trying to hold their hands outstretched with their eyes closed, patients with severe impairments to their joint position sense may show slow, continuous movement of their fingers (known as pseudoathetoid movement). Although this is not strictly true for vibration, for clinical purposes both the sense of joint position and the capacity to perceive vibration are thought to depend on fibers carried in the posterior columns of the spinal cord.

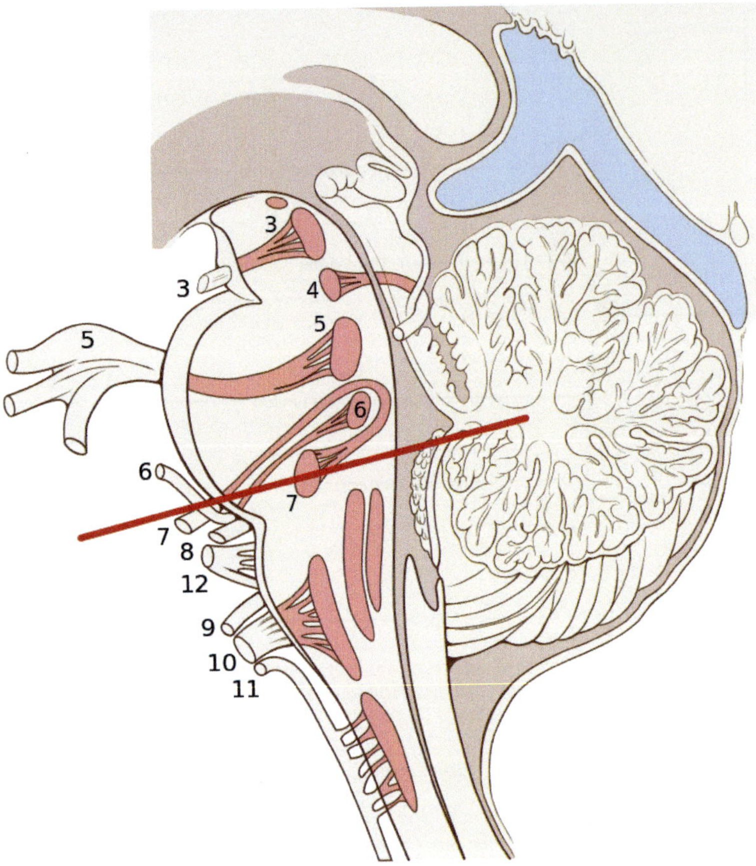

Figure 9.3. Sensory pathways in the brainstem. In the medulla, spinothalamic fibers conveying pain and temperature sensation are widely separated from medial lemniscal fibers mediating touch and pressure; these pathways converge as they ascend in the pons and midbrain.

Source: By Patrick J. Lynch, medical illustrator - Patrick J. Lynch, medical illustrator, CC BY 2.5, https://commons.wikimedia.org/w/index.php?curid=1496662.

9.1.3.2. Complex Sensory Functions

- **Romberg Test:** The patient stands with their feet together, arms extended, and eyes closed in a steady stance. They are then watched for any signs of swaying or falling. If eye closure significantly increases unsteadiness—as it does, for example, in tabes dorsalis—the test is positive (abnormal). A positive test result indicates severely compromised leg joint position sense.
- **Two-Point Discrimination:** The degree of separation between the two points, the part of the body being stimulated, and the integrity of the central and peripheral nervous systems all affect one's capacity to discriminate between simultaneous touch at two nearby points. The patient indicates whether one or both of the compass points are touching him or her, and the distance between the points is adjusted to find the minimum distance at which they can be distinguished from one another. The two-point

discrimination threshold may be several centimeters on the back and roughly 4 mm at the fingertips. Impaired two-point discrimination indicates a disorder affecting the sensory cortex when peripheral sensory function is unaffected.

- **Graphesthesia, Stereognosis, and Barognosis:** Agraphesthesia, which is the inability to recognize a number traced on the hand's palm skin despite having normal cutaneous sensation, suggests a contralateral parietal lobe lesion. This also applies to the impaired ability to discriminate between different weights (abarognosis) and the inability to distinguish different shapes or textures by touch (astereognosis).
- **Bilateral Sensory Discrimination:** Simultaneous stimulation of the two sides of the body reveals apparent neglect of (or inattention to) sensation from one side in certain patients with apparently normal sensation; this is typically due to an underlying contralateral cerebral lesion.

9.1.4. Sensory Changes and Their Significance

It is necessary to ascertain the type and extent of any sensory alteration. If clinical evidence of sensory loss is not found in patients exhibiting sensory symptoms, this does not always mean that the symptoms are psychogenic. Frequently, sensory symptoms appear long before sensory signs do.

9.1.4.1. Peripheral Nerve Lesions

- **Mononeuropathy:** The anatomical prediction of sensory loss in patients with a single peripheral nerve lesion is typically not met due to overlap from neighboring nerves. Furthermore, a sensory nerve's fibers may be impacted differently based on the kind of lesion. For example, compressive lesions typically target the large fibers that support touch more strongly.
- **Polyneuropathy:** Sensory loss in patients with polyneuropathies is typically symmetric and more pronounced distally than proximally (also known as length-dependent neuropathy or stocking-and-glove sensory loss). Usually, the loss has advanced nearly to the knees before it affects the hands. This could lead to a motor impairment and modifications in reflexes along with sensory loss. Small nerve fibers that serve pain and temperature perception are preferentially involved in diabetes mellitus, amyloidosis, and some other metabolic disorders (such as Tangier disease, a recessive trait marked by the nearly complete absence of high-density lipoproteins). In a pure small-fiber sensory neuropathy, tendon reflexes are unaffected, and no motor deficit occurs.

9.1.4.2. Root Lesions

When nerve roots are involved, the cutaneous sensation is impaired in a segmental pattern (Figure 9.4), but unless two or more adjacent roots are affected, there is typically no sensory loss due to overlap. Compressive root lesions frequently present with pain. Loss of tendon reflexes (C5–C6, biceps and brachioradialis; C7–C8, triceps; L3–L4, knee; S1, ankle) may occur, depending on the level affected. If the anterior roots are also affected, weakness and muscle atrophy may also manifest.

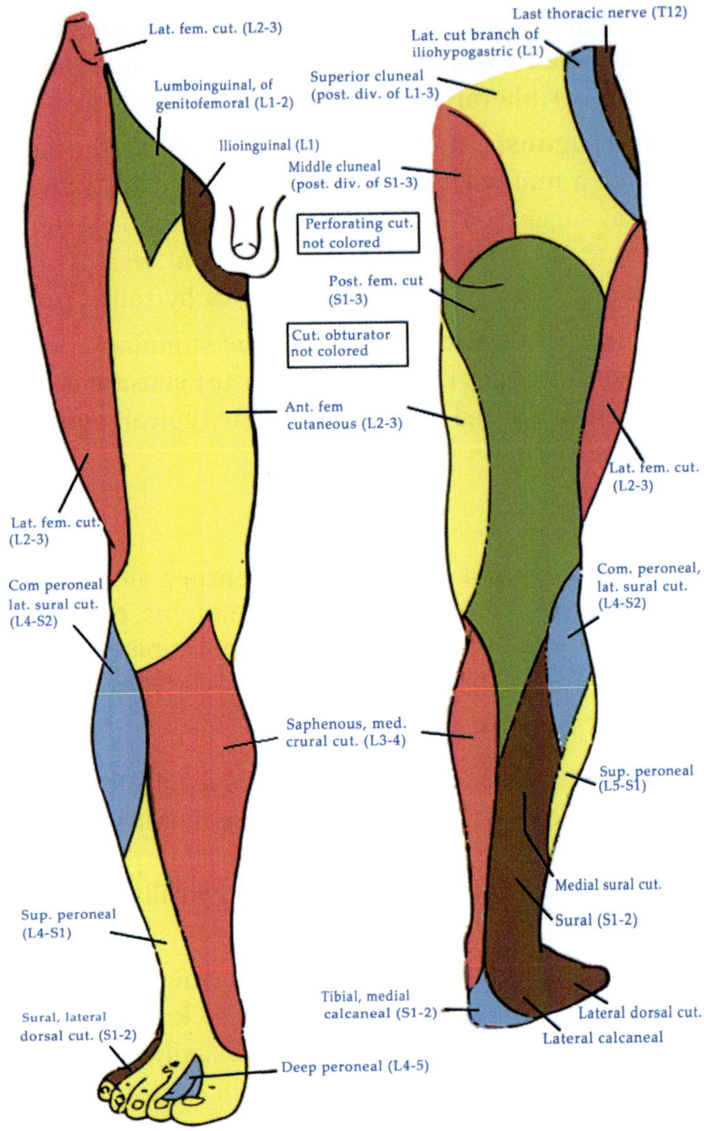

Figure 9.4. (A) Cutaneous innervation.

Source: By Henry Vandyke Carter – Henry Gray (1918) Anatomy of the Human Body (See "Book" section below)Bartleby.com: Gray's Anatomy, Plate 826, Public Domain, https://commons.wikimedia.org/w/index.php?curid=3429653.

9.1.4.3. Spinal Cord Lesions

A transverse sensory level may be present in patients with spinal cord lesions. However, there are physiological sites of increased sensitivity in the groin, over the breasts, and at the costal margin; these should not be interpreted as aberrant. Therefore, careful sensory testing over the back, as opposed to the chest and abdomen, is the best way to assess the degree of a sensory deficit affecting the trunk.

- **Central Cord Lesion:** A central cord lesion, like the one seen in syringomyelia, after trauma, and with some tumors, is characterized by a loss of feeling of pain and temperature while leaving other modalities intact. This loss results from the disruption of nerve fibers that carry temperature and pain signals from one side of the spinal cord to the other, the spinothalamic tract. Such a loss primarily affects the fibers of the affected segments, is typically bilateral, and may be asymmetric. It can also be accompanied by a deficit in the pyramidal and posterior columns beneath the lesion, as well as lower motor neuron weakness in the muscles supplied by the affected segments (Figure 9.5).
- **Anterolateral Spinal Cord Lesion** In segments below the level of the lesion, contralateral impairment of pain and temperature perception can result from lesions affecting the lateral spinothalamic tract, which is the anterolateral portion of the spinal cord. The fibers from the sacral segments are the outermost in the laminate that is the spinothalamic tract. Sacral fibers are frequently spared from intrinsic cord (intramedullary) lesions, but these fibers as well as those originating from more rostral levels are typically involved in extramedullary lesions, which compress the cord.
- **Anterior Spinal Cord Lesion:** When the front part of the spinal cord is damaged, it can lead to impaired pain and temperature sensation below that level due to the involvement of the lateral spinothalamic tract. Additionally, weakness or paralysis in muscles controlled by the affected segments of the cord can occur from damage to anterior horn cells. In more severe cases, the corticospinal tracts in the lateral funiculi may also be affected, causing a pyramidal deficit below the lesion. The posterior column function is relatively preserved. Ischemic myelopathies, resulting from occlusion of the anterior spinal artery, manifest as anterior spinal cord lesions.
- **Posterior Column Lesion:** When there is a posterior column lesion, a patient may experience paresthesias (which feel like electric shocks) that radiate down their extremities when they bend their neck, as well as a tight or band-like sensation in the areas that correspond to the degree of spinal involvement (Lhermitte sign). Below the level of the lesion, there is a loss of joint position sense and vibration, but other sensory modalities are preserved. The deficiency might be similar to that caused by big fiber involvement in the posterior roots.
- **Spinal Cord Hemisection:** Brown-Séquard syndrome is caused by spinal cord hemisection at the lateral end. Below the lesion, there is a loss of pain and temperature appreciation on the contralateral side, which starts two or three segments below the lesion, as well as an ipsilateral pyramidal deficit and disturbed appreciation of

vibration and joint position sense (Figure 9.5). Sometimes ipsilateral hyperalgesia and spontaneous pain are noticeable.

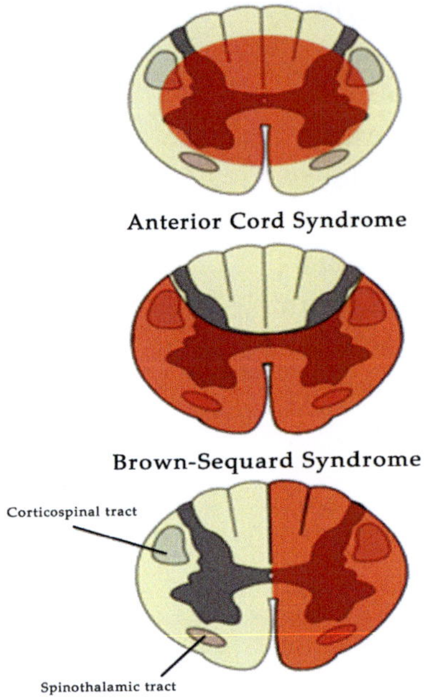

Figure 9.5. Central cord lesions: Less extensive lesions impair pain and temperature response by interrupting incoming sensory fibers as they cross to the contralateral spinothalamic tract; involvement of anterior horn cells causes lower motor neuron weakness. These deficits are restricted to dermatomes and muscles innervated by the involved spinal cord segments. More extensive lesions also produce disturbances of touch, pressure, vibration, and joint position sense because of involvement of the posterior columns and cause pyramidal signs because of corticospinal tract involvement, especially affecting the arms. These deficits occur below the level of the lesion.

9.1.4.4. Brainstem Lesions

Sensory disturbances associated with brainstem lesions may include cranial nerve palsies, cerebellar signs, and motor deficit.

The opposite side of the body's limbs and trunk lose their ability to perceive pain and temperature when there are lesions affecting the spinothalamic tract in the dorsolateral medulla and pons. In addition to usually affecting the spinal trigeminal nucleus, a medullary lesion of this type impairs sensation of temperature and pain on the same side of the face as the lesion. The ipsilateral face and contralateral limbs are affected by the resulting crossed sensory deficit. By contrast, the face, limbs, and trunk contralateral to the lesion are affected by spinothalamic lesions above the spinal trigeminal nucleus. On the other side of the body, lesions affecting the medial lemniscus cause loss of proprioception and touch. Because the spinothalamic tract and medial lemniscus run parallel in the upper brainstem, a single lesion may result in the loss of all deep and superficial sensation on the body's contralateral side (Figure 9.3).

9.1.4.5. Thalamic Lesions

On the contralateral side of the body, thalamic lesions may result in loss or impairment of all forms of sensation, and this may occur in a different location than the area of symptomatic involvement. On the affected side, spontaneous pain is possible; occasionally, it may have an especially unpleasant aspect. Patients frequently struggle to characterize the pain, although they may describe it as burning, tearing, knifelike, or stabbing. It is possible for any type of cutaneous stimulation to cause uncomfortable or painful feelings. Lesions in the spinal cord or in the parietal lobe's white matter can also occasionally cause a thalamic syndrome similar to this one (Dejerine-Roussy syndrome).

9.1.4.6. Lesions of the Sensory Cortex

Disease confined to the sensory cortex affects the opposite side of the body's ability to discriminate between senses. Patients may experience difficulties identifying the location of various body parts or localizing stimuli on the affected side. They might not be able to estimate an object's size, weight, consistency, or texture, nor can they recognize an object by touch. Compared to the trunk or the proximal regions of the limbs, cortical sensory abnormalities are typically more noticeable in the hands.

9.1.5. Distinction Between Organic and Psychogenic Sensory Disturbances

Psychogenic sensation disturbances have been linked to psychiatric disorders like conversion disorder. Although they can take on any shape, they are typically limited to loss of skin feeling. There might be multiple distinguishing characteristics. Nonorganic sensory loss does not follow a particular neuroanatomic pattern in its distribution. It could encircle a bony landmark or pertain to a region delineated by surface landmarks instead of innervation. Although organic sensory loss with a margin like that is uncommon, it is not uncommon for there to be an apparent loss of sensation in one or more extremities, with circumferential margins in the axilla or groin. Due to overlap in the innervation on the two sides, organic peripheral sensory loss over the trunk or face typically stops 3 to 5 cm before the midline; in the case of nonorganic disturbances, apparent sensory loss typically ends exactly at the midline. Nonorganic sensory loss can abruptly change to normal sensation, while organic disturbances typically have an area of altered feeling between insensitive and normal sensibility areas.

It can be challenging to interpret a dissociated loss in nonorganic disturbances from an anatomical perspective. For instance, the ability to appreciate pinpricks may completely disappear while the sense of temperature is retained. Furthermore, the patient might still be able to walk normally, maintain an extended arm range without difficulty, or perform pseudoathetoid movements even though there appears to be a loss of posterior column function.

The ability to perceive vibration on one side of a bony midline structure, like the sternum or skull, but not the other, may be compromised in nonorganic sensory disturbances. In patients with organic sensory disorders, the vibrations are perceived on either side despite a hemisensory disturbance because the vibrations are actually conducted to both sides by the bone.

Lastly, it should be mentioned that the examiner's own expectations frequently lead the patient to believe that there are sensory disturbances. These results may be neuroanatomically correct, which makes them especially deceptive. Before conducting formal sensory testing, it can be beneficial to have the patient describe on their body the degree of any perceived sensory disturbance.

9.2. Peripheral Nerve Lesions

When a patient has peripheral nerve lesions, sensory symptoms are typically a noticeable characteristic (Table 9.1). Patients with polyneuropathies may experience sensory impairment in a distal stocking-and-glove pattern, while those with mononeuropathies may experience sensory impairment according to the pattern of individual peripheral nerves (Figure 9.4).

9.2.1. Classification

- **Mononeuropathy Simplex:** This term signifies involvement of a single peripheral nerve.
- **Mononeuropathy Multiplex:** Numerous individual nerves are impacted by this disorder, usually randomly and noncontiguously. A clinical examination indicates a deficit that can be attributed to one or more isolated peripheral nerves, unless there is a significant multiplex mononeuropathy and the resulting deficits become confluent.

Table 9.1. Causes of Peripheral Neuropathy

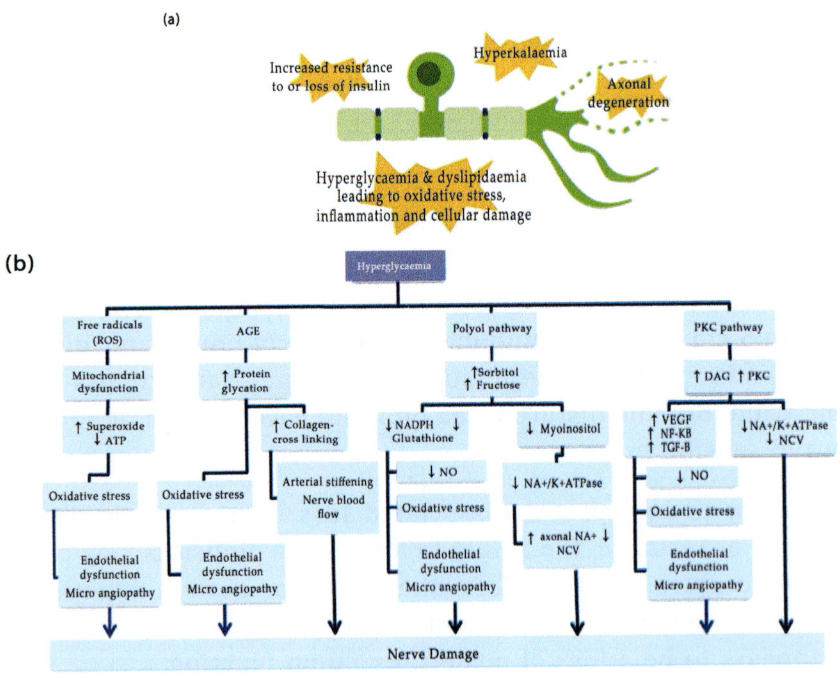

Source: Chiang JCB, Arnold R, Dhanapalaratnam R, Markoulli M, Krishnan AV. Current and Emerging Pharmacotherapeutic Interventions for the Treatment of Peripheral Nerve Disorders. *Pharmaceuticals.* 2022; 15(5):607. https://doi.org/10.3390/ph15050607.

- **Polyneuropathy:** A disorder known as polyneuropathy refers to a situation in which multiple peripheral nerves are simultaneously affected in function. Loss of tendon reflexes results, with the exception of situations in which small fibers are specifically involved, in a deficit that is primarily distal and symmetric. Depending on the primary site of nerve damage, polyneuropathies can occasionally be divided into smaller groups.

  The axon is the primary pathologic target in distal axonopathies, also known as axonal neuropathies; the majority of polyneuropathies fall into this group.

Myelin sheath disorders, also known as demyelinating neuropathies, affect the axon's myelin sheath. These disorders comprise the following: metachromatic leukodystrophy, Krabbe disease, types 1 and 3 Charcot-Marie-Tooth hereditary motor and sensory neuropathy (CMT-1 and 3), acute idiopathic polyneuropathy (Guillain-Barré syndrome), chronic inflammatory demyelinating neuropathy, diphtheria, certain paraneoplastic and paraproteinemic states.

Lastly, some conditions known as neuronopathies primarily impact nerve cell bodies in the dorsal root ganglion or anterior horn of the spinal cord. Examples include certain paraneoplastic syndromes, pyridoxine-induced neuropathy, and type 2 CMT hereditary motor and sensory neuropathy.

9.2.2. Clinical Findings

- **Sensory Disturbances:** When sensory fibers are involved, abnormal spontaneous sensations like pain and paresthesias, distorted sensations like hyperpathia (an exaggerated reaction to a normally painful stimulus), and numbness and impaired sensation can result.
    - **Pain:** One obvious sign of some neuropathies is pain, particularly if the affected nerve fibers are small. It's unclear exactly how it originated. Fabry disease, diabetes, alcoholism, porphyria, amyloidosis, rheumatoid arthritis, acquired immunodeficiency syndrome (AIDS), dominantly inherited sensory neuropathy, and paraneoplastic sensory neuronopathy are among the polyneuropathies linked to prominent pain. Numerous entrapment neuropathies and idiopathic brachial plexopathy also exhibit pain.
    - **Dissociated Sensory Loss:** Dissociated sensory loss is the loss of certain sensory modalities (pain, temperature, vibration) while maintaining other modalities (light touch, vibration, joint position sense). Dissociated sensory loss can occur in peripheral neuropathies when there is selective involvement of peripheral nerve fibers of a certain size, as in the case of hereditary sensory neuropathy, amyloid neuropathy, or leprous neuritis, although it also frequently indicates a spinal cord lesion. Autonomic dysfunction, spontaneous pain, and disproportionate impairment of pain and temperature perception are frequently linked to small fiber

disease. Large fiber disease, on the other hand, causes early loss of tendon reflexes, prominent motor symptoms, and impaired touch, vibration, and joint position sense.

- **Motor Deficits:** Lesions to the peripheral nerve can result in weakness of the muscles that the nerve innervates, and in more severe cases, wasting and fasciculation. The inability to perform fine motor skills may be exacerbated by any associated sensory loss. The distribution of these signs and the presence of concomitant sensory and reflex alterations suggest that the clinical findings, which point to a lower motor neuron deficit, may be the result of peripheral nerve involvement.
- **Tendon Reflexes:** If either the afferent or efferent side's reflex arcs (C5–C6, biceps and brachioradialis; C7–C8, triceps; L3–L4, knee; S1, ankle) are disrupted, these are compromised or lost. In patients with polyneuropathies, the ankle reflexes typically disappear first, though they can also disappear in older, healthy subjects.
- **Autonomic Disturbances:** Some peripheral neuropathies, such as Guillain-Barré syndrome and those caused by diabetes, renal failure, porphyria, certain paraneoplastic disorders, and amyloidosis, are characterized by autonomic disturbances that are particularly noticeable. Postural hypotension, tachycardia, cold extremities, reduced thermoregulatory sweating, bowel and bladder dysfunction, and impotence are among the symptoms.
- **Enlarged Nerves:** The possibility of leprosy, amyloidosis, hereditary motor and sensory neuropathies, Refsum disease, acromegaly, or chronic inflammatory demyelinating polyneuropathy is increased in cases of palpably enlarged peripheral nerves.

9.2.3. Evaluation of Patients

- **Time Course:** Acute polyneuropathy, such as that seen in Guillain-Barré syndrome, typically arises from an inflammatory process over the course of a few days. It might also be connected to an underlying tumor, infections like diphtheria, metabolic conditions like acute intermittent porphyria, or exposure to harmful substances like triorthocresyl phosphate or thallium. Chronic inflammatory demyelinating polyneuropathy shares characteristics with many hereditary or metabolic polyneuropathies, including a chronic course that evolves gradually over several years.

  When mononeuropathy develops gradually, it is more likely to be related to entrapment (i.e., compression by surrounding anatomic structures) or recurrent minor trauma. Acute mononeuropathy is likely to be traumatic or ischemic in origin.
- **Age at Onset:** Childhood or early adulthood-onset polyneuropathy is frequently inherited, though it can also be associated with an underlying inflammatory disease.

Polyneuropathy that manifests later is more likely to be caused by an underlying neoplasm or by a metabolic, toxic, or inflammatory disorder.

When mononeuritis appears in the neonatal period, it usually has a developmental origin or is related to birth injury; when it appears later in life, it may be related to entrapment or injury, which is frequently determined by one's occupation.

- **Occupational History:** Peripheral neuropathy can result from exposure to several industrial pollutants, such as DDT, arsenic, lead, thallium, methyl bromide, n-hexane, carbon disulfide, ethylene oxide, acrylamide, triorthocresyl phosphate, and some other organophosphates. Mononeuropathy may develop in response to entrapment or recurrent minor occupational trauma, but it can also occur as the initial clinical manifestation of a polyneuropathy related to the workplace. For instance, carpal tunnel syndrome is more common in people who perform heavy manual labor or who suffer from repetitive motion injuries from using computer terminals. Similarly, a lesion of the deep palmar branch of the ulnar nerve may be related to repeated pressure on the hand's palm from activities like using a pneumatic road drill or forcefully punching down on a stapler.
- **Medical History**
    - **Metabolic Disorders:** Metachromatic leukodystrophy, Fabry disease, diabetes mellitus, uremia, liver disease, myxedema, and acromegaly are some metabolic disorders that may be associated with peripheral neuropathy. Diabetes-related mononeuropathy is particularly significant and can manifest as autonomic neuropathy, subacute proximal motor polyradiculoplexopathy (diabetic amyotrophy), distal sensorimotor polyneuropathy, entrapment mononeuropathy, or acute ischemic mononeuropathy.
    - **Neoplasm:** Primary tumors or metastatic lymph nodes may extend and compress peripheral nerves, spinal nerves, and limb plexuses. Lambert-Eaton syndrome and nonmetastatic (paraneoplastic) sensory or sensorimotor polyneuropathy can also result from neoplastic disease.
    - **Connective Tissue Disorders:** Mononeuropathy multiplex, polyneuropathy, and cranial neuropathy can be associated with Polyarteritis nodosa, rheumatoid arthritis, Churg-Strauss syndrome, and granulomatosis with polyangiitis (formerly Wegener granulomatosis). Systemic lupus erythematosus more commonly presents with polyneuropathy. Focal entrapment or compressive mononeuropathies near affected joints can occur with rheumatoid arthritis.
    - **AIDS:** A distal, symmetric, predominantly sensory polyneuropathy is frequently

linked to acquired immune deficiency syndrome (AIDS). Acute or chronic inflammatory demyelinating polyneuropathy, polyradiculopathy, mononeuropathy multiplex, or autonomic neuropathy are less commonly linked to AIDS. Additionally, asymptomatic HIV-1 infection and HIV-1 seroconversion are associated with neuropathies.

- **Drug and Alcohol History:** A selection of medications that selectively affect motor or sensory fibers is shown in Table 9.2, which includes some of the medications that cause peripheral neuropathy.

9.2.4. Differential Diagnosis

A motor, sensory, or combined deficit may result from peripheral neuropathies. The motor deficit resulting from pure pyramidal lesions, spinal muscular atrophies, myopathies, or disorders of neuromuscular transmission can be distinguished from that resulting from peripheral nerve involvement by the preservation of sensation and tendon reflexes.

Distal sensory loss and a pyramidal deficit below the level of the lesion are characteristics of myelopathies. Examination reveals additional stigmas associated with syphilis. A history of syphilitic infection is common in cases of tabes dorsalis. Furthermore, tactile perception is maintained.

Table 9.2. Summary of Antineoplastic and Neurotoxic Mechanisms in Chemotherapy-Induced Peripheral Neurotoxicity. DRG: Dorsal Root Ganglia; NGF: Nerve Growth Factor; TRP: Transient Receptor Potential Channels

Chemotherapy Agent	Antineoplastic Mechanisms	CIPN Pathophysiology
Taxanes	Microtubule damage that impairs mitotic spindle formation in cancer cells [4–6].	Activation of caspases, oxidative stress on peripheral neuronal and non-neuronal cells, mitotoxicity, inhibition of anterograde fast axonal transport, prevention of microtubule disassembly, alteration of both activity and expression of voltage-gated ion channels in the DRG; immune activation in the DRG and peripheral nerves, and microglial activation in the spinal cord; TRP upregulation in DRG [7–12].
Vinca alkaloids	Binding to free tubulin dimers close to the GTP-binding sites and induction of cell death by inhibition of microtubule assembly [13, 14].	Increase of microtubule depolymerization and inhibition of the hydrolysis of GTP; membrane excitability, inflammation, axonal transport impairment; mitochondria and glial function alterations; differential expression of voltage-gated ion channels, alteration of neurotransmission, impairment of axonal transport, increased production and release of proinflammatory cytokine and chemokines [8, 9, 11, 12, 15].

Eribulin	Suppression of microtubule dynamic instability at low concentration and promotion of microtubule disassembly at high concentration [16].	Reduction of anterograde fast axonal transport; reduction of kinesin-dependent transport in axon [17].
Epothilones	Stabilization of microtubules, leading to apoptosis in cancer cells [18].	Microtubule stabilization; reduction of kinesin-dependent transport [17].
Platinum compounds	Platinum-DNA adduct formation, alterations in transmembrane receptors and channels that lead to cell cycle arrest and apoptosis [19, 20].	Accumulation of platinum atom in the DRG sensory neurons, nuclear and mitochondrial DNA damage, oxidative stress and channellopathy; TRP channels affected; axonal transport impairment; activation of caspases and protein kinase, glial cell activation, increased production and release of proinflammatory cytokine and chemokines [7–12, 21].
Proteasome inhibitors	Inhibition of proteasome activity, which results in protein aggregate accumulation in tumor cells, cell cycle arrest and apoptosis [22, 23].	Protein aggregate accumulation in soma neurons, alteration of physiological turnover of axonal proteins, axonal transport impairment; damage to neuronal mitochondria and organelles and Schwann cell microtubule stabilization, oxidative stress; activation of TRP channels; inflammation and glial cell activation; alterations of neurotransmission [9–12, 15].
Thalidomide	Immunomodulation and antiangiogenic effects, down-regulation of tumor necrosis factor alpha (TNFα) [24].	Capillary damage due to its antiangiogenic activity in nerve fibers; downregulation of TNFα and inhibition of NF-κB that interferes with NGF activity [10, 21].

Source: Malacrida A, Meregalli C, Rodriguez-Menendez V, Nicolini G. Chemotherapy-Induced Peripheral Neuropathy and Changes in Cytoskeleton. *International Journal of Molecular Sciences.* 2019; 20(9):2287. https://doi.org/10.3390/ijms20092287.

The distribution of motor or sensory deficits distinguishes radiculopathies from peripheral neuropathies (Figure 9.4). A radicular distribution of neck or back pain radiating to the extremities is another indication of a root lesion.

9.2.5. Investigative Studies

The goal of laboratory testing on peripheral neuropathy patients is to confirm the diagnosis and identify any underlying causes.

Electromyography can be used to assess whether any motor units are still capable of being controlled voluntarily and can also show signs of denervation in the affected muscles. Conduction velocity in motor and sensory fibers can be measured thanks to research on nerve conduction. Peripheral neuropathies can be classified as demyelinating or axonal neuropathies based on electrodiagnostic or histopathologic investigations.

Electromyography usually shows little to no evidence of denervation in demyelinating neuropathies, but affected nerves exhibit conduction block or a marked slowing of their maximal conduction velocity. Electromyography reveals denervation in axonal neuropathies, particularly in the distal extremities, but the maximal nerve conduction velocity is either normal or only slightly slowed.

The diagnosis of a peripheral nerve disorder may be made with the aid of a chest X-ray, erythrocyte sedimentation rate, serum urea nitrogen and creatinine, serum protein, protein electrophoresis and immunoelectrophoresis, serum vitamin B12, liver and thyroid function blood tests, and serologic tests for syphilis (FTA or MHA-TP), rheumatoid factor, and antinuclear antibody. Serologic testing for hepatitis, HIV infection, Lyme disease, or paraneoplastic antibodies may be necessary, depending on the clinical situation. Further genetic studies might be required following appropriate genetic counseling.

If toxic causes are suspected, samples of hair and fingernail clippings can be tested for arsenic, and a 24-hour urine collection followed by a heavy metal analysis may be useful. When porphyria is suspected, a fresh specimen of urine must be examined for δ-aminolevulinic acid and porphobilinogen.

9.2.6. Treatment

- **Disease-Specific Treatment:** Treating the underlying cause of the neuropathy may stop it from getting worse or even reverse it. Treatments particular to each disease are covered under individual disorders later on.
- **Ventilatory Assistance:** It is important to keep an eye on respiratory function, especially in cases of acute idiopathic polyneuropathy (Guillain-Barré syndrome), chronic inflammatory demyelinating polyneuropathy, and diphtheritic neuropathy. If the forced vital capacity falls below 15 mL/kg, the mean inspiratory force falls below -40 mm Hg, dyspnea appears, or the arterial blood's oxygen saturation starts to drop, ventilation assistance should be prepared.
- **Trauma Prevention:** Nursing care is essential to preventing joint contractures, decubitus ulcers, and further compressive peripheral nerve damage in patients with severe motor or sensory deficits. A cradle, or metal bar frame, can be used to prevent bedclothes from touching delicate skin in patients suffering from severe dysesthesia.

It is necessary to protect extremities with sensory loss from recurrent minor trauma, such as thermal injury, which can cause tissue destruction. To avoid scalding, water heater settings should be lowered and the temperature of heated surfaces should be tested using a body part that retains feeling. The nails and skin need to be properly taken care of.

- **Pain Relief:** Individuals with sensory disorders may experience exceptionally intense pain, which can negatively impact their quality of life. It's critical that this pain be treated.

Both venlafaxine and duloxetine are selective serotonin and norepinephrine reuptake inhibitors that are frequently helpful. Venlafaxine can be titrated up to 75 mg twice or three times daily in the standard formulation, or as the equivalent dose once daily in the extended-release formulation. Neuropathic pain is also alleviated by pregabalin (150 mg, increasing to 300 mg daily in divided doses after 1 week; maximum, 600 mg daily).

Certain neuropathies can occasionally be made to stop the lancinating pain by taking 300 mg/d of phenytoin, up to 1200 mg/d of carbamazepine, or 600–900 mg/d of mexiletine. Amitriptyline 25 to 100 mg before bed is frequently beneficial, as are other tricyclic medications, if the pain is persistent, burning, or dysesthesia.

Treatment for different neuropathic pain disorders with gabapentin (300 mg three times a day, with further increases based on response and tolerance) is successful; less research has been done on the effects of lamotrigine, topiramate, or sodium valproate on pain. To prevent skin rashes and other side effects, lamotrigine dosages must be gradually increased.

For neuropathic pain (such as diabetic neuropathy or postherpetic neuralgia), a combination of gabapentin and nortriptyline may be more beneficial than either medication used alone. For patients who need more pain relief and show a partial response to either medication when taken alone, this combination of drugs is advised. Another useful treatment for neuropathic pain syndromes is topical capsaicin.

- **Autonomic Disturbances:** In certain polyneuropathies, particularly diabetic polyneuropathy, dysautonomic symptoms can be problematic. Postural hypotension may be treated with waist-high elastic stockings, dietary salt supplementation, and oral fludrocortisone dosages of 0–0.5 mg/d; however, the patient needs to be closely watched to avoid recumbent hypertension. Moreover, clonidine, midodrine, dihydroergotamine, octreotide, or β-blockers might be beneficial. Because dysautonomic patients frequently cannot conserve salt and water when recumbent, it is beneficial to instruct the patients to sleep semierect rather than recumbent.

9.3. Polyneuropathies

9.3.1. Idiopathic Inflammatory Neuropathies

9.3.1.1. Acute Idiopathic Polyneuropathy (Guillain-Barré Syndrome)

Acute or subacute polyneuropathy, Guillain-Barré syndrome can develop after minor infectious diseases, vaccinations, or surgical procedures, or it can develop without any clear cause. Evidence from clinical and epidemiologic studies points to a correlation with a prior infection with *Campylobacter jejuni*. Although the exact cause is unknown, immunologic factors are probably involved. There are two types: demyelinating and axonal, each with unique clinical and electrophysiologic characteristics. In the US, the demyelinating neuropathy is more prevalent, but axonal variants, such as acute motor sensory axonal neuropathy, are also occasionally seen. A related axonal form known as acute motor axonal neuropathy is common in northern China.

- **Clinical Features:** Table 9.3 provides a summary of the diagnostic features. Patients typically exhibit symmetrical ascending weakness that usually starts in the legs, is more noticeable close to the source than farther away, and can even be fatal if it affects the swallowing or breathing muscles. If there has been axonal degeneration, muscle atrophy results. Even though they are typically milder than motor symptoms, sensory complaints are nonetheless common. Usually, the deep tendon reflexes are not present. Significant autonomic dysfunction may be present, along with other anomalies such as paralytic ileus, tachycardia, cardiac irregularities, labile blood pressure, disturbed sweating, and impaired pulmonary function.
- **Investigative Studies:** The cerebrospinal fluid (CSF) frequently exhibits cytoalbuminologic dissociation, which is an elevated protein concentration with a normal cell count; however, abnormalities may not appear during the first week. Electrophysiologic studies may demonstrate a discernible slowing down of sensory and motor conduction velocity, as well as signs of axonal loss and denervation. It's not always the case that clinical advancements coincide with the electrophysiologic changes' time course. Serologic testing should be carried out when HIV-1 infection is suspected due to high-risk factors or the clinical setting in which the neuropathy first appeared.

Table 9.3. Features of GBS Subtypes

Type	Symptoms	Pathology
AIDP	Most common variant (85% of cases). Primarily motor inflammatory demyelination ± secondary axonal damage. Maximum of four weeks of progression.	Macrophages invade intact myelin sheaths and denude the axons.
AMAN	Motor only with early and severe respiratory involvement. Primary axonal degeneration. Often affects children, young adults. Up to 75% positive *Campylobacter jejuni* serology. Often positive for anti-GM1, anti-GD1a antibodies.	Macrophages invade the nodes of Ranvier where they insert between the axon and the surrounding Schwann-cell axolemma, leaving the myelin sheath intact.
AMSAN	Motor and sensory affection with critical course of respiratory and bulbar involvement. Primary axonal degeneration with poorer prognosis.	Similar to AMAN but also involving vetral and dorsal roots.
MF	Ophthalmoplegia, sensory ataxia, areflexia. 5% of all cases. 96% positive for anti-GQ1b antibodies.	Abnormality in sensory conduction, although the underlying pathology is not clear.

Source: Torres-Vásquez M, Chávez-Bosquez O, Hernández-Ocaña B, Hernández-Torruco J. Classification of Guillain–Barré Syndrome Subtypes Using Sampling Techniques with Binary Approach. *Symmetry.* 2020; 12(3):482. https://doi.org/10.3390/sym12030482.

Key:

- Acute Inflammatory Demyelinating Polyneuropathy (AIDP)
- Acute Motor Axonal Neuropathy (AMAN)
- Acute Motor Sensory Axonal Neuropathy (AMSAN)
- Miller–Fisher Syndrome (MF)
- **Treatment:** Plasmapheresis seems to shorten the time needed for recuperation and may lessen the possibility that neurologic deficits will persist. It is recommended for patients with a severe or quickly progressing deficit or respiratory compromise, and it is best to start as soon as possible. If an adult or child has cardiovascular instability, intravenous immunoglobulin (400 mg/kg/d for 5 days) seems to be as effective as plasmapheresis; the two treatments are not complementary.

  The goal of therapy, which is otherwise symptomatic, is to avoid complications like vascular collapse or respiratory failure. Because of this, patients who are seriously impacted are best cared for in intensive care units, where resources for monitoring and assisted respiration are available if needed (e.g., if the patient experiences dyspnea, the mean inspiratory force drops to –40 mm Hg, the forced vital capacity reaches 15 mL/kg, or the blood oxygen saturation decreases). To counteract hypotension, volume replacement or pressor agent therapy may be necessary. Low-dose heparin may also help prevent pulmonary embolism. Corticosteroids are not advised because they could have a negative effect or prolong the healing process.
- **Prognosis:** By around four weeks into the illness, the symptoms and indicators stop getting worse. The illness is self-limiting, and weeks or months after onset are when improvement happens. 70% of patients fully recover, 25% have mild neurologic deficits, and five percent pass away, usually from respiratory failure. Axonal degeneration is the predominant pathology, and a longer course and less complete recovery are also likely when there is evidence of prior Campylobacter jejuni infection. These factors contribute to a worse prognosis. A worse prognosis may also be predicted by advanced age, the need for ventilatory support, or earlier onset of symptoms.

9.3.1.2. Chronic Inflammatory Demyelinating Polyneuropathy

Clinically, chronic inflammatory demyelinating polyneuropathy is comparable to Guillain-Barré syndrome, with the exception that it progresses chronically or relapses frequently and shows no improvement within six months of onset. The cause of it is unknown. Table 9.4 provides a summary of its clinical characteristics.

Results from a CSF examination are similar to those seen in Guillain-Barré syndrome. The electrophysiologic results show axonal degeneration superimposed on a demyelinating neuropathy.

Treatment with corticosteroids (prednisone 60–100 mg/d for 2–4 weeks, then tapered to 5–20 mg every other day) is often effective in treating the disorder and may be necessary in the long run. Intravenous immunoglobulin therapy is also effective as initial or follow-up therapy (1 g/kg daily for 2 days with a single additional infusion at 3 weeks, or 400 mg/kg/d for 5 consecutive days for a total of 2 g, with subsequent courses as needed to maintain benefit). It is more expensive than prednisone but has fewer side effects when used as initial therapy. Its exact mechanism of action is unclear. Although it is more difficult to administer, plasma exchange is another efficient immunomodulator therapy. Treatment with azathioprine or cyclophosphamide may be beneficial in nonresponsive patients; however, claims of benefit from cyclosporine, interferon-β, or interferon-α, as well as from these agents, need to be verified by randomized trials.

Table 9.4. Clinical Features of Chronic Inflammatory Demyelinating Polyneuropathy (CIDP)

Typical CIDP		
	Signs	Symptoms
	Absent or reduced tendon reflexes in all limbs	Gradual or recurring, similar weakening of muscles in both the upper and lower limbs, affecting the closer and farther parts of the limbs, accompanied by sensory issues in at least two limbs
Atypical CIDP		
Variant	Signs	Symptoms
DADS	Normal or low DTR in proximal areas	Distal sensory loss and muscle weakness, predominantly in the lower limbs
Multifocal CIDP	Tendon reflexes may be normal in unaffected limbs	Loss of sensation and muscle weakness occur in multiple areas, often with uneven distribution, typically showing a preference for the upper limbs and affecting more than one limb
Focal CIDP	Low DTR	Loss of sensation and muscle weakness restricted to a single limb
Motor CIDP	Low DTR	Symptoms related to movement and physical indications without any associated sensory issues
Sensory CIDP	Absent or low DTR inall limbs	Sensory indications and signs present without any associated involvement of movement or motor functions

Source: Tsoumanis P, Kitsouli A, Stefanou C, Papathanakos G, Stefanou S, Tepelenis K, Zikidis H, Tsoumani A, Zafeiropoulos P, Kitsoulis P, et al. Chronic Inflammatory Demyelinating Polyneuropathy and Evaluation of the Visual Evoked Potentials: A Review of the Literature. *Medicina*. 2023; 59(12):2160. https://doi.org/10.3390/medicina59122160.

9.3.2. Metabolic and Nutritional Neuropathies

9.3.2.1. Diabetes Mellitus

Diabetes frequently results in peripheral nerve involvement, which can manifest in a variety of ways (Table 9.5) and happen singly or in combination. The degree of diabetes control, which should always be optimized, may have an impact on the incidence of peripheral nerve involvement.

- **Clinical Features:** The most prevalent symptom is distal polyneuropathy, which can be mostly sensory (30%) or mixed (sensory, motor, and autonomic; 70% of cases). The symptoms, which include paresthesias, pain, and numbness, are typically more prevalent in the legs than the arms. Depressed tendon reflexes and reduced ability to perceive vibration in the legs can be used as presymptomatic indicators. Severe cases involve some accompanying motor disturbance and distal sensory loss in all limbs.

Numerous symptoms, such as postural hypotension, cardiac rhythm abnormalities, reduced thermoregulatory sweating, and problems with the bladder, bowel, stomach, and sexual organs are caused by diabetic dysautonomia.

Diabetic mononeuropathy multiplex is characterized by pain and weakness, often with a vascular cause. The specific clinical symptoms depend on which nerves are affected. Diabetic amyotrophy can be caused by radiculoplexopathy, polyradiculopathy, or polyradiculoneuropathy, resulting in pain, weakness, and muscle atrophy in the pelvic girdle and thigh muscles, as well as diminished quadriceps reflexes and minimal sensory loss. Diabetic mononeuropathy simplex typically has a sudden onset and is often painful. An increased concentration of CSF protein is usually seen in cases of diabetic polyneuropathy and mononeuropathy multiplex.

Table 9.5. Diabetic Mononeuropathy and Other Complications

Category	**Etiology**	
Diabetes	Diabetes mellitus type 1, type 2	
Alcohol	Alcohol consumption	
Toxins	Lead, mercury, arsenic, acrylamide, thallium, organic solvent	
Thyroid	Myxedema (hypothyroidism)	
Connective tissue disease	Systemic lupus erythematosus, Sjögren syndrome, systemic sclerosis, vasculitis	
Infections	HIV, leprosy, Lyme borreliosis	
Systemic disease	Liver failure (cirrhosis), renal failure (uremia), acromegaly, amyloidosis, Sarcoidosis	
Vitamin deficiency	Vitamin B12 (distal sensitive deficit), pyroxidin overdose, thiamine (alcohol, malnutrition), malabsorption syndrome	
Paraneoplastic	Lymphoma, paraproteins (combined with POEMS, CANOMAD syndromes)	
Hereditary	Charcot-Marie-Tooth disease, hereditary sensitive and autonomic neuropathy, family amyloid polyneuropathy, distal hereditary motoric neuropathy	
Spinal cord	Trauma, tumor, infection	
Idiopathic	About 25% of patients	
Medication	Class	Medication
	Chemotherapy	Quinecin, bortezomib, platinum, (carboplatin, cisplatin), suramin, taxol (docetaxel, paclitaxel), vincristine
	Antibiotics	Ethambutol, isoniazid, metronidazole, misonidazol, nitrofurantoin, dapson

	Anticonvulsants	Phenytoin
	Antiarrhythmic	Amiodarone
	Antirheumatics	Chloroquine, gold
	Vitamins	Pyridoxine (vitamin B6)
	Toxins (may be found in homeopathic medication)	Lead, mercury, arsenic, acrylamide, thallium, organic solvent, organophosphates

Source: Volmer-Thole M, Lobmann R. Neuropathy and Diabetic Foot Syndrome. *International Journal of Molecular Sciences*. 2016; 17(6):917. https://doi.org/10.3390/ijms17060917.

- **Treatment and Prognosis:** Diabetes-related peripheral nerve problems have no particular treatment, with the possible exception of entrapment neuropathy, in which case a decompressive procedure may be beneficial. The earlier section covered the treatment of pain or autonomic disturbances. Diabetic amyotrophy typically gets better on its own. Optimizing the management of diabetes is crucial.

9.3.2.2. Other Endocrinopathies

- **Hypothyroidism:** Though it rarely results in polyneuropathy, hypothyroidism is linked to entrapment neuropathy, particularly carpal tunnel syndrome (median nerve entrapment). Patients with delayed relaxation of tendon reflexes, a classic sign of hypothyroidism that is distinct from neuropathy, or those with proximal limb weakness from hypothyroid myopathy may be misdiagnosed with polyneuropathy. Additional neurological symptoms of hypothyroidism include cerebellar ataxia, dementia, and an acute state of confusion.
- **Acromegaly:** Moreover, this frequently results in polyneuropathy and, less frequently, carpal tunnel syndrome. Since many patients with acromegaly also have diabetes, it can be challenging to identify which condition is primarily to blame for polyneuropathy in a particular patient.

9.3.2.3. Uremia

Uremia may cause a symmetric sensorimotor polyneuropathy, primarily of the axonal type. It is more prominent distally than proximally, primarily affecting the legs as opposed to the arms, and it is related to the degree of impaired renal function. Burning feet, cramping in the muscles, and restless legs could be related. Renal transplantation may significantly ameliorate the neuropathy. In addition to developing distal to the arteriovenous fistulas inserted in the forearm to provide access during hemodialysis, carpal tunnel syndrome can also be associated with renal disease. It is frequently associated with amyloidosis and β2-microglobulin accumulation in patients receiving chronic hemodialysis.

9.3.2.4. Liver Disease

It is possible for primary biliary cirrhosis to cause axonal-type sensory neuropathy. With chronic liver disease, a predominantly demyelinating polyneuropathy may develop. The degree of the hepatic dysfunction does not seem to be correlated with the neurologic findings.

9.3.2.5. Vitamin B12 Deficiency

Loss of tendon reflexes, symmetric distal sensory impairment, and mild motor impairment are linked to vitamin B12 deficiency. Vitamin B12 deficiency is discussed in more detail later, in the section on myelopathies, due to disagreement regarding the relative contributions of polyneuropathy and myelopathy in the development of this syndrome. Following bariatric surgery, polyradiculoneuropathy, polyneuropathy, and myelopathy may occur. These conditions are associated with deficiencies in certain nutrients, such as vitamin B12.

9.3.3. Infective and Granulomatous Neuropathies

9.3.3.1. AIDS

A common consequence of HIV-1 infection is neuropathy (Table 9.6); about 40% of AIDS patients have peripheral nerve involvement during autopsy. It could have an immunologic basis, be related to medication or nutritional deficiencies, be the result of HIV infection, or be a secondary infection with another organism (such as the cytomegalovirus, varicellazoster virus, or Treponema pallidum).

Table 9.6. Neuropathies Associated With AIDS

Demographic Risk Factors	Genetic Risk Factors
Low nadir $CD4^+$ T-cell count HIV duration Age Height High plasma HIV RNA Diabetes mellitus Malnutrition Neurotoxic drugs • NRTI: stavudine, didanosine • Protease inhibitors: indinavir, ritonavir, saquinavir	Race (more common in African populations) Polymorphisms in • Mitochondrial DNA (mtDNA) • HFE (affecting iron metabolism) • Cytokine genes (IL4, IL10, IL12B) • TNF gene block (central MHC) • P2X4R, P2X7R (purinergic receptors) • CAMKK2 (affecting neuronal repair)

Source: Octaviana, F., Yanuar Safri, A., Imran, D., & Price, P. (2019). HIV-Associated Sensory Neuropathy. IntechOpen. doi: 10.5772/intechopen.81176.

HIV-1-associated distal symmetric sensorimotor or predominantly sensory polyneuropathy is the most prevalent neuropathy. Myelin is not the main target; axons are. The exact cause is unknown, however, in certain patients, exposure to neurotoxic medications (which should be avoided) or a vitamin B12 deficiency may be partially to blame. It is necessary to rule out other causes of neuropathy. Seldom is HIV-1 found in the damaged nerves. The majority of symptoms are sensory, with pain and paresthesias primarily affecting the feet. Weakness is a subtle or developed trait. There is a lack of ankle and occasionally knee reflexes. Usually, the course is progressive. Enhancement of sensory function could be facilitated by combination antiretroviral therapy (cART). As previously mentioned, pharmacological means can be employed to manage pain. Plasmapheresis has no advantages.

Early on in HIV-1 infection, inflammatory demyelinating polyneuropathy may develop and may progress either acutely or chronically. Immune-mediated neuropathy is possible, but direct secondary viral infections, like those caused by cytomegalovirus, can also cause neuropathy. It is typified by areflexia or hyporeflexia, proximal weakness with less severe sensory disturbances, and occasionally distal weakness. Unlike the results in patients without HIV-1 infection who have chronic inflammatory demyelinating polyneuropathy or Guillain-Barré syndrome, the CSF is aberrant, with an increased protein concentration and frequently a lymphocytic pleocytosis. While some patients respond to intravenous immunoglobulin, plasmapheresis, or corticosteroids, others may improve on their own or stabilize.

Late in the course of HIV-1 infection, lumbar polyradiculopathy typically manifests in individuals who have previously experienced opportunistic infections. The cause, at least in some cases, is cytomegalovirus infection. Clinical features include diffuse, progressive leg weakness, back pain, painful paresthesias of the feet and perineum, lower extremity areflexia, and early urinary retention. These features typically appear over a few weeks. The course can occasionally be more benign, particularly when the etiology is unknown, but it can also be fulminant, with ascending paralysis leading to respiratory failure. Increased protein concentration, decreased glucose, and mononuclear or polymorphonuclear pleocytosis are among the CSF findings; additional support comes from a positive polymerase chain reaction test for cytomegalovirus. Excluding meningeal lymphomatosis, cord compression, or syphilis as the underlying cause is always crucial because these conditions have different treatment needs and have an impact on prognosis. Individuals infected with the cytomegalovirus may benefit from ganciclovir injections 2 × 10^5 mg/kg every 8 hours for 10 days, followed by 7 ± 5 mg/kg/d for 5 days per week. Foscarnet is an alternate method; in extreme circumstances, both medications are administered. It is not a sign of treatment failure if there is some worsening during the first two weeks of ganciclovir therapy. After three weeks, the CSF should be reexamined to see if the polymorphonuclear cell count has decreased; if not, ganciclovir should be switched out for foscarnet.

Multiple cranial and peripheral nerves are affected by mononeuropathy multiplex, which causes focal weakness and sensory loss. This could stem from vasculopathy, neoplastic, infectious, or autoimmune causes (e.g., cytomegalovirus infection). Mononeuropathy multiplex in the early stages of HIV-1 infection may be a self-limited condition affecting only one limb that resolves on its own or stabilizes spontaneously. Multiple limbs may gradually become affected in the latter stages of AIDS. When HIV-1 infection is first developing, mononeuropathy simplex typically manifests acutely and resolves on its own. A vascular cause seems likely.

Autonomic neuropathy typically manifests towards the end of HIV-1 infections and can cause syncopal episodes, orthostatic hypotension, sphincter or sexual function disturbances, poor thermoregulatory sweating, and diarrhea. Central or peripheral pathology may be connected to dysautonomia. Symptomatic treatment is applied.

Treatment with the antiretroviral medications stavudine (d4T), didanosine (ddI), and zalcitabine (ddC) may cause medication-related neuropathy after about 4 months unless the patient has other coexisting conditions that make them more susceptible. It is an axonal sensory neuropathy that manifests as pain, numbness, and distal tingling. Other medications such as isoniazid, ethambutol, vincristine, vinblastine, Taxol, thalidomide, and statins may also be linked to neuropathy in AIDS patients.

9.3.3.2. Leprosy

Peripheral neuropathy is frequently caused by leprosy, according to global statistics. On the other hand, neuropathy is the most incapacitating leprosy symptom. The skin and peripheral nerves are affected by Mycobacterium leprae due to its ability to grow in cooler temperatures found at the skin's surface.

The immune system responds to tuberculoid leprosy well enough to limit the infection to one or more small skin patches and the cutaneous and subcutaneous nerves that supply them. This results in a hypopigmented macule or papule that impairs feeling, most notably in the areas of pain and temperature perception. The autonomic fibers are involved in anhidrosis. While motor findings are typically associated with involvement of the ulnar or fibular (peroneal) nerve, sensory deficits are most frequently found in the distribution of the digital, sural, radial, and posterior auricular nerves. The nerves involved are frequently enlarged.

A more common form of lepromatous leprosy causes a symmetric, mostly sensory polyneuropathy that disproportionately impairs the senses of pain and temperature. Its distribution is unique in that it preferentially affects exposed areas of the body, such as the nose, cheeks, ears, forearms, and feet, as well as the lateral parts of the legs. Leprosy-related polyneuropathies, in contrast to most others, typically spare the tendon reflexes. Resorption of the fingers, trophic ulcers, cyanosis and anhidrosis of the hands and feet are associated findings.

9.3.3.3. Diphtheria

The upper respiratory tract tissues are infected by Corynebacterium diphtheriae, which also produces a toxin that demyelinates peripheral nerves. Patients may experience a notable impairment in their ability to accommodate their eyes due to cranial motor neuropathy within a month of infection. The most common presenting complaint is blurred vision. The pupillary light reflex is unaffected, but extraocular muscles, the face, palate, pharynx, and diaphragm may also be impacted. Usually, recovery takes several weeks. A more delayed syndrome manifests as a symmetric distal sensorimotor polyneuropathy and typically appears two to three months after the initial infection. The majority of patients fully recover.

9.3.3.4. Sarcoidosis

Rarely, polyneuropathy or mononeuropathy may result from sarcoidosis. Cranial nerves, particularly the facial nerve, are frequently affected by mononeuropathy. A small-fiber neuropathy can occasionally cause autonomic involvement, pain, and dysesthesias. Sarcoidosis can be diagnosed with the aid of clinical assessment for extraneural disease, X-rays of the lungs and bones, CSF examination, and measurement of angiotensin-converting enzyme serum levels. Prednisone therapy, administered orally at a dose of 60 mg/d, may expedite recuperation.

9.3.3.5. Sepsis and Multiorgan Failure

Patients with sepsis and multiorgan failure may develop a critical illness polyneuropathy.

9.3.4. Neuropathies in Vasculitis and Collagen Vascular Disease

Systemic vasculitis and collagen-related vascular pathologies can lead to polyneuropathy, mononeuropathy simplex, mononeuropathy multiplex, or entrapment neuropathy (Table 9.7).

9.3.5. Systemic Necrotizing Vasculitis

This comprises granulomatosis (Churg-Strauss syndrome), allergic angiitis, and polyarteritis nodosa. About 50% of patients develop neuropathy, most commonly as mononeuropathy multiplex, which can cause acute pain in one or more cranial or peripheral nerves. It is less common to have distal symmetric sensorimotor polyneuropathy. As soon as a diagnosis is made, treatment should start. Oral prednisone dosages range from 60 to 100 mg/d and cyclophosphamide dosages from 2 to 3 mg/d.

- **Granulomatosis with Polyangiitis (Wegener Granulomatosis):** Up to 30% of cases have polyneuropathy or mononeuropathy multiplex. The course of treatment for systemic necrotizing vasculitis is the same.
- **Giant Cell Arteritis:** Mononeuropathy affecting cranial nerves innervating the extraocular muscles is seen here.
- **Rheumatoid Arthritis:** About 45% of patients with rheumatoid arthritis experience entrapment neuropathy, which most often affects the median nerve, and about 30% experience distal symmetric sensorimotor polyneuropathy. A common feature in cases complicated by necrotizing vasculitis is mononeuropathy multiplex.
- **Systemic Lupus Erythematosus:** Up to 20% of patients experience neuropathy. A distal, symmetric sensorimotor polyneuropathy is the most typical pattern. An ascending polyneuropathy, primarily motor (Guillain-Barré syndrome; see earlier) may also manifest, as can simplex or multiplex mononeuropathy, which frequently affects the sciatic, ulnar, radial, or fibular (peroneal) nerves.

Table 9.7. Neuropathies Associated with Vasculitis and Collagen Vascular Disease

Disease	Polyneuropathy	Mononeuropathy Simplex or Multiplex[1]	Entrapment Neuropathy[1]
Vasculitis			
Systemic necrotizing vasculitis[2]	+	+	–
Granulomatosis with polyangiitis	+	+	–
Giant cell arteritis	–	+ (III, VI, IV)	–
Collagen vascular disease			
Rheumatoid arthritis	+	+	+ (M, U, R)
Systemic lupus erythematosus	+	+	–
Sjögren syndrome	+	+ (V, III, VI)	+ (M)
Progressive systemic sclerosis	–	+ (V)	–
Mixed connective-tissue disease	+	+ (V)	–

[1]Commonly affected nerves: III, oculomotor; IV, trochlear; V, trigeminal; VI, abducens; M, median; R, radial; U, ulnar.

[2]Includes polyarteritis nodosa and Churg-Strauss syndrome.

+, present; –, absent.

Source: https://dl.mehrsys.ir/pdf-books/Clinical%20Neurology%209%20Edition%20(www.myuptodate.com).pdf.

- **Sjögren Syndrome:** About 20% of cases of Sjögren syndrome involve the peripheral nerves. The most prevalent type of polyneuropathy is distal symmetric sensorimotor polyneuropathy; entrapment neuropathy, which primarily affects the median nerve, is also common; and mononeuropathy multiplex can also happen.
- **Scleroderma and Mixed Connective tissue Disease:** Cranial mononeuropathy, most commonly affecting the trigeminal (V) nerve, can result from mixed connective tissue disease and progressive systemic sclerosis (scleroderma).

9.3.6. Neoplastic and Paraproteinemic Neuropathies

- **Compression and Infiltration by Tumor:** One common side effect of multiple myeloma, lymphoma, and carcinoma is nerve compression. Cancers such as leukemia, lymphoma, and pancreatic or breast carcinoma can all cause tumorous invasion of the epineurium.
- **Paraneoplastic Syndromes:** Based on the finding of autoantibodies to neuronal antigens in multiple cases, neuropathies related to cancer (particularly small-cell lung cancer) and lymphoma may be immunologically mediated.
    - **Sensory or Sensorimotor Polyneuropathy:** Both lymphoma and carcinoma exhibit this. It is occasionally asymmetrical, can be acute or chronic, and may be accompanied by noticeable pain. Although the CSF is normally acellular, there may be a slight increase in protein concentration. About 10% of patients with a chronic sensorimotor polyneuropathy of unknown etiology have a monoclonal gammopathy; many of these patients go on to develop a hematologic malignancy, as will be covered later. The neuropathy might get better if the cancer is treated.
    - **Sensory Neuronopathy:** Additionally, carcinoma can result in sensory neuronopathy, which is primarily related to the presence of anti-Hu (or ANNA-1) antibodies and affects the cell bodies of sensory neurons in the dorsal root ganglion. This unusual ailment might be cancer's initial symptom. Pain and numbness usually start out distally, but they can also occasionally start proximally or in the face. The illnesses frequently worsen over a few days or weeks, resulting in pronounced sensory ataxia and impairment of all senses. Autonomic dysfunction is rare, and motor involvement occurs later. There might be an inflammatory formula in the CSF. Usually, treating the underlying tumor is not fruitful.
    - **Motor Neuronopathy, Guillain-Barré Syndrome, and Other Motor Disorders:** Anterior horn cell disorders such as motor neuronopathy

can exacerbate lymphoma. Guillain-Barré syndrome is occasionally linked to Hodgkin's disease and angioimmunoblastic lymphadenopathy. Patients with this syndrome respond to treatment similarly to those who do not have cancer. These and additional paraneoplastic motor disorders (such as neuromyotonia, stiff-person syndrome, and Lambert-Eaton myasthenic syndrome).

    - **Autonomic Neuropathy:** As a paraneoplastic condition, autonomic neuropathy is possible, particularly in small-cell lung cancer patients. The most common association is with anti-Hu antibodies, although anti-nAChR (anti-ganglionic acetylcholine receptor) antibodies can also cause it. It has a poor prognosis, is underdiagnosed, and frequently occurs in conjunction with other paraneoplastic syndromes. Sleep apnea, gastroparesis, intestinal pseudo-obstruction, hypotension, orthostatic hypotension, hypoventilation, abnormal thermoregulatory sweating, and cardiac arrhythmias are among the symptoms that can occasionally result in sudden death. Even after the underlying tumor has been treated, immunotherapy does not help the affected patients.

- **Paraproteinemias:** Malignant plasma cell dyscrasia may be present in patients with paraproteinemic demyelinating neuropathy, particularly in chronic distal sensory neuropathy. When the paraprotein is an immunoglobulin (Ig)M, the neuropathy is probably caused by it. If the neuropathy is caused by IgG or IgA, it may resemble chronic inflammatory demyelinating polyradiculoneuropathy in both its response to treatment and clinical and electrophysiological characteristics.

One typical multiple myeloma complication is polyneuropathy. The majority of lytic myeloma patients are male. A distal symmetric sensorimotor polyneuropathy is the clinical picture. Pain is a common occurrence, all sensory modalities are compromised, and the reflexes are weak. Typically, the illness worsens over time and results in death in two years.

A chronic demyelinating polyneuropathy may coexist with sclerotic myeloma. The predominant involvement is motor; however, there may also be deficiencies in vibration and position sense, and a depression of the reflexes. Compared to lytic myeloma neuropathy, pain is less common, and symptoms may get better with underlying cancer treatment or plasmapheresis.

Skin abnormalities, M protein, organomegaly, polyneuropathy, and endocrinopathy, or POEMS syndrome, can exacerbate plasma cell dyscrasias, particularly osteosclerotic myeloma. The sensorimotor polyneuropathy frequently improves with treatment and may exhibit some characteristic electrophysiologic features, such as conduction slowing that is more pronounced in intermediate than distal nerve segments. Melphalan, with or without corticosteroids, should be taken into consideration, as should localized radiation therapy or resection of an isolated plasmacytoma.

Benign monoclonal gammopathy and Waldenström macroglobulinemia can also cause a sensorimotor polyneuropathy akin to that seen in lytic myeloma. Immunosuppressive medication and plasmapheresis therapy can occasionally be beneficial.

- **Amyloidosis:** Primary generalized amyloidosis, a form of nonhereditary amyloidosis, can manifest as an isolated disorder or in patients with multiple myeloma. It may also be linked to polyneuropathy. Another characteristic of hereditary amyloidosis is polyneuropathy. Amyloid neuropathies are discussed in the hereditary neuropathies section after this.

9.3.7. Drug-Induced and Toxic Neuropathies

- **Alcoholism:** One of the most frequent neurologic side effects of long-term alcohol abuse is polyneuropathy, which can happen on its own or in conjunction with other alcohol-related neurologic conditions like Wernicke encephalopathy or the Korsakoff amnestic syndrome. There is debate over the relative roles that alcohol's direct neurotoxicity and related nutritional deficiencies, particularly thiamine deficiency, play in the development of polyneuropathy.

A symmetric distal sensorimotor neuropathy is commonly observed in alcoholic polyneuropathy. The most affected areas are the legs, leading to impaired sensation of touch and vibration as well as diminished or nonexistent ankle reflexes. There are instances where distal weakness is severe and autonomic dysfunction can happen. When pain arises, it might react to the earlier-discussed treatment for painful neuropathy. Reducing alcohol intake and supplementing with thiamine can stop the symptoms from getting worse.

- **Other Drugs:** Many medications have the potential to cause neuropathies, as shown in Table 9.2, and the majority don't need further discussion here. The polyneuropathy is primarily related to isoniazid-induced impairment of pyridoxine metabolism, a commonly used anti-tuberculous drug. This complication is predisposed by high doses, genetic variations in drug metabolism, and malnourishment. When the medication is stopped, improvements happen on their own. Pyridoxine 100 mg/d can be taken orally concurrently with isoniazid to prevent isoniazid-induced neuropathy.

A sensory neuronopathy that disproportionately affects vibration and position sense may result from pyridoxine (vitamin B6) toxicity. Patients with this disorder typically take at least 200 mg of pyridoxine daily, which is about 100 times the daily minimum required. Common findings include sensory ataxia, the Romberg sign, the Lhermitte sign, and ankle areflexia. Both pain and motor involvement are uncommon. If the abuse stops, the symptoms usually go away over the course of months or years, but high doses of pyridoxine given intravenously have also been linked to an irreversible syndrome.

- **Toxins:** Hexacarbons found in solvents and glues (such as n-hexane and methyl n-butyl ketone) and organophosphates used as plasticizers or insecticides (such as triorthocresyl phosphate) are among the organic compounds linked to polyneuropathy. In contrast to triorthocresyl phosphate neuropathy, which primarily affects motor nerves, n-hexane neuropathy exhibits the most notable sensory involvement.

Polyneuropathy may also be caused by heavy metals. Both cisplatin, an analog of platinum with anticancer activity, and gold, which is used to treat rheumatoid arthritis, have the potential to cause symmetric polyneuropathy and sensory neuropathy.

9.3.8. Hereditary Neuropathies

9.3.8.1. Hereditary Motor and Sensory Neuropathies

These are known as hereditary neuropathies of Charcot-Marie-Tooth (CMT). These disorders share a common clinical phenotype despite being genetically diverse in nature. The distal muscles of the limbs weaken and deteriorate, either with or without sensory loss; pes cavus and diminished or nonexistent tendon reflexes also happen. They fall into two categories: demyelinating (CMT-1) and neuronal (CMT-2), the latter of which resembles progressive spinal muscular atrophy while sparing sensory neurons. Although cases seem to be random, both types have an autosomal dominant pattern of inheritance.

CMT-1 begins in the first decade of life, progresses slowly over time, and has varying degrees of severity. The nerves are frequently noticeably thicker. There is a noticeable decrease in nerve conduction speeds. Genetic research allows for the division of CMT-1 into several forms, the most prevalent of which is caused by mutations or duplications in the peripheral myelin protein-22 (PMP22) gene. When compared to CMT-1, CMT-2 is typically less severe, does not result in nerve enlargement, and is linked to normal or nearly normal nerve conduction velocities. The genes encoding mitofusin 2 (MFN2) and kinesin family member 1B (KIF1B) are the most frequently mutated. There have also been reports of autosomal recessive (CMT-4) and X-linked dominant (CMT-X) variants.

Dejerine-Sottas disease (HMSN3; CMT-3) is characterized by severe sensorimotor neuropathy that often extends to the proximal muscles and is associated with skeletal abnormalities such as scoliosis. The disease usually manifests as delayed motor milestones by the time the child is two years old. The nerves have severe demyelination. It is inherited either dominantly or recessively by autosomal recessive mutations involving the same genes as CMT-1.

9.3.8.2. Hereditary Sensory and Autonomic Neuropathies

These neuropathies can also manifest in different ways. A slowly progressive course beginning in early adulthood, dominant inheritance, symmetric loss of distal pain and temperature perception, and relative preservation of light touch are characteristics of hereditary sensory and autonomic neuropathy (HSAN) type I. Both painless infections of the extremities and perforating ulcers over pressure points are frequent. There is minimal, if any, motor disruption despite the depressed tendon reflexes. Mutations in the genes encoding DNA methyltransferase 1 (DNMT1), the GTPase atlastin family (ATL1 and ATL3), or the serine palmitoyltransferase long-chain subunits (SPTLC1 and SPTLC2) are linked to this phenotype.

HSAN type II is characterized by recessive inheritance, slow progression, onset in infancy or early childhood, impairment of all sensory modalities, variable autonomic involvement, and loss of tendon reflexes. Lysinedeficient protein kinase 1 (WNK1), family with sequence similarity 134, member B (FAM134B), and kinesin family member 1A (KIF1A) are the genes that are impacted.

Familial dysautonomia, also known as HSAN type III (Riley-Day syndrome), is a progressive recessive disorder that starts in infancy and is more common in Ashkenazi Jews. Conspicuous autonomic dysfunction (labile blood pressure and temperature, absent tearing), impaired pain and temperature perception, and areflexia are its defining characteristics. The disorder is associated with mutations in the gene for inhibitor of kappa light polypeptide gene enhancer in B cells, kinase complex-associated protein (IKBKAP). The disorder is more common in individuals of Ashkenazi Jewish descent.

HSAN type IV has been linked to recessive mutations in the gene encoding a receptor tyrosine kinase for nerve growth factor (NTRK1), which is linked to congenital insensitivity to pain and absent sweating. Cognitive dysfunction is prevalent in these patients. Hyperpyrexia may result in death. Although type V HSAN is similar to type IV, there are no cognitive abnormalities. The nerve growth factor β-subunit gene (NGFB) is the site of the mutation.

9.3.8.3. Amyloidosis

Both hereditary and nonhereditary forms of amyloidosis can result in polyneuropathy. Pain and temperature perception, as well as autonomic functions, are significantly impacted because small-diameter sensory and autonomic nerve fibers are particularly likely to be affected. Distal paresthesias, dysesthesias, and numbness, postural hypotension, impaired thermoregulatory sweating, and abnormalities in the bladder, bowel, or sexual function are typical clinical presentations. At some point, distal weakness and wasting happen. Until a comparatively late stage, tendon reflexes are frequently maintained. Amyloid buildup may result in entrapment neuropathy, particularly carpal tunnel syndrome.

Finding amyloid deposits in the tissues is how primary amyloidosis is diagnosed; the first step in this process is typically to examine an aspirate of abdominal fat. Alkylating drugs and autologous peripheral blood stem cell transplantation have been used as forms of treatment. When diagnosing hereditary (familial) amyloidosis, tissue analysis for amyloid deposition is less helpful than genetic testing for transthyretin (TTR) mutations. Orthotopic liver transplantation is a successful form of treatment.

9.3.8.4. Friedreich Ataxia

Friedreich's ataxia is primarily inherited by autosomal recessive means, though dominant inheritance can also happen on occasion. An enlarged GAA trinucleotide repeat in a noncoding region of the mitochondrial protein gene frataxin (FXN) is typically the cause. A clumsy gait and other symptoms of cerebellar dysfunction appear first, then ataxic gait. Depressed or absent tendon reflexes and sensory deficits in the limbs are caused by peripheral sensory fiber involvement. Additionally, due to central motor involvement, there may be extensor plantar responses and leg weakness.

9.3.8.5. Hereditary Neuropathy with Liability to Pressure Palsies

This disorder is genetically diverse, with a common cause being a deletion in the peripheral myelin protein 22 (PMP22) gene. With varying expression, inheritance is an autosomal dominant trait. Patients may exhibit one or more simple or multiple mononeuropathies, which are caused by mild nerve stretching or pressure. Electrophysiologic studies show that abnormalities are more common than are shown clinically.

9.3.8.6. Metabolic Disorders

The first neurologic symptom of acute intermittent porphyria, which is inherited recessively, is frequently a polyneuropathy that primarily affects motor fibers rather than sensory ones. It is possible for sensory symptoms and signs to be primarily distal or proximal. Variegate porphyria can also affect the peripheral nerves.

There are two autosomal recessive lipidoses linked to polyneuropathy, which usually manifests in early childhood or infancy. These include arylsulfatase A deficiency, which causes metachromatic leukodystrophy, and galactocerebroside β-galactosidase deficiency, which causes Krabbe disease.

Abetalipoproteinemia, linked to acanthocytosis, malabsorption, retinitis pigmentosa, and cerebellar ataxia, and Tangier disease, resulting in cataracts, tonsil discoloration, and hepatosplenomegaly, are two examples of lipoprotein deficiencies that cause polyneuropathy. These disorders are recessive autosomal.

A genetic disorder known as refsum disease is caused by a defective phytanic acid metabolism and is inherited recessively. It causes ichthyosis, polyneuropathy, retinitis pigmentosa, and cerebellar ataxia. Reducing the amount of phytol in the diet is the treatment. At the start of treatment, plasmapheresis to lower phytanic acid stores in the body may also be beneficial.

Fabry disease is a recessive X-linked deficiency of the α-galactosidase-A enzyme. It causes angiokeratomas, painful sensory and autonomic neuropathy, cardiac and renal disease, and a higher risk of stroke. Brain MRI results may show white matter lesions. It is the α-galactosidase-A (GLA) gene that is impacted. In males, a low level of α-galactosidase-A activity in leukocytes or plasma can confirm the diagnosis. To diagnose female carriers, mutation analysis is necessary. Both pharmacologic (discussed previously) and enzyme replacement therapy (agalsidase β or α, a recombinant human α-galactosidase A enzyme) may be useful in the treatment of pain. The latter should be administered indefinitely and helps to stabilize or improve renal and cardiac function.

9.4. Entrapment Neuropathies

At weak points, some peripheral nerves are especially prone to mechanical damage. When a nerve is so severely compressed, stretched, or angulated by surrounding anatomic structures that dysfunction results, the condition is referred to as entrapment neuropathy. There are many different types of entrapment neuropathies, and pain or sensory symptoms are frequently the first or most noticeable clinical complaints.

9.4.1. Upper Limb Entrapment Syndromes

9.4.1.1. Median Nerve Compression

In the carpal tunnel at the wrist, compression of the median nerve is frequently observed. Pregnancy can cause carpal tunnel syndrome, which can also result from trauma, degenerative arthritis, tenosynovitis, diabetes mellitus, myxedema, and acromegaly. The thumb, index, and middle fingers as well as the lateral half of the ring finger are the main areas of pain and paresthesia that are restricted to the hand's median nerve distribution in the early stages of the condition. Forearm and, in rare cases, more proximally located pain may be experienced. Nighttime symptoms can be especially bothersome and cause the patient to wake up. The thenar muscles may eventually become weak and atrophy as the neuropathy progresses.

Upon examination, the hand's median nerve distribution exhibits reduced cutaneous sensation, and the abductor pollicis brevis and opponens pollicis muscles show signs of weakness and wasting. Positive results from the Phalen maneuver (flexion of the wrist for one minute exacerbates or reproduces symptoms) or a positive Tinel sign (percussion of the wrist nerve causes paresthesias in its distribution) could be present.

Electrophysiologic studies can typically confirm the diagnosis. Surgical decompression of the carpal tunnel may be required if simple measures like wearing a nocturnal wrist splint or local corticosteroid injections are ineffective in treating the symptoms.

9.4.1.2. Interdigital Neuropathy

Examination reveals hyperpathia or impaired cutaneous sensation in the appropriate distribution of the affected nerve or nerves. Interdigital neuropathy can cause pain in one or both fingers. Such neuropathy can be caused by arthritis, tenosynovitis, direct trauma, or entrapment in the hand's intermetacarpal tunnel.

In some cases, local corticosteroid infiltration therapy is beneficial; however, in more extreme situations, neurolysis might be required.

9.4.1.3. Ulnar Neuropathy

Paresthesias, hypesthesia, and nocturnal pain in the little finger and ulnar border of the hand are caused by dysfunction of the ulnar nerve at the elbow. Elbow pain is another possible symptom. Using the arm or bending the elbow can exacerbate symptoms.

An examination may reveal a weakness in the adductor pollicis, the deep flexor muscles of the fourth and fifth digits, and the intrinsic hand muscles, as well as sensory loss on the ulnar aspect of the hand. The lesion could be caused by a cubitus valgus deformity causing a chronic stretch injury to the nerve, entrapment within the cubital tunnel, or external pressure. The lesion may be localized with electrodiagnostic studies.

It is sometimes enough to halt progression and relieve symptoms to avoid applying pressure to the elbow or to perform repetitive flexion and extension. In certain cases, this is also accomplished by splinting the elbow in an extended position. Depending on the origin, extent, and duration of the lesion, surgical decompression or ulnar nerve transposition to the flexor surface of the arm may also be beneficial.

Furthermore, arthritis, compression from ganglia or benign tumors, or repetitive trauma to the wrist or palm can all result in an ulnar nerve lesion. A more proximal palmar lesion affects the latter muscles as well; there is no sensory deficit. In contrast, the involvement of the deep terminal branch in the palm causes a motor deficit in ulnar-innervated hand muscles other than the hypothenar group. Both sensory and motor changes in the hand occur when lesions at the wrist involve the ulnar nerve itself or its deep and superficial branches. However, because the cutaneous branch to the dorsal surface of the hand arises proximal to the wrist, sensation over this area remains intact. Compression caused by a benign tumor or ganglion can be relieved surgically.

9.4.1.4. Radial Neuropathy

Crutch pressure or other external factors can compress the radial nerve in the axilla; this condition is commonly observed in alcoholics and drug addicts who have fallen asleep with their arm resting on a hard surface (a condition known as "Saturday night palsy"). The resulting deficit is primarily motor, causing weakness or paralysis in the muscles that the nerve supplies. However, sensory abnormalities may also arise, particularly in the small area on the hand's back between the thumb and index finger. Preventing additional nerve compression is the goal of treatment. Except for cases where axonal degeneration has been caused by an extremely serious injury, recovery usually happens completely on its own. Until healing takes place, physical therapy and a wrist splint might be beneficial.

9.4.1.5. Thoracic Outlet Syndrome

The lower portion of the brachial plexus may be compressed by a cervical rib, band, or other anatomical structure. Pain, paresthesias, and numbness in the C8 and T1 distributions are among the symptoms (see Figure 9.4). Diffuse weakness of the intrinsic hand muscles is possible; this mimics carpal tunnel syndrome and frequently involves the muscles in the thenar eminence.

9.4.2. Lower Limb Entrapment Syndromes

- **Fibular (Peroneal) Neuropathy:** Lesions of the fibular (peroneal) nerve can result from pressure or trauma around the knee at the fibular head. Impaired sensation over the dorsum of the foot and the lower anterior aspect of the leg coexists with the ensuing weakness or paralysis of foot and toe extension—and foot eversion. Both the foot inversion reflex and the ankle reflex are intact.

  The only kind of treatment is supportive. The nerve needs to be shielded from additional harm or compression. Individuals who have foot drop might need to wear a brace while they heal. With time and unless the injury was severe enough to cause noticeable axonal degeneration, recovery happens on its own.
- **Tibial Neuropathy:** The tarsal tunnel, which is situated at the ankle directly behind and below the medial malleolus, has a ligamentous roof that can compress the posterior tibial nerve or any of its branches. Typically, people complain of burning in their feet, especially at night, and occasionally they also experience weakness in their intrinsic foot muscles. Electrical diagnosis confirmation is typically possible. Surgical decompression may be required if corticosteroid injections administered locally prove to be ineffective.
- **Femoral Neuropathy:** The following conditions may be linked to isolated femoral neuropathy: diabetes mellitus, vascular disease, bleeding disorders (such as hemophilia or anticoagulant medication therapy), and retroperitoneal neoplasms. A diminished or absent knee reflex is a sign of quadriceps weakness, and sensory abnormalities may also affect the medial portion of the lower leg and the anterior and medial aspects of the thigh. The underlying cause is treated.
- **Saphenous Neuropathy:** The medial aspect of the leg around and below the knee receives cutaneous sensation from the saphenous nerve, which is the femoral nerve's terminal sensory branch (see Figure 9.4). Patients who experience pain or diminished sensation in the nerve's distribution are said to have suffered a mechanical injury to the

nerve at various stages during its course. Involvement of the femoral rather than the saphenous nerve is indicated by weakness in quadriceps function, or the ability to extend at the knee. Although there isn't a specific treatment, the nerve needs to be shielded from more harm.

- **Lateral Femoral Cutaneous Neuropathy:** The outer border of the thigh receives sensation from the lateral femoral cutaneous nerve. Excessive angulation or compression from adjacent anatomic structures can impair its function, particularly during pregnancy or other conditions that result in an exaggerated lumbar lordosis. Examination reveals impaired sensation in the lateral thigh, which results in pain and paresthesias. The best way to treat this syndrome, also known as meralgia paresthetica, is with symptomatic treatments like oral simple analgesics. It usually runs its course on its own, but sometimes it spreads to a permanent, painless numb patch.
- **Obturator Neuropathy:** An obturator nerve injury, such as from a surgical procedure or a pelvic fracture, can cause pain to radiate down the inner aspect of the thigh from the groin. An obturator hernia or osteitis pubis may be the cause of a related condition in which the adductor thigh muscles are weak.

9.5. Root and Plexus Lesions

9.5.1. Compressive and Traumatic Lesions

The symptoms of cervical spondylosis, traumatic plexopathy, neuralgic amyotrophy, acute intervertebral disk prolapse, and cervical rib syndrome. Patients with metastatic cancer may also experience trauma from radiation therapy or develop lesions in the plexus or roots as a result of tumor compression.

When neoplastic meningitis is present, root lesions are usually compressive in nature. Tumor infiltration, particularly from lung or breast cancer, can cause brachial plexopathy, which can cause excruciating arm pain and occasionally dysesthesia. Since the lower trunk of the plexus is most frequently involved, symptoms typically arise in the C8 and T1 dermatomes, and in about 50% of cases, Horner syndrome is present. When the upper trunk of the brachial plexus (the C5 and C6 nerve roots) is affected, weakness is a prominent presenting symptom, arm swelling occurs, or symptoms appear within a year of finishing radiation therapy with a total dose exceeding 60 Gy, radiation injury should be suspected instead of direct tumor invasion. A radiation-induced plexopathy is supported by MRI findings of thickening and diffuse enhancement of the brachial plexus without a focal mass lesion, as well as by electromyography findings of myokymic discharges.

Patients with colorectal, cervical, uterine, or ovarian carcinoma or sarcoma typically experience lumbagosacral plexopathy. Early and severe pain, unilateral involvement, leg swelling, and a palpable rectal mass are clinical features that point to tumor invasion. Radiation injury is more frequently linked to bilateral symptoms and early, noticeable leg weakness.

9.5.2. Tabes Dorsalis

The main symptoms and indicators of this kind of neurosyphilis, which is currently uncommon, are sensory symptoms and indicators that point to significant involvement of the posterior roots, particularly in the lumbosacral region, with subsequent degeneration in the posterior columns of the spinal cord. Urinary incontinence, abrupt, lancinating somatic pains, and unsteadiness are common complaints. There are also visceral crises, which are typified by severe abdominal pain.

Examining the legs reveals a significant impairment in joint position and vibration perception, along with an ataxic gait and the Romberg sign. Although superficial pain perception is often retained, deep pain perception is compromised. Overflow incontinence results from the bladder's flaccidity and insensitivity, which can frequently be felt as a palpable enlargement. The limbs are hypotonic and lack tendon reflexes. Hypertrophic (Charcot) joints can result from sensory loss and hypotonicity. Additional symptoms of neurosyphilis in many patients include ptosis, optic atrophy, Argyll Robertson pupils, variable ophthalmoplegia, and in certain cases, pyramidal and mental abnormalities due to cerebral involvement (taboparesis). Therapy is given to the underlying infection.

9.5.3. Lyme Disease

Similar to syphilis, Lyme disease is a spirochetal infection that causes illness of the central and peripheral nervous systems. Meningitis or meningoencephalitis are symptoms of involvement of the central nervous system. Inflammatory mono- or polyradiculopathy, brachial plexopathy, mononeuropathy (including facial palsy), and mononeuropathy multiplex are further conditions linked to Lyme disease. In addition to focal weakness, the radiculopathy causes pain, sensory loss, or dysesthesia in the impacted dermatomes. There could be involvement with one or more cervical, thoracic, or lumbar nerve roots. Radiculopathy can be verified by electromyography, and Lyme disease is proven to be the cause by serologic testing.

9.6. Myelopathies

Myelopathies can cause motor abnormalities, pain, or a variety of sensory complaints. The lesion's level should be indicated by the clinical findings, but more research is required to fully characterize and define it.

9.6.1. Syringomyelia

Spinal cord cavitation is known as syringomyelia. Hydrodynamic disorder of the CSF pathways, communicating syringomyelia is characterized by communication between the cavity and the central canal of the cord. Cystic dilation of the cord, which is not in communication with the CSF pathways, is present in noncommunicating syringomyelia.

The site of cavitation determines the ensuing clinical disturbance. At the level of the lesion, there is typically a dissociated sensory loss; light touch perception is preserved but pinprick and temperature appreciation are compromised (Figure 9.5). The presence of painless skin ulcers, scars, edema, hyperhidrosis, neuropathic joints, resorption of the terminal phalanges, and other abnormalities may indicate sensory loss. Because the anterior horns of the spinal cord are involved, weakness and muscle wasting happen at the lesion level (Figure 9.5).

Sometimes, below the level of the lesion, gliosis or compression of the descending corticospinal pathways results in a pyramidal deficit and sphincter disruptions. Due to disruption of their afferent, central, or efferent pathways, the tendon reflexes may be enhanced below the lesion and depressed at its level. Cord cavitation is frequently accompanied by scoliosis.

Cavitation usually affects the cervical region; involvement of the T1 segment often results in ipsilateral Horner syndrome. The condition causes a capelike distribution of sensory loss over one or both shoulders, diffuse neck pain, and radicular pain in the arms. In addition to ipsilateral tongue wasting, palatal weakness, vocal cord paralysis, dissociated trigeminal sensory loss, and other signs of brainstem involvement, there may be syringobulbia, or lower brainstem cavitation.

Chronic arachnoiditis of the basal cisterns or developmental abnormalities of the brainstem and foramen magnum region are frequently linked to communicating syringomyelia. The Arnold-Chiari malformation may cause one or more of the following conditions: hydrocephalus, cerebellar ataxia, abnormalities of the lower cranial nerves, and pyramidal and sensory deficits in the limbs. A small posterior fossa and an enlarged foramen magnum are visible on CT scans; additional skeletal abnormalities at the base of the skull and upper cervical spine may also be present. The syrinx and the Arnold-Chiari malformation are visible on an MRI, along with the fourth ventricle's caudal displacement and the herniation of cerebellar tonsils through the foramen magnum.

Spinal arachnoiditis, intramedullary tumors, and trauma are common causes of noncommunicating syringomyelia (Figure 9.6). Rarely, posttraumatic syringomyelia develops after only a few months in patients who already have significant neurologic deficits from spinal trauma, but it usually happens after a few years. Presentation is with a worsening of a formerly stable deficit; prominent symptoms include weakness, impaired sensation, and spasticity, as well as potentially upsetting radicular pain. Patients with cavitation due to prior injuries or intramedullary neoplasms show focal cord enlargement on MRI.

Therapy is based on the underlying reason. A temporary benefit might result from the decompression of a distended syrinx. Sometimes, amputation of the cerebellar tonsils and removal of the posterior rim of the foramen magnum are beneficial in cases of communicating syringomyelia linked to Arnold-Chiari malformation. Once the cord cavity has been emptied, the fourth ventricle may need to have an outlet created. Surgery is used to treat posttraumatic syringomyelia if it results in unbearable pain or a progressive neurological deficit. Numerous surgical techniques have been employed, such as myelotomy, different cord cavity draining techniques, and the creation of surgical meningocele. In general, radicular pain and sensory disruptions are alleviated, while spasticity responds less well.

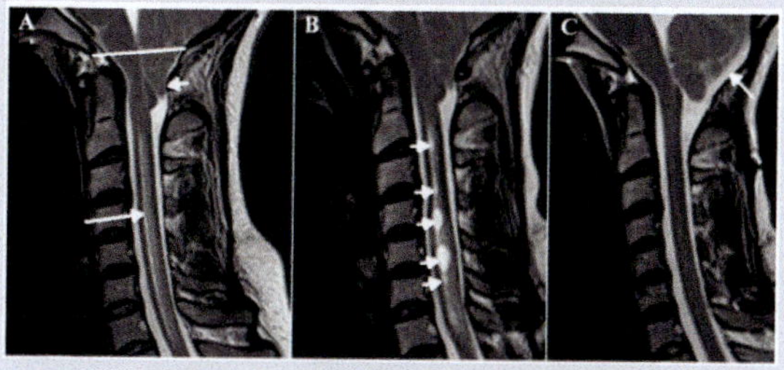

Figure 9.6. The progression of edema in syringomyelia. A T2 weighted sagittal MRI of the neck in a 28-year-old female patient who presented with headache on bending and coughing. There is a Chiari 1 malformation with significant cerebellar tonsil herniation (small white arrow) below the foramen magnum (white line) leading to reduced spinal compliance. There is spinal cord edema from C2 to T1 (long arrow) (A). One year later, following conservative management, there were multiple cystic cavities developing (arrows) (B). Following posterior fossa decompression (arrow), there is now improved compliance in the spinal canal with the resolution of the edema and the cystic cavities previously noted (C).

Source: Bateman GA, Bateman AR. Syringomyelia Is Associated with a Reduction in Spinal Canal Compliance, Venous Outflow Dilatation and Glymphatic Fluid Obstruction. *Journal of Clinical Medicine*. 2023; 12(20):6646. https://doi.org/10.3390/jcm12206646.

9.6.2. Subacute Combined Degeneration

Vitamin B12 deficiency (Figure 9.7) can be caused by a strictly vegetarian diet, gastrointestinal surgery, sprue, infection with fish tapeworms, or impaired absorption by the gastrointestinal tract, as in the case of pernicious anemia. Subacute combined degeneration of the lateral and posterior columns of the spinal cord can result from a vitamin B12 deficiency.

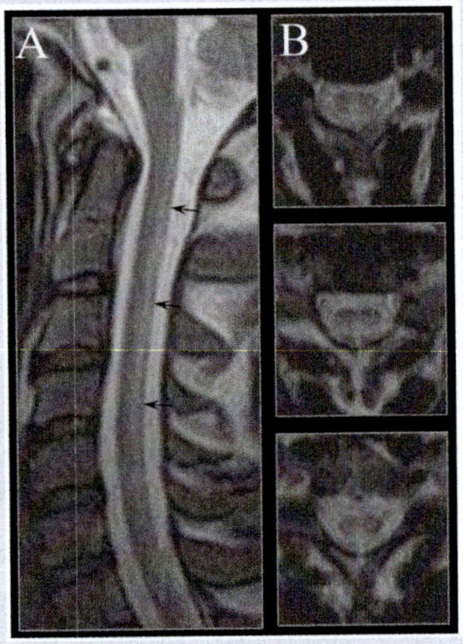

Figure 9.7. Cervical spinal cord MRI in a 49-year-old male presenting with subacute combined degeneration due to a deficit of B12. (A) The midsagittal T2 weighted image shows linear hyperintensity in the posterior portion of the cervical tract of the spinal cord (black arrows). (B) Axial T2 weighted images reveal the selective involvement of the posterior columns.

Source: Briani C, Dalla Torre C, Citton V, et al. Cobalamin deficiency: clinical picture and radiological findings. Nutrients. 2013;5(11):4521–4539. Published 2013 Nov 15. doi:10.3390/nu5114521.

Clinical manifestations include distal paresthesias, weakness in the extremities (hand involvement occurs relatively early), and ataxia due to impaired leg postural sensation. Spastic paraparesis then develops. Examination reveals a combined posterior column (vibration and joint position sense) and pyramidal deficit in the legs, with a possible presence of Lhermitte sign. Extensor plantar responses occur, but depending on the location and degree of involvement, depressed or increased tendon reflexes may occur. Signs of involvement of the spinal cord may be associated with peripheral neuropathy, behavioral or mental abnormalities, optic atrophy or centrocecal scotoma due to involvement of the optic (II) nerve. Although it is not always the case, macrocytic megaloblastic anemia frequently coexists with the neurologic symptoms.

In untreated cases, serum homocysteine and methylmalonic acid levels are elevated, and the level of vitamin B12 is low. Gastritis is a common symptom of pernicious anemia, and the diagnosis is confirmed by antibodies against gastric parietal cells and anti-intrinsic factor. However, hematologic results could be normal, particularly if folic acid supplements have been administered. Peripheral nerve involvement may be confirmed by electrophysiologic studies, and abnormalities suggestive of posterior column dysfunction may be seen in somatosensory evoked potentials derived from the median or tibial nerve. An occasional spinal MRI reveals anomalies in the posterior columns.

Vitamin B12 is administered intramuscularly as an injection every day (1,000 μg) for two weeks, then weekly (100 μg) for another two months, and finally monthly (100 μg) after that. It should be noted that folic acid supplements may conceal related anemia but do not treat the neurologic condition.

Abuse of nitrous oxide can cause vitamin B12 to become inactive, which can lead to a similar disorder. The management strategy is centered on limiting future nitrous oxide exposure. Subacute combined degeneration can also result from a copper deficiency. Complete parenteral hyperalimentation, enteral feeding-induced copper insufficiency, malabsorption, gastric surgery, or excessive zinc consumption, which prevents intestinal copper absorption, can all lead to copper deficiency. The diagnosis is supported by low levels of copper excreted in the urine, ceruloplasmin, and copper in the serum. The goal of treatment is to stabilize the neurologic deficit by modifying risk factors and supplementing with copper.

A Closer Look

Anosmia

Partial or total loss of smell is called anosmia. Anosmia may be a transient or ongoing ailment. When the mucous membranes in your nose become inflamed or clogged—as they can during a severe cold or sinus infection, for example—you may lose some or all of your sense of smell.

However, you ought to consult a physician if your loss of smell isn't caused by a sinus infection or cold, or if it doesn't go away when your congestion goes away. It might be a sign of something else.

Since a diminished sense of smell can result in poor appetite and malnutrition, particularly in the elderly, it is important for overall health and nutrition. A changed sense of smell could be the cause of additional health issues. Individuals suffering from anosmia may inadvertently ingest rancid or sour food items due to their inability to recognize the telltale smells of spoiling. People who suffer from anosmia might not even be aware that they are breathing in smoke, pollution, or hazardous materials. Congenital anosmia is the term for the rare condition in which a person is born devoid of sense of smell. This happens when the olfactory system—the body's sense of smell—develops abnormally either before birth or as a result of an inherited genetic disorder. Regretfully, congenital anosmia cannot be cured.

Numerous negative consequences may arise from anosmia. Food may not seem as appetizing to those with sudden onset anosmia, though congenital anosmics seldom complain of this and none report losing weight. The inability to detect gas leaks, fires, and spoiled food is another reason why losing one's sense of smell can be dangerous. Patients with anosmia may find it more challenging to receive the same medical care as those who have lost other senses, like hearing or sight, due to the widespread perception that the condition is insignificant. Many people have a unilateral loss of smell, which is frequently the consequence of mild head trauma. Usually, this kind of anosmia can only be identified through separate testing of the two nostrils. When testing each nostril independently, it is frequently possible to detect a reduced or absent sense of smell in one or both nostrils—a finding that is frequently hidden when testing both nostrils at once.

Losing a familiar and meaningful scent memory (e.g., It has been observed that certain smells, such as those of grass, the grandparents' attic, a certain book, loved ones, or oneself, can induce depressive symptoms. Libido loss may result from loss of smell, but this is not usually the case for people who have olfactory dysfunction from birth. People who are born deaf frequently report that as children, they pretended to smell because they didn't understand the concept of smell or didn't want to stand out from the crowd. They also told stories about thinking that only older, more mature people could smell. As kids get older, they frequently come to the realization—and often to their parents' surprise—that they don't really have a sense of smell.

Summary

- Dorsal root ganglia are home to the cell bodies of first-order sensory neurons originating from the limbs and trunk.
- Pain, unusual sensations, or loss of feeling are examples of sensory disturbances. While dysesthesia refers to any unpleasant sensation caused by a normally painless stimulus, paresthesia refers to abnormal spontaneous sensations like burning, tingling, or pins and needles.
- The patient stands with their feet together, arms extended, and eyes closed in a steady stance. They are then watched for any signs of swaying or falling.
- The anatomical prediction of sensory loss in patients with a single peripheral nerve lesion is typically not met due to overlap from neighboring nerves.
- A transverse sensory level may be present in patients with spinal cord lesions. However, there are physiological sites of increased sensitivity in the groin, over the breasts, and at the costal margin; these should not be interpreted as aberrant.
- Psychogenic sensation disturbances have been linked to psychiatric disorders like conversion disorder.
- A disorder known as polyneuropathy refers to a situation in which multiple peripheral nerves are simultaneously affected in function.
- Dissociated sensory loss is the loss of certain sensory modalities (pain, temperature, vibration) while maintaining other modalities (light touch, vibration, joint position sense).
- Acute polyneuropathy, such as that seen in Guillain-Barré syndrome, typically arises from an inflammatory process over the course of a few days.
- Guillain-Barré syndrome can develop after minor infectious diseases, vaccinations, or surgical procedures, or it can develop without any clear cause.
- Diabetes-related peripheral nerve problems have no particular treatment, with the possible exception of entrapment neuropathy, in which case a decompressive procedure may be beneficial.
- Both lymphoma and carcinoma exhibit this. It is occasionally asymmetrical, can be acute or chronic, and may be accompanied by noticeable pain.
- Pregnancy can cause carpal tunnel syndrome, which can also result from trauma, degenerative arthritis, tenosynovitis, diabetes mellitus, myxedema, and acromegaly.

References

1. Aminoff, M. J., & Josephson, S. A. (Eds.). (2014). *Aminoff's Neurology and General Medicine* (5th ed.). San Diego: Elsevier.
2. Arnold, A. C., & Shibao, C. (2013). Current concepts in orthostatic hypotension management. *Curr. Hypertens. Rep., 15*, 304–312.
3. Benarroch, E. E. (2014). The clinical approach to autonomic failure in neurological disorders. *Nat. Rev. Neurol., 10*, 396–407.

4. Benson, M. D., & Kincaid, J. C. (2007). The molecular biology and clinical features of amyloid neuropathy. *Muscle. Nerve., 36*, 411–423.
5. Bouche, P. (2013). Compression and entrapment neuropathies. *Handb. Clin. Neurol., 115*, 311–366.
6. Finnerup, N. B., Sindrup, S. H., & Jensen, T. S. (2013). Management of painful neuropathies. *Handb. Clin. Neurol., 115*, 279–290.
7. Charnogursky, G., Lee, H., & Lopez, N. (2014). Diabetic neuropathy. *Handb. Clin. Neurol., 120*, 773–785.
8. Finnerup, N. B., Sindrup, S. H., & Jensen, T. S. (2010). The evidence for pharmacological treatment of neuropathic pain. *Pain, 150*, 573–581.
9. Freeman, R. (2007). Autonomic peripheral neuropathy. *Neurol. Clin., 25*, 277–301.
10. Gwathmey, K. G., Burns, T. M., Collins, M. P., & Dyck, P. J. (2014). Vasculitic neuropathies. *Lancet Neurol., 13*, 67–82.
11. Halperin, L. L. (2003). Lyme disease and the peripheral nervous system. *Muscle Nerve, 28*, 133–143.
12. Harrison, T. B., & Smith, B. (2011). Neuromuscular manifestations of HIV/AIDS. *J. Clin. Neuromuscul. Dis., 13*, 68–84.
13. Jaiser, S. R., & Winston, G. P. (2010). Copper deficiency myelopathy. *J. Neurol., 257*, 869–881.
14. Karam, Y., Hitchon, P. W., Mhanna, N. E., et al. (2014). Post-traumatic syringomyelia: Outcome predictors. *Clin. Neurol. Neurosurg., 124*, 44–50.
15. Krishnan, A. V., & Kiernan, M. C. (2007). Uremic neuropathy: Clinical features and new pathophysiological insights. *Muscle Nerve, 35*, 273–290.
16. Kumar, N. (2014). Neurologic aspects of cobalamin (B12) deficiency. *Handb Clin. Neurol., 120*, 915–926.
17. Kwan, J. Y. (2007). Paraproteinemic neuropathy. *Neurol. Clin., 25*, 47–69.
18. Lehmann, H. C., Hughes, R. A., & Hartung, H. P. (2013). Treatment of chronic inflammatory demyelinating polyradiculoneuropathy. *Handb Clin. Neurol., 115*, 415–427.
19. O'Connor, A. B., & Dworkin, R. H. (2009). Treatment of neuropathic pain: An overview of recent guidelines. *Am. J. Med., 122*(suppl), S22–S32.
20. Rossor, A. M., Polke, J. M., Houlden, H., & Reilly, M. M. (2013). Clinical implications of genetic advances in Charcot-Marie-Tooth disease. *Nat. Rev. Neurol., 9*, 562–571.
21. Said, G., & Krarup, C. (Eds.). (2013). *Peripheral Nerve Disorders*. Handbook of Clinical Neurology, Vol 115. Amsterdam: Elsevier.
22. Said, G. (2007). Diabetic neuropathy – a review. *Nat. Clin. Pract. Neurol., 3*, 331–340.
23. Sax, T. W., & Rosenbaum, R. B. (2006). Neuromuscular disorders in pregnancy. *Muscle Nerve, 34*, 559–571.
24. Sharp, L., & Vernino, S. (2012). Paraneoplastic neuromuscular disorders. *Muscle Nerve, 46*, 841–850.

25. Stewart, J. D. (2010). *Focal Peripheral Neuropathies* (4th ed.). West Vancouver, Canada: JBJ Publishing.

26. Vallat, J. M., Mathis, S., & Funalot, B. (2013). The various Charcot-Marie-Tooth diseases. *Curr. Opin. Neurol., 26*, 473–480.

27. van den Berg, B., Walgaard, C., Drenthen, J., et al. (2014). Guillain-Barré syndrome: Pathogenesis, diagnosis, treatment and prognosis. *Nat. Rev. Neurol., 10*, 469–482.

28. Vandertop, W. P. (2014). Syringomyelia. *Neuropediatrics, 45*, 3–9.

29. Wilbourn, A. J. (2007). Plexopathies. *Neurol. Clin., 25*, 139–171.

INDEX

B

C

I

J

L

M

N

O

P

R

S

T

U

V

W

X

Printed and bound by CPI Group (UK) Ltd, Croydon, CR0 4YY
18/09/2026
14965061-0006